Ernst Lehnhardt

Clinical Aspects of Inner Ear Deafness

With 52 Figures

Springer-Verlag
Berlin Heidelberg New York
London Paris Tokyo

Professor Dr. Dr. ERNST LEHNHARDT
Medizinische Hochschule Hannover
Hals-Nasen-Ohrenklinik
Konstanty-Gutschow-Str. 8
D-3000 Hannover 61

Translators:
Dr. CHARLES LANGMAID, Cardiff
and Dr. KATRIN LUETGEBRUNE, Hannover

German Edition:
Ernst Lehnhardt: Klinik der Innenohrschwerhörigkeiten
In: Verhandlungsbericht 1984 der Deutschen Gesellschaft
für Hals-Nasen-Ohren-Heilkunde, Kopf- und Hals-Chirurgie
Teil I: Referate

Library of Congress Cataloging-in-Publication Data. Lehnhardt, Ernst. Clinical aspects of inner ear deafness. Translation of: Klinik der Innenohrschwerhörigkeiten. Originally published in: Verhandlungsbericht 1984 of the Deutsche Gesellschaft für Hals-Nasen-Ohrenheilkunde, Kopf- und Halschirurgie, T. 1. Bibliography: p. 1. Deafness–Etiology. 2. Labyrinth (Ear)–Wounds and injuries. 3. Labyrinth (Ear)–Diseases. 4. Diseases–Complications and sequelae. I. Title. [DNLM: 1. Deafness. 2. Labyrinth–injuries. 3. Labyrinth Diseases. WV 270 L5235k] RF290.L44 1986 617.8′8 85-27793
ISBN-13: 978-3-642-70931-9 e-ISBN-13: 978-3-642-70929-6
DOI: 10.1007/978-3-642-70929-6

Typesetting, printing and bookbinding: Brühlsche Universitätsdruckerei, Giessen
2125/3130-543210

Preface

The work on clinical aspects of inner ear deafness started out in 1983/1984 as a general review conceived by the Deutsche Gesellschaft für Hals-Nasen-Ohren-Heilkunde, Kopf- und Hals-Chirurgie (German Society for Oto-Rhino-Laryngology and Head and Neck Surgery) under the presidency of Professor Harald Feldmann, Münster. My task was to sift through the literature available at that time, to record the current status of knowledge, and if appropriate to describe existing new tendencies and potential developments.

It was a conscious decision that the subject matter should extend to the entire field of inner ear deafness, though without reproducing too much of the detail given in the reviews already available, such as those by Vosteen (1961) on the biology of the inner ear, Beckmann (1962) on deafness in children, and Lehnhardt (1965) on industrial otopathies. The text contains only brief references to these, followed by more detailed expositions of what has come to light in the interim.

In keeping with the broadness of the topic the list of references is extremely long, though we are aware that it is still not absolutely comprehensive. It is intended to give readers interested in specific topics an idea of the literature available and to provide a point of departure for further work. Scientific research is progressing and news insights appearing so fast, however, that the topicality of the material will be limited.

I am indebted to my staff: Mrs. M. Pitschmann for her help in collecting the literature and preparing the manuscript; Mrs. D. Becker for collecting the audiometrically typical syndromes; and Mr. W. Zimmermann for drawing the graphs ready for the press. Thanks are also due to Dr. Charles Langmaid and Dr. Katrin Luetgebrune for their translation of the original German text.

Hannover ERNST LEHNHARDT

Contents

1 Introduction and Definitions

In spite of the apparently clear task which has been set, the structure of any report on the clinical aspects of inner ear (sensorineural) deafness must put up with certain logical contradictions. It is impossible to find a classification purely according to the etiology or only according to the type of reaction of the inner ear, or perhaps only according to age. Although infantile deafness and senile deafness will be discussed separately, low tone deafness, too, will be dealt with in a separate chapter, and etiologic distinctions will be made between ototoxic, metabolic and noise-induced deafness. The report is to refer to

- *deafness* as a symptom of disease of the inner ear
- the *inner ear* as the origin of deafness.

Vertigo and tinnitus as well as those types of deafness located beyond the inner ear are therefore deliberately neglected. The clinical study of sensorineural deafness requires a differential diagnosis of all those disturbances of hearing based on identical values for the thresholds of bone- and airconduction. This is assumed in all following audiograms too. The term sensorineural deafness implies mainly those functional disturbances which involve the organ of Corti, regardless of whether they originate primarily in the hair cells or arise secondarily as a result of a metabolic or electrolyte disturbance of the stria vascularis or of the lymph. The functional lesions of the auditory nerve, too, are often classed with sensorineural deafness in its *wider* sense. It would be logically more consistent if one took the trouble to distinguish between sensory, ganglionic and neural deafness.[1]

This report will only deal with inner ear deafness in its narrower sense, i.e. the sensory and the ganglionic disturbances of hearing, as far as this latter may at all be recognized as such.

Even today many investigators unfortunately diagnose inner ear deafness only on the basis of the pure tone audiogram. This can be explained, among other things, by the endeavour (basically to be welcome), to portray the results of speech audiometry, too, in a *diagrammatic form* – a procedure that in many places has become too expensive, with the result that it is difficult for us to compete with the international standards. In diagnostic audiometry abroad the *speech diagram* has now been almost completely dispensed with, in favor of merely two values, namely the speech discrimination threshold and the percentage of mono-syllable discrimination at one given loudness. However, in many countries these two parameters are integral components of *every* audiometric test. Though this may be regretted with regard to the more significant *speech diagram* it must be admitted that the two single values are sufficient for the great majority of audiometric findings and, in any case, are more informative than no speech audiogram at all. What the speech audiogram means for the recording of the deafness pattern as a whole, does the measurement of impedance mean for the diagnosis of disturbances of middle ear function and of the *neural or central neural conduction*. Diagnostics of inner ear deafness without registration of the middle ear pressure and the stapedius reflex threshold (contra- *and* ipsi-lateral) is nowadays no longer imaginable. The comprehensive evidence of the complicated findings can, nevertheless, only be fully exploited if they are illustrated in clearly arranged scheme.

[1] It would be better to substitute the Anglo-American term sensorineural by sensoriganglionic

2 General Features

2.1 Essential Physiological Data

The physiology of the inner ear and the knowledge of its pathology are the basis of inner ear diagnostics. Unfortunately – with all our knowledge of the physiology – we have a rather limited idea about audition in the *diseased* inner ear.

There is no doubt about the *arrangement of frequencies* along the basilar membrane, that is, that the lower frequencies are perceived at the apex of the cochlea and the higher ones near the windows. The distribution of the individual pitches on the 32 mm long membrane is also sufficiently known. It is therefore quite reasonable that with a high tone loss the injury should be localised in the basal turn and with a low tone *deafness* in the apical turn.

It may also be regarded as an established fact that – largely independent of the type of injury – first of all the *outer* and only later the *inner* hair cells are affected. This concept has recently been confirmed again in an extensive, very thorough study (Stebbins et al. 1979). Within the outer hair cells, the row located next to the tunnel of Nuel degenerates first. Finally, there has not yet been any dispute about the observation that the extent of the hearing loss at the individual frequencies correlates well with the number of non-functioning hair cells in the related part of the basilar membrane (Nomura and Kitamura 1979).

As regards the two populations of hair cells it has been assumed until now that both types of cell function largely independent of each other, namely the outer hair cells responding to slight and the inner ones only to great sound intensities (e.g. Spoendlin 1975); meanwhile the conviction prevails that both populations contribute to every impression of loudness, so that the characteristic curve of the increase in loudness in its flat initial part is not exclusively determined by the outer, and in its steep end portion not only by the inner ones. While the type of combined action of both cell populations is still being discussed it is established that a threshold difference of 50 dB exists between the outer and inner hair cells (Ryan and Dallos 1975, Stebbins et al. 1979). Elevations of threshold by <50 dB affect only the outer hair cells. Only with hearing losses of >50 dB the inner hair cells, too, are involved in the failure. This pattern of injury has been confirmed in various species.

In recent years further knowledge has been added to the concepts on recruitment and on the ability of the inner ear to resolve frequencies. They concern, on the one hand, the validity of the duplicity theory and, on the other, the "second filter" i.e. the question whether the sharp tuning curves of the ear are neural in origin or whether they actually arise from the inner ear. It appears that a common answer has been found to both these hitherto controversial questions.

The duplicity theory had its anatomical basis in the observation that the *outer* hair cells and the *spiral* fibers emerging from them might degenerate on their own while at the same time the *inner* hair cells with their appertaining *radial* fibers remain intact (Meyer zum Gottesberge 1948, Ranke 1953, Davis 1957, Yoshie 1968). On the other hand could a recruitment also have existed, when for example in Menière's disease the outer haircells had remained widely intact (Lindsay

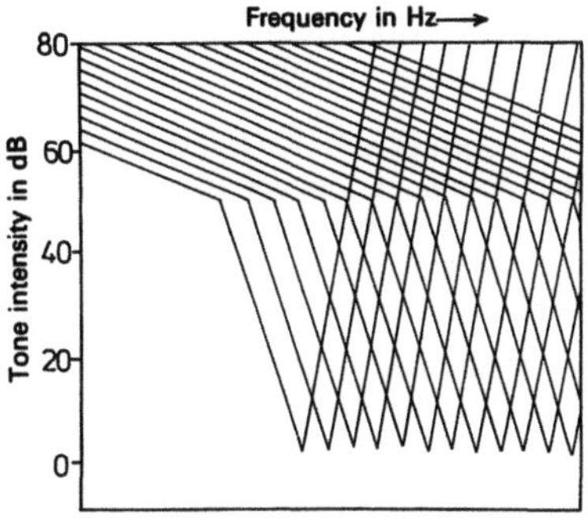

Fig. 1. Schematic diagram of frequency-specific threshold sensitivity (tuning curve) of single fibers of the cochlear nerve, with overlapping tracings. The pointed, sharply tuned part of each curve reaches the hearing threshold i.e. the few respective fibers are already stimulated by the threshold intensity. A greater intensity reaches the flat part of the curve of many fibers – namely, even those whose "best frequency" is higher than the stimulation frequency; at the same time loudness and loudness discrimination increase rapidly. (From Evans 1975)

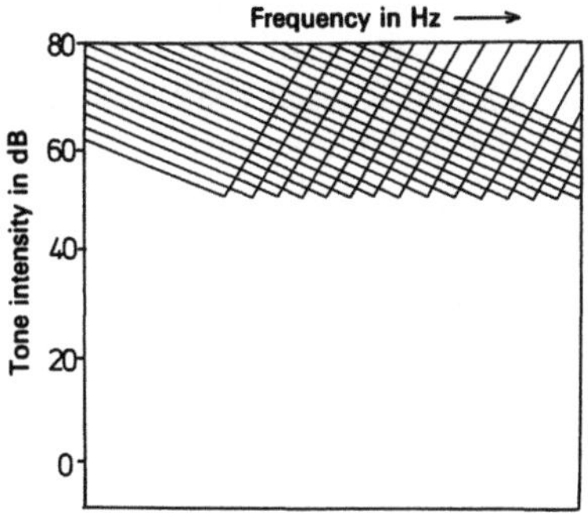

Fig. 2. Theory of recruitment according to Evans, assuming here an inner ear deafness around 50 dB. The frequency-specific threshold sensitivity of the single fibers has lost the sharply tuned part of the curve. The fibers are only stimulated with more than 50 dB but then loudness and loudness discrimination increase steeply, corresponding to the flat running "low frequency tail". (From Evans 1975)

1968, Schuknecht 1968, 1974). In addition Kiang et al. (1970) were able to show that in ears damaged by ototoxic agents, fibers with a high threshold had degenerated, while those with a lower threshold still reacted normally.

Although Evans (1972, 1975) confirmed that among the single fibers led to date there are some with a low and some with a high threshold he pointed out that all of them reflect the behavior of the *inner* hair cells. The recruitment phenomenon could already be explained by the mere tuning curves of these fibers (Fig. 1). With increasing deafness the sharply tuned portion of the respective fiber would become smaller and broader, and would completely disappear with hearing losses of >50 dB (Fig. 2). While in the normal ear threshold intensities stimulated only single fibers, greater volumes also reached the flat running portion of many other fibers. With inner ear deafness of >50 dB the situation is the same, namely the stimulation of many fibers by great sound intensities. The schematic representation of several tuning curves within one diagram reveals at the same time that with great intensity loudness discrimination is better, corresponding to the large number of stimulated fibers, and must increase steeply with growing intensity of stimulus – in the healthy as well as the diseased ear.

These findings collected in the first place under physiological conditions have also been confirmed in hypoxemic animals (Evans 1974) and in those damaged by Kanamycin (Evans 1979), as well as by electrocochleography (ECochG) in recruitment deaf patients (Eggermont 1977). In all cases a flattening and broadening of the tuning curves was shown, regularly in ears damaged by ototoxic agents but only at particular stages in patients with sudden hearing loss. In retrocochlear deafness the tuning curves behaved the same as in the healthy ear.

Galetti et al. (1981) developed another interpretation of the recruitment phenomenon. In their opinion it does not arise in the hair cells but in the spiral ganglion by inadequate inhibition of the presynaptic connections between the axons. Though this concept has not yet been proved it would explain why ganglionic deafness evidently cannot be distinguished by audiometry from hair cell deafness.

If the recruitment behaviour of the damaged inner ear was to be explained by the findings described, even without having to fall back on the duplicity theory, it still remains an open question whether the tuning curves are exclusively neural in origin or if the same information is already contained in the hair cells or even in the mechanical pattern of oscillation. In order to answer this question it was necessary to record the potentials of single hair cells. Meanwhile this has successfully been accomplished not only for the inner hair cells (Russell and Sellick 1978, Sellick and Russell 1980) but also for the outer hair cells (Dallos and Santos-Sacchi 1982). The measurements produced tuning curves with a tuning as sharp as had so far only been recorded from nerve fibers. The frequency selectivity also known from psychoacoustic tests is thus already existent in the sensory cell.

Khanna and Leonard (1982) successfully accomplished the hitherto last step of these experiments. By means of a laser-interferometer and tiny mirrors on the basilar membrane they were able to record even here tuning curves with a steepness corresponding to that of the sensory cells and the nerve fibers (Fig. 3). Only the height of the sharply tuned portion stayed behind that of the comparable curves, an effect which the authors explain by the inner ear alteration associated with the experiment. The steepness towards the low frequencies amounted to 86 dB, that towards the higher tones was actually 538 dB/octave! It reflects a micromechanism whose non-linearity might be explained by the rigidity of the stereocilia of the outer hair cells (Allen 1980). In this way the site of origin of the tuning curve was explained; the basilar membrane and the organ of Corti are the supposed second filter.

Further understanding has followed from these results. The sharpness of resonance of the basilar membrane cannot be explained only by a *passive* hydrodynamic model of the cochlea. One therefore assumes an *active* non-linear amplifier in the inner ear which is particularly effective near the threshold of hearing. The phenomenon of cochlear echo discovered by Kemp (1978,

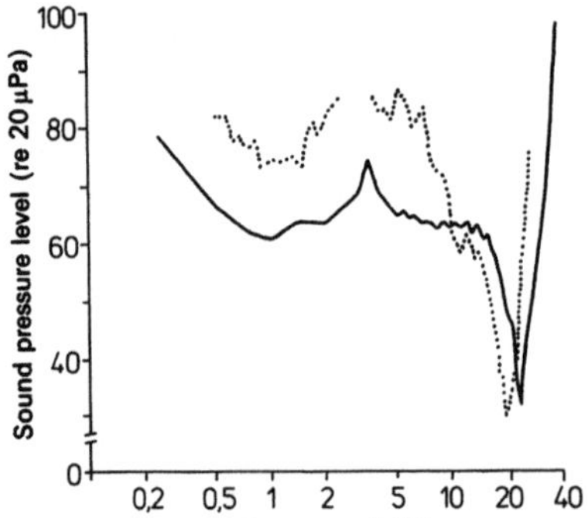

Fig. 3. The continuous line reproduces the oscillation amplitude of vibration of the basilar membrane upon the corresponding frequency-specific stimulation, the dotted line the *neural* tuning curve. The smaller difference between the peak and the horizontal portion of the curve for the basilar membrane is explained by the authors as the result of damage associated with the experiment. The basic agreement in the steep portion of the two curves is decisive for the physiological evidence. (From Khanna and Leonard 1982)

1979, 1982) has also contributed to this conclusion. It appears as the response of the inner ear to definite tone stimuli, after an interval of about 5 ms and it can be recorded for a few ms in the external auditory meatus. As it corresponds to the ingoing frequency and is thus reflected as a tone, too, *it must* originate in the basilar membrane or in the hair cells and, indeed, with the same sharp tuning as for the afferent transformation of the stimulus. The echo is absent in disturbances of inner ear function. In this respect it also supports the idea that some active micro-*mechanism* is involved in the process of hearing in the healthy ear.

Besides the recruitment due to irreversible decay of sensory cells, a recruitment caused only by a temporary reversible dysfunction of the hair cells gains in importance. It is mainly to be expected in low tone deafness and probably also in the reversible disturbances of hearing caused by loop diuretics or salicylates. These two types of recruitment can scarcely be distinguished from one another by audiometry. In the discussion of the ECochG as well as of the types of deafness already mentioned they will be dealt with in more detail.

The old assumption, that the *efferent nerve fibers* were involved in the phenomenon of recruitment or adaptation, did not seem to be confirmed. It is true that the efferences insert in each hair cell with at least one synapse and as the division of the Rasmussen bundle leads to a disappearance of the acetylcholine-esterase in all four rows of hair cells (Schuknecht et al. 1959) it may be assumed that the efferences normally decompose the stimulator substance acetylcholine. Klinke and Galley (1974) assume the own voice to induce this process suggesting that during speech hearing impressions from without were suppressed. Yet even this effect cannot be lasting, since patients with a neurectomy of the vestibular and thus of the efferent nerve have not made corresponding complaints (Pfalz 1983).

By and large, the *clinical* significance of the olivocochlear bundle is therefore regarded as trifling.

Among the *fluid spaces* of the inner ear, the one for the endolymph is secluded while the perilymph communicates with the CSF through the aquaeductus cochleae (Fig. 4). In addition, a communication exists between the perilymph and the CSF through the perineural and perivascular spaces of the internal auditory meatus (Galle and Siegel 1979, Salt and Stupp 1979, Kaupp and Giebel 1980, Asher and Sando 1981). Both pathways – through the aquaeductus cochleae and through the internal auditory meatus – are evidently functionally effective also in man; all the more as they are even permeable for erythrocytes (Palva et al. 1979). Moreover, the perilymph is said to flow away from the inner ear into the lymphatic spaces of the bone as well as of the mucous membrane of the middle ear (Arnold 1972), although, in view of the tight cell junctions in all boundaries of the perilymphatic space (Franke 1979), this idea does not seem very plausible.

The *lymph from the tunnel of Nuel* and the organ of Corti (Corti-lymph, Wittmaack 1936) communicates with the perilymph, among other ways, via the habenula perforata along the nerve fibers leading to the hair cells (v. Ilberg 1980). As the Corti-lymph also rinses the basal surface of the outer hair cells (Ryan et al. 1979 and many others) it seems likely that oxygen and glucose also arrive there by this route – that is through the perilymph (Smith 1954, Vosteen 1961, Rauch 1964). This implies that the sensory endings of the organ of Corti are only able to function electrophysiologically in an environment rich in sodium and poor in potassium. From recordings of the intracellular resting potential and the endocochlear sustained potential it has nevertheless been inferred that the organ of Corti is supplied with O_2 via the perilymph as well as via the endolymph (Nuttall and Lawrence 1979).

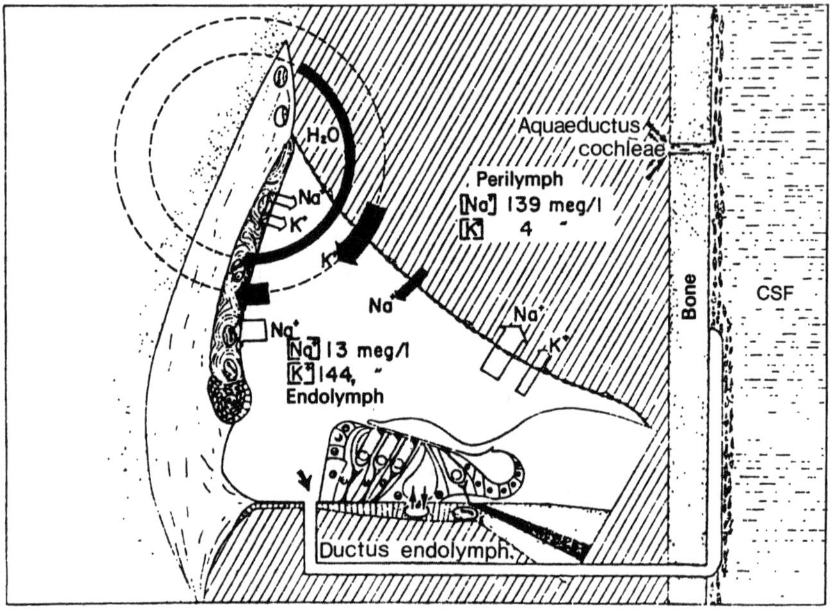

Fig. 4. Schematic representation of the ion exchange in the inner ear. On the one hand, this occurs continuously along the ductus cochlearis, while at the same time the endolymph moves slowly towards the ductus and saccus endolymphaticus. (From Lawrence 1980)

An exceptional position is apparently occupied by the *subtectorial fluid* in the sulcus internus. On the one hand, its O_2 tension corresponds to that of the Corti-lymph (Lawrence 1974), on the other hand, the parameters measured here are different from those found in other parts of the scala media. As, according to more recent ultrastructural investigations and intravital observations, at least the outer hair cells are firmly attached to the tectorial membrane (Lit. quoted by Arnold and Vosteen 1979), one should for the present regard the subtectorial fluid as Corti-lymph, though evidently with a relatively high potassium content (compare Fig. 7).

The endolymph is largely a product of the stria vascularis, which is also involved in the spiral longitudinal diffusion gradient towards the site of resorption of the endolymph in the saccus endolymphaticus, as shown by the rising potassium content (Miyamoto and Morgenstern 1979, 1980, Kimura et al. 1980). The movements of fluid and the exchange of individual substances from the serum within the cochlea do not only vary between the endolymph and the perilymph but also between the basal and the apical portions (Giebel 1982). The perilymph serves as a water reservoir for the endolymph (Kley 1951, Jahnke and Gorgas 1974) depending on the electrolyte concentration of both fluids (Vosteen 1976).

As a result of the movements of the electrical charges through the adjoining membranes the endolymph shows a DC potential of +80 mV as compared with the perilymph (endocochlear potential, EP; v. Békésy 1951).The electrolyte gradient is maintained by the electropositive potassium pump in the stria vascularis and the electronegative sodium-potassium pump of Reissner's membrane. In cases of anoxic breakdown a positive diffusion of potassium may also become effective (Arnold and Vosteen 1979). As compared with the *perilymph* a negative

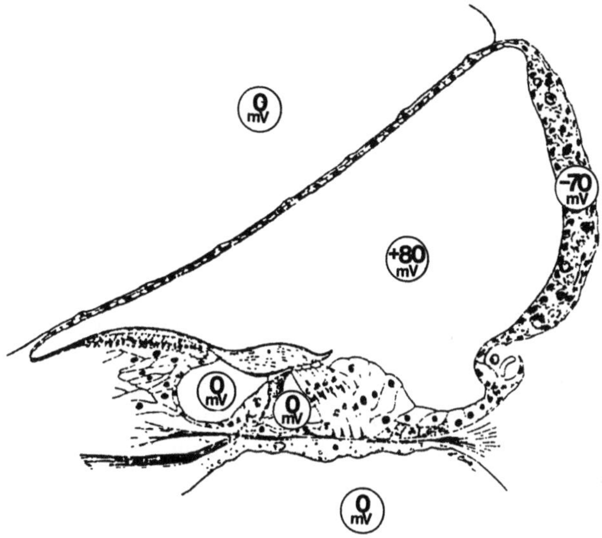

Fig. 5. Semischematic representation of the ductus cochlearis and the sustained potentials. A difference in potential of 150 mV exists between the stria vascularis and the endolymph, and one of 80 mV between the potassium-rich endolymph and sodium-rich perilymph as well as between the endolymph and the Cortilymph. (After Lawrence et al. 1974)

potential gradient of up to 70 mV predominates in the stria vascularis (Chou and Hellenbrecht 1979) – (Fig. 5).

Injury to the hair cells may have occurred directly, for example *mechanically* by blast or explosion trauma, by metabolic exhaustion after excessive noise stress or by ototoxic aminoglycoside antibiotics. Or the injury results from changes in the lymph surrounding the hair cells, e.g. a shift in the electrolyte balance, a hindrance of the oxygen and glucose transport or changes in viscosity or pressure. These are mostly caused by a disturbance of the stria vascularis whereas *deafness* does not arise but in the affected sensory cell, even if this is not definitely damaged. The cells of the *spiral ganglion* may also be the site of deafness. They might be damaged by toxic agents or viral infections without the endolymphatic system with the organ of Corti being involved. Circulatory disturbances of the inner ear however, are only exceptionally expected to cause *isolated* damage of the ganglion cells but rather of the organ of Corti *and* the spiral ganglion.

2.2 Differential Audiometry

As far as the supra-threshold tests are concerned, one must proceed from the recruitment and its equivalents as for hair cell deafness, from Fowler's recruitment as for deafness differing on the two sides, and otherwise from loudness discrimination or the stapedius reflex threshold, which – in spite of the hearing loss – are still normal or approximately normal. In this connection it may be assumed for exclusive hair cell deafness (with normal middle ear function), that up to a hearing loss of about 50 dB the stapedius reflex threshold remains at about 80 dB HL and only shows a linear rise with further increase in hearing loss (Lehnhardt 1976, Hyde et al. 1980). This behaviour is also in accordance with the observation that the stapedius reflex threshold does not correlate with the subjective loudness (Martin and Brunette 1980), or with the threshold of discomfort (Tabo and Rainville 1976).

Even in noise masking as a recruitment equivalent (Langenbeck's test) hair cell deafness reacts in accordance with the norm – in contrast to neural deafness which is associated with increased masking. When recording the tuning curves, patients with inner ear deafness show a reduced ability to distinguish frequencies in the impaired tone levels (Zwicker and Schorn 1978, Bonding 1979, Fastl and Schorn 1981, Schorn 1981, Helle 1983).

Speech audiometry also belongs to the suprathreshold tests, at least as far as monosyllable discrimination is concerned. It should *in no case* be dispensed with in the diagnosis of inner ear deafness if only for reasons of control. The discrimination of monosyllables correlates very well with the tone threshold in inner ear deafness (Lehnhardt 1978, Battmer and Lehnhardt 1984), but not in neural deafness or in psychogenic hearing disturbances. In cases of acoustic neurinoma or multiple sclerosis for example the monosyllable discrimination may be extremely poor and/or the curve shows a "roll over" – a finding that was formerly ascribed to recruitment deafness but does nowadays no longer appear on account of the more sophisticated techniques of amplification (Bess et al. 1979, Hannley and Jerger 1981). Psychogenic hearing disturbances are surprising because of their "too good" monosyllable discrimination (Lehnhardt 1973, 1974).

Objections were repeatedly brought forward against the inner ear specificity of the recruitment phenomenon and its equivalents. They refer above all to the observation that "neural" hearing disturbances, too, may show a positive recruitment (Sanders and Bess 1981). It would be more correct to call them "disturbances of hearing which have arisen as a result or side effect of pathological changes in the vicinity of the auditory nerve." If then the recruitment phenomena are actually the expression of a dysfunction in the organ of Corti or if neural dysfunctions may also have the character of recruitment, this question cannot be decided in the particular case – probably not even in general.

If *recruitment phenomena thus do not rule out a neural hearing defect* it may on the other hand be considered as valid that (sensory) *inner ear deafness always shows a positive recruitment* – provided that the testing conditions are correct. This subtle distinction in the form of the statement is of significance in the evaluation of the results of suprathreshold tests (Lamoré and Rodenburg 1980). Isolated hair cell damage and *ganglionic* dysfunction (occasionally additional) cannot yet be distinguished by suprathreshold tests, at least not without being forced to give speculative explanations (Fig. 6).

Objections to *all* suprathreshold tests – even to electrocochleography (q.v.) – in the sense that, particularly in patients with inner ear diseases further damage can be produced by the test are only justified if great tone intensities are applied indiscriminately and senselessly. Twenty dB SL will at the least cause no damage, if the threshold had been correctly determined. If, however, this had already been assessed too high by e.g. 20 dB the patient will probably express discomfort or pain sensation, signs which should already suffice for classification of the deafness as sensory. It goes without saying that further tests should then be prohibited, even very brief ones.

The appropriate limitation applies in the same way to speech audiometry and the stapedius reflex threshold, which should be measured only up to a maximum of 115 dB HL, naturally only proceeding from the least to greater intensities and only until the threshold value is reached, but not beyond it (Lenarz and Gülzow 1983).

The *high or highest tone audiometry* has been developed into a reliable technique in recent years (Dieroff 1976, 1982, Osterhammel 1979, 1980). Up to the present, however, it has only been used by a few investigators. Its results will be dealt with in connection with the various clinical

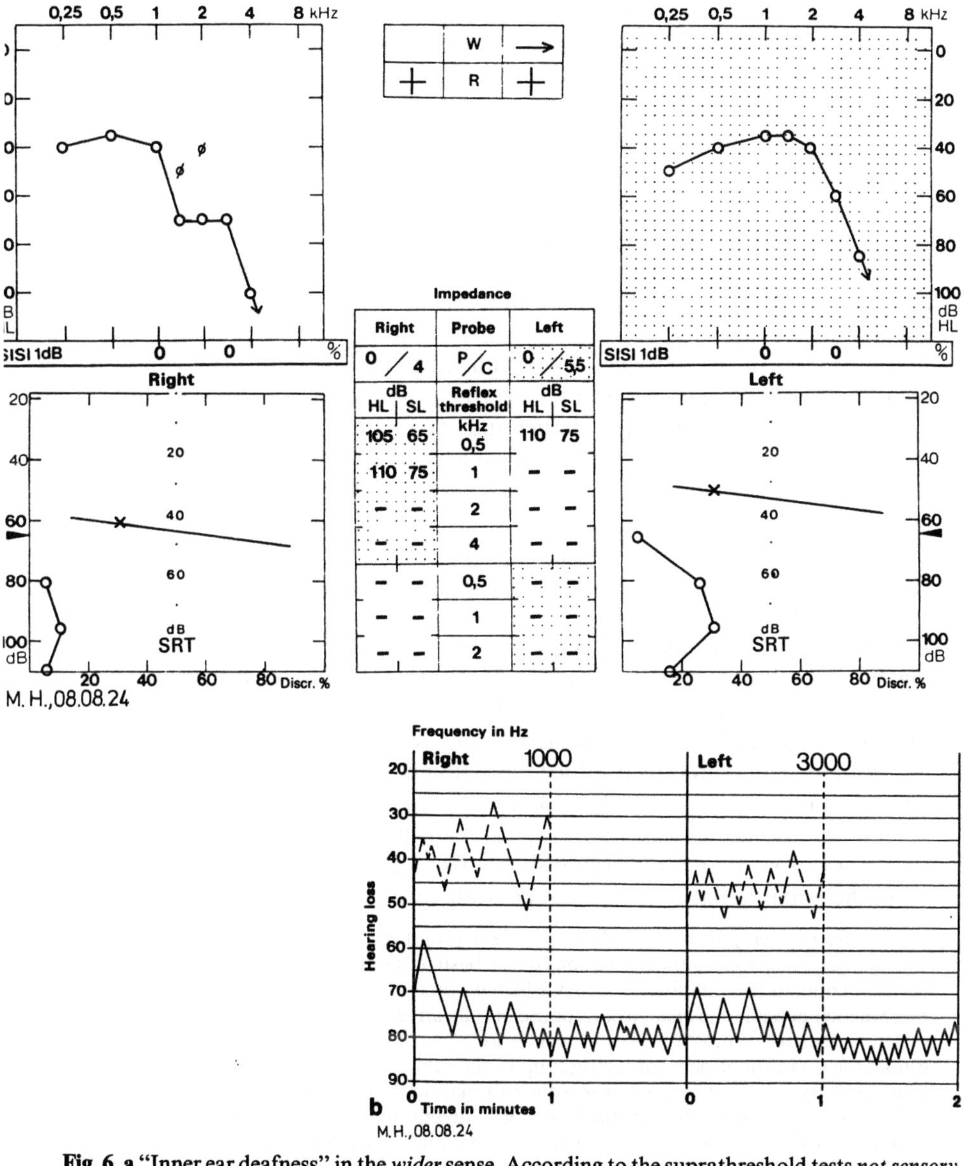

Fig. 6. a "Inner ear deafness" in the *wider* sense. According to the suprathreshold tests *not sensory* in origin. SISI = 0%. Stapedius reflex threshold markedly raised or reflex not elicitable. Extremely poor monosyllable discrimination. The brain stem responses were markedly delayed. Hardness of hearing since childhood. Diagnosis not elucidated. In this audiogram and the following ones the area for the left ear is dotted, in order to refer to the impedance results. Therefore, also those areas are dotted in which the threshold of the stapedius reflex elicited from the left ear is noted down – for the contralateral recording (right) as well as for the ipsilateral recording (left). P/C in the impedance field stands for pressure and compliance; dB HL represents the reflex threshold above the general hearing threshold and dB SL above the individual hearing threshold at the respective frequencies. In the speech audiogram x means speech threshold (ST) for numbers, o means discrimination of monosyllable words. **b** In the Békésy audiogram there is dissociation of the continuous tone and the pulsed tone curves by about 30–40 dB, relatively large amplitudes. Good agreement of all the audiometric results with each other. Here and in all following audiograms only air conduction is noted. BC = AC

pictures. It must, however, be mentioned that the results are largely age-dependent to such an extent that the clinical application of the method remains problematic (Osterhammel and Osterhammel 1979).

The adaptation and fatigue tests are applicable in inner ear diagnostics, in the sense that an extreme hearing fatigue is not to be expected here, that is, that with a constant amplitude of recording there is no unlimited (> 30 dB) dissociation of the continuous and the pulsed tone thresholds. Apart from this negatively defined symptom complex all the others are evidently unspecific. Diminution of the recording amplitude with and without separation, or constant amplitudes without or with only limited (< 30 dB) separation occur in hair cell deafness as well as in ganglionic or neural deafness. In general, the (pathologic) adaptation seems to reflect a process in the inner ear whereas hearing fatigue indicates a defect in the neural part of the auditory system. Nevertheless, in the Anglosaxon literature this distinction is mostly neglected (Jerger and Jerger 1983).

Nowadays, any report on the clinical aspects of inner ear deafness is bound to deal also with *electrocochleography (ECochG)*. Though it is not yet an integral part of clinical diagnostics it can obviously provide insights into the process of disease which have so far been missing. However, conventional audiometry will still remain the basis even of electrocochleographic evidence.

In the ECochG leads will either be made from the promontory (Aran and Portmann 1971, and many others) or from the depth of the external auditory meatus (Elberling and Salomon 1973, Humphries et al. 1977, Walter and Blegvad 1981, Mori et al. 1980, and others). The hair cells "respond" by the cochlear microphonics (CM), the basilar membrane generates the summation potential (SP) and the ganglion cells produce the action potential (AP). These three potentials from the inner ear may be separated from each other by different forms of stimulation, polarities and following rates or indeed displayed superimposed in such a way that they are distinguishable from each other. The technical details of all these manipulations shall not be dealt with here.

The *microphone potentials* (CM) reproduce the stimulation current (Ranke 1943) of the sensory cells as a response to the oscillations of the basilar membrane. They have a sinusoidal form corresponding to the stimulus frequency which is applied; for this reason, it is difficult to recognize whether actually the *biological* response or only an *electrical* artefact was recorded. This uncertainty demands utmost reserve in the interpretation of the findings (Hoke 1973, 1976). In addition, the CM cannot be recorded right up to the subjective threshold, although the outer hair cells evidently contribute more towards their formation than the inner ones (Sellick and Russell 1980). Since, in addition to this, the lead is not directly made from the relevant portion of the cochlea, but from the promontory or the external auditory meatus, the response includes the phase differences with which the CM are generated along the basilar membrane (v. Békésy 1951).

The significance of the CM is therefore limited (Aran and Charlet de Sauvage 1976). This is regrettable since they would have been expected to answer the question whether, with damage of the ganglion cells, responses to stimulation of the sensory cells, i.e. the CM, can still be recorded or not (Beagley 1974, Elberling and Salomon 1973, Nishida 1977). The CM may still function in spite of deafness, provided that the lesion is located beyond the hair cells – possibly in the spiral ganglion; in animal experiments this symptom complex is seen for example in lesions caused by loop diuretics (Klinke et al. 1981). On the other hand, the failure of the CM naturally causes an interruption of all the potentials which result from it, i.e. the SP, the AP and the brain stem potentials.

The *summation* potential does not represent the response of a biological generator, but merely results from the fact that the basilar membrane oscillates asymmetrically, namely with a greater amplitude towards the scala tympani than towards the scala vestibuli. For the most part the SP has a negative polarity. The audiometric value of the SP lies in the fact that it is particularly clear if the basilar membrane is additionally affected by an endolymphatic hydrops and then "swings out" with an even greater asymmetry towards the scala tympani (Eggermont 1976a–c, Nishida 1977, Beagley and Gibson 1978, Moffat 1978, Moffat et al. 1978, Rietema 1979, Morrison et al. 1980, Gibson 1980). The increase of the SP may therefore be judged as evidence of a hydropic dysfunction of the organ of Corti. The technical assessment of *the size* of the SP, however is difficult; moreover the SP is only produced by very loud stimuli ($\geqq 80$ dB), as only these lead to asymmetric oscillations of the basilar membrane.

Occasionally the SP was used for demonstrating a high tone loss because at the start of the deterioration there is a reversal of polarity in the SP from negative to positive (Eggermont 1976a). It is only in exceptional cases that this finding is of any significance in auditory diagnostics. The interpretation of a reversal of polarity becomes complicated if one follows Zwislocki (1975) who attributes the negativity of the SP to the outer and the positivity to the inner hair cells.

The *action*-potential (AP) of the ganglion cells can be recorded nearly up to the subjective threshold of hearing. Its amplitude and latency are clearly dependent on the loudness of the stimulus above the subjective threshold. As the clinical ECochG does not reproduce the action of the individual nerve fiber, but only the sum of the potentials in the high frequency range one should rather speak of the Compound Action Potential (CAP).

The CAP consists of two subsequent portions, N_1 and N_2. At great intensities only N_1 is shown and only with decreasing intensity of stimulus does N_2 appear, in order to take over the lead near the hearing threshold. This behaviour suggests that N_1 refers to the function of the inner hair cells and N_2 to that of the outer hair cells or their respective transition of stimulus to the auditory nerve fiber. What does also contribute to this effect is the fact that with very loud stimuli the responses from the basal turn prevail whereas with decreasing intensity of stimulus the middle turn of the cochlea is also involved in the formation of the CAP – an observation which among others resulted from ECochG findings in low tone and middle tone deafness.

The CAP serves first of all for the *verification* of the subjective tone threshold, although valid only for the high frequencies. In addition, the CAP helps to determine the recruitment for amplitude and latency, is used in the plotting of tuning curves, and finally it can give hints as to the adaptation behaviour of the inner ear (Eggermont and Odenthal 1974). The *amplitude-* or *latency-input-output* function is recorded in input-output curves, whose steepness reflects the recruitment, similar to the loudness-intensity function of subjective audiometry.

The tuning curves can only be plotted with an extraordinary expenditure in apparatus and time (Eggermont et al. 1973, Eggermont 1976a, Eggermont 1977a). They are designed to give information on the acuteness of the frequency tuning in the inner ear, i.e. on Δf. As the acuteness of tuning is already given in the basilar membrane, as explained above, changes in its microme-

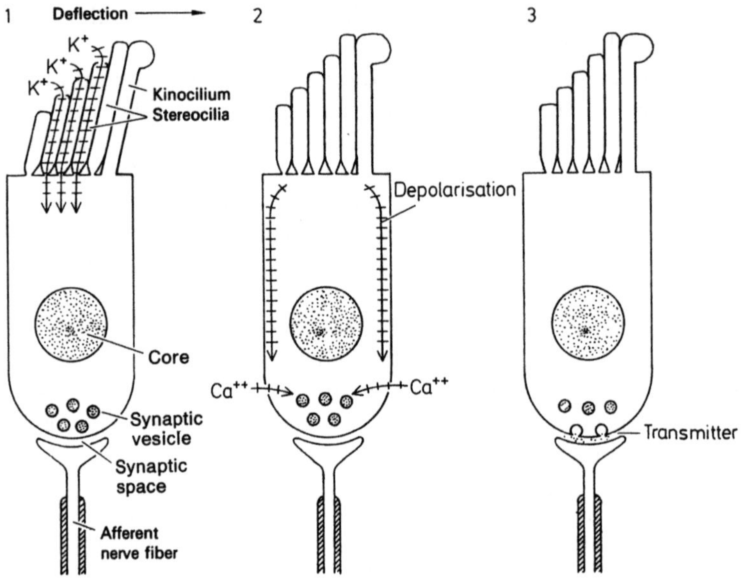

Fig. 7. Function of the hair cell – schematic. The deflection of the cilia allows potassium ions to flow into the cell (*1*). The resulting decrease of the membrane potential leads to an immigration of calcium ions (*2*), which cause the neurotransmitters in the base of the cell to empty themselves via the cell wall (*3*) and to diffuse in the afferent endings of the cochlear nerve fiber. (From Hudspeth 1983)

chanics e.g. as a result of an endolymphatic hydrops, must lead to a broadening of the tuning curves. However, their evaluation, particularly in the differential diagnosis of hydropic and degenerative recruitment, seems only possible in consideration *of the SP* (Kumagami and Miyazaki 1983).

The *adaptation* behaviour of the inner ear is determined by the stimulus transition from the hair cell to the afferent synapse. This process requires a certain amount of time (Fig. 7). It is therefore not possible to work with unlimitedly high following rates unless the rate is to be determined at which *stimulus transition* is no longer synchronous. In patients with normal hearing e.g. the CAP becomes increasingly smaller and from 70/second onwards finally disappears completely (Eggermont 1974). In the light of these considerations, ECochG could fill a gap, where subjective tests have until now largely failed, because they do not reveal with sufficient reliability, in which portion of the hearing pathways from the sensory cells to the cortex the psychoacoustic phenomenon has its origin. Electrocochleographic findings, however, would actually refer to reactions *in the inner ear*.

For the present, however, the long duration of such tests as well as the necessarily great intensities of stimulus (>70 dB) will prevent most investigators from exposing inner ear patients to such a strain and to the risk of additional hearing impairment.

The brain stem and the cortical ERA can hardly be expected to provide information for the differentiation of inner ear dysfunctions. Only Yamada et al. (1979) think that in cases of endolymphatic hydrops they have observed a particularly steep climb of the latency curve for the V wave (P_6) immediately above the stimulation response threshold.

So far no other techniques are available for inner ear diagnostics in man, apart from radiography for the illustration of bony abnormalities. The removal of perilymph for biochemical analysis remains restricted to special intra-operative situations. In this context the procedure of Nagahara et al. (1983) is of interest. They have performed direct measurements of the perilymphatic O_2-tension in diseased inner ears, by means of micropolarography through a perforation in the footplate of the stapes. These measurements showed low initial values but a normal reaction to CO_2 inhalation in *sudden* hearing loss, and normal initial values with a slight reaction to CO_2 inhalation in *chronic* progressive inner ear deafness.

Scintigraphy is unsuccessful in inner ear diagnostics on account of the poor resolution capability – except for otosclerotic foci which can now be demonstrated by cochleotympanic scintigraphy (Bornemann et al. 1983). Certain hopes may be placed on nuclear spin tomography with its possibilities of an in vivo molecular biology.

Laboratory (*biochemical*) investigations may contribute to the etiological diagnosis in a few types of deafness, as e.g. in certain kidney, thyroid and metabolic diseases. The special clinical features and the audiometric and cochleographic findings will have to be dealt with in the relevant chapters.

2.3 The Differentiation of Various Types of Inner Ear Deafness by Means of the Sound Threshold Curves

As regards the tone threshold curve, it is to be distinguished between

- High tone deafness with high tone dip, oblique or steep fall
- Middle tone deafness
- Low tone deafness and the
- Pantonal deafness, the flat curve

The terms baso- medio- apico- and panchochlear should no longer be used because on the one hand, they require the translation of the audiogram into the anatomy of the cochlea and, on the other hand, because the suffix-"cochlear" anticipates the site of origin of the disturbance. Deafness with identical bone and air conduction need not be localised in the inner ear and thus need not be *cochlear*. It would thus be a *contradiction in terms* to speak of an apico*cochlear neural* deafness e.g. in an acoustic neurinoma or of a pan*cochlear* brain stem deafness in a disturbance of the central auditory pathways.

The causal specificity of a high tone dip[2] consists in the fact that, though acoustic traumata do not necessarily cause dips, there are only a few cases where the dip is of non-traumatic genesis. Glorig (1973) nevertheless called it a myth that the 4000 Hz dip should be pathognomonic for noise injury.

The site of the maximum dip is determined within narrow limits by the frequency pattern of the acoustic noxa to the effect that the high frequency noises (for example in smithies), or bangs, tend to cause injury around 6000 Hz whereas low tone noises (e.g. in weaving mills) involve the frequencies around 3000 Hz. In addition to that, individual factors related above all to the middle ear appear to play a part, in particular the function of the middle ear muscles (Lehnhardt 1965, Borg et al. 1983).

---

[2] The term "dip" should be restricted to those thresholds patterns in which the hearing threshold approaches normal values again above the frequency of the maximum nearing loss.

Among the many explanations for the phenomenon of the dip which have so far been presented the one referring to the hydrodynamics of the inner ear has up to now remained uncontradicted (Meyer zum Gottesberge 1960, Lehnhardt 1966). According to it, the summation effect of the various noise components leads to a maximum consumption of energy around 4000 Hz that is around the upper frequency limit of optimum hearing (1000–4000 Hz). This interpretation takes into consideration the observation that even after experimental narrow band stress the maximum dip regularly lies about half an octave above the upper frequency limit of the stress noise (Davis et al. 1950), however, only up to 4000 Hz, since above this frequency the threshold sensitivity of the ear decreases steeply (Meyer zum Gottesberge 1960).

Tonndorf (1979) recently again referred to the length of the external auditory meatus as the factor which influences the position of the dip, but this is only *one* causal factor for the frequency access of the *whole* ear and thus for the range of optimum hearing at the upper limit of which the drop originates.

The dip in high tones may arise in the same way as the sequel to noise- or *explosion* stress, as well as after a blunt cranial trauma (Escher 1948). Wittmaack (1932) suspected a "fluid pressure wave" to be the cause of the resulting dip or the high tone drop. Schuknecht and Tonndorf (1960) ascribed it to non-linear distortions of extreme amplitudes at the stapes; on account of their short time constant these would become effective in the transitional zone between the middle and upper third of the basal turn, all the more since further towards the windows the sensitivity of the inner ear decreases again. This implies at the same time that the sequels to a blast or a blunt cranial trauma cannot be distinguished basically from those to noise stress.

In addition, a so-called *extra high tone loss* with a steep drop of the hearing threshold above 6000 Hz is occasionally observed as a residue of an exposure to *blast*, above all in the case of soldiers after gun-fire. There seems to exist an individual predisposition, as only some of those taking part at any one time are affected. The extremely high sound of particular light weapons appears to be responsible for this special type of blast trauma.

In general, however, the steepness of the high tone loss is not the expression of a particular genesis of deafness, that is to say not every steep high tone loss must be traumatic in origin. Below 1500 Hz for example, the steep drop of the hearing threshold is for the most part hereditary or infantile in origin (Rösler and Anderson 1978).

The steepness of the drop in the high and middle tone region can amount to several hundred dB per octave, and in the low tone region to 70–90 dB. Another possible cause of this *steep* fall off, independent of its relation to frequencies, is meningitis, not only the bacterial but also the viral one. The specificity of this clinical picture, however, is not great enough to permit any definite conclusions regarding the cause of deafness in the individual patient (Rösler and Anderson 1978).

The *oblique high tone loss* is the most frequent type of inner ear deafness. Behind this type of curve, very diverse etiological and genetic factors may be concealed. These will be dealt with in the discussion of the individual clinical pictures.

Although the explanation seems reasonable that acoustic and mechanical factors preferentially damage the high tone region it is indeed difficult to understand why circulatory or metabolic disturbances and toxic causes lead to identical audiometric findings. No differentiation seems to be possible on the basis of the audiometric findings alone, neither regarding the hearing threshold curve, not the related speech discrimination nor the pattern of the supra-threshold test results. Even the course of the continuous tone threshold has so far not shown any binding regularity: In the Békésy test small amplitudes with or without separation of the continous and the pulsed tone threshold are found in all etiologically different forms of high tone loss – or not.

The non-specificity of the high tone loss also applies to those types of deafness which develop in early childhood as well to the hereditary or constitutional forms – independent of whether they are stationary or progressive. The question whether "presbyacusis" is to be distinguished from all these causes of high tone loss in advanced age, requires detailed discussion (see Chap. 3.7).

With the flattening of the threshold curve towards the *high tone diagonal loss* noise damage as the exclusive etiology becomes increasingly doubtful. On the other hand, limited [85 to 90 dB (A)] and uniform noise may occasionally also result in relatively flat high tone losses, as for example in textile workers. The same pattern of the threshold is again part of the genetically unclear types of deafness, including the so-called presbyacusis, for the most part with all signs of recruitment and with a speech discrimination that corresponds to the pure tone hearing loss.

There is more specificity in the *middle tone dip* or *"trough."* This is in most cases of endogenous hereditary origin. With increasing age or under other forms of stress, the trough develops into a high tone loss commencing already at 500–1000 Hz, and therefore loses its characteristic threshold picture (cf. Fig. 24). Occasionally an acoustic neurinoma may be recognised by a middle tone dip, certainly not frequently, but the irregularity is precisely the characteristic feature in the differential diagnosis of this tumor-induced type of deafness.

It is common to all *high* tone and *middle* tone hearing losses that only exceptionally they are reversible. Among the exceptions there are for example the deafness in Cogan's syndrome, in syphilis, in some cases of sudden hearing loss or as a sequel to raised intracranial pressure (Hommerich 1963). In general, however, improvements can scarcely be expected in the many cases of high tone deafness caused by noise, circulatory or metabolic disturbances or toxic agents.

In contrast to this, *low tone* deafness does not reflect a primary degeneration of the sensory cells but an initially reversible disturbance of the osmotic and electrolyte balance in the endolymphatic system. This is at least an attempt to understand the clinical picture of the *fluctuating hearing impairment*. It is, for the most part, limited to the low and middle tone range; in contrast to this, significant fluctuations of hearing are rare in the high (and middle) tone levels.

Pantonal deafness has occasionally developed from a low tone deafness, that is to say by the involvement of the originally unaffected frequencies above 2000 Hz, or a low tone deafness is added to the high tone loss. More frequently it will have extended over all the frequencies from the beginning. Only exceptionally it is of exogenous origin, i.e. caused by noise (Chung et al. 1980), blast, mechanical trauma or intoxication; for the most part pantonal deafness is endogenous in origin.

Almost all patterns of the hearing threshold can be the expression not only of a sensory but also of a neural or central-neural deafness. The only exception seems to be the low tone deafness. Its tone threshold pattern is the only one, which is not met with in acoustic neurinomas and cerebello-pontine angle tumors. The audiograms *can* therefore provide evidence as to the etiology and origin of the various forms of inner ear deafness, *scarcely one, however, is on its own specific for a certain illness*. Additional information is necessary in the individual case, in order to be able to classify the respective impairment of hearing with the appropriate clinical picture. This refers above all to the anamnesis and to the findings of internal medical examination as well as of laboratory diagnostics.

3 Special Features

3.1 Traumatic Inner Ear Deafness

3.1.1 Noise and Blast Injury

The last two decades have yielded only a few new discoveries about the pathology and clinical features of noise-induced deafness. It is still being assumed that a minimum level must have had an effect *over several years* in order to leave *a permanent* loss of hearing. In the Federal Republic of Germany the legislator and the Employer's Liability Insurance Associations nowadays regard a person-related assessment level of ≧85 dB (A) already as noxious (Memorandum issued by the Federal Minister of Labour on 20.7.77, cf. VB 21/78 HVBG – VB 59/78 of 13.4.78) as compared with the earlier limit of 90 dB (A) which for example still applies today in France (Duclos and Dubreuil 1979). The justification for the German level has in the meantime been confirmed by 25,000 audiograms from noise-exposed Austrian workers (Schwetz et al. 1980).

In dealing with the *Temporary Threshold Shift* (TTS) a new concept has appeared: Asymptotic Threshold Shift (ATS). This *saturation* value of noise-induced threshold shift is said to correspond to the *maximum* damaging effect of a particular sound independent of the duration of occupational exposure (Henderson and Hamernik 1982). If for example after an exposure over ten days to 113 dB p.e. SPL the TTS has reached an asymptotic course at 40 dB, this *temporary* hearing loss of 40 dB would be expected to be *permanent* hearing damage at the frequency concerned after many years of occupational noise exposure (Fig. 8).

The ATS – in contrast to the TTS – is said to be largely independent of any pre-existing hearing loss (Humes and Koval 1981); however, up to now all statistics are based exclusively on animal experiments. The values found cannot therefore be transferred to man, but only their basic tendencies (Bohne and Clark 1982).

The determination of the ATS is not regarded as a test for the individual noise-sensitivity or -resistance either. The ATS is particularly suitable, however, for the assessment of *impulse*-containing noise. This could mean an important progress in so far as the impulse peaks show intensities of 130 to 150 dB and more, and therefore can only be recorded by apparatus which are able to register such levels and have a time constant of 35 ms.

The possibility of recording the CM, with the necessary precautions, even in man has been made use of by Pratt et al. (1978) in order to determine the site of the threshold shift. According to their findings, it does not affect the CM but rather the AEP[3] of the brain stem. Apparently the *reversible* decrease of the threshold after noise stress, originates in the synaptic junction between the sensory cells and the nerve fibers. However, the reservations as to the assessment of the CM were pointed out above.

---

[3] Acoustically evoked potentials.

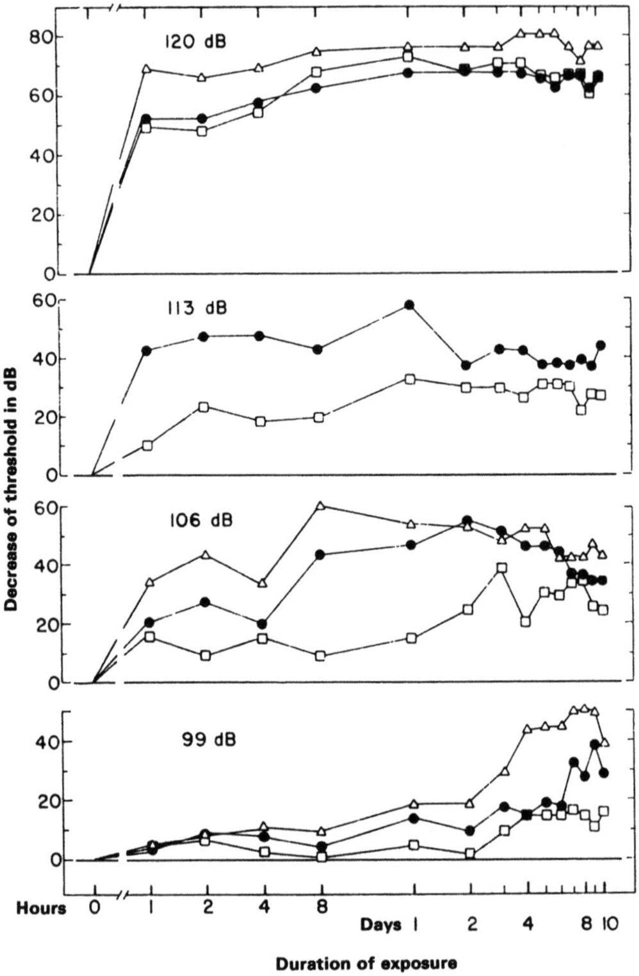

Fig. 8. *Asymptotic* threshold shift (ATS). Increase of the average threshold decay during ten days of noise exposure to 99, 106, 113, and 120 dB peak SPL in the chinchilla. *Squares* for 0.5, *triangles* for 2, and *circles* for 8 kHz. The asymptote has already been reached after one day with 113 and 120 dB. (From Henderson and Hamernik 1982)

The mechanical destruction of hair cells as well as disturbances of microcirculation in the cochlea are considered to be special noxae of *pulsed* noise (Kellerhals 1972). In the cytocochleogram, pulsed noise stress is striking because of the extremely sharp transition from the intact hair cell pattern to the area of complete degeneration (Johnsson and Hawkins 1976). In the audiogram this picture corresponds to the extremely steep high frequency drop (Dieroff 1979). However, this is not specific for pulsed noise since some hereditary hearing defects show exactly the same picture.

In general the *audiometric differential diagnosis* of noise-induced deafness continues to cause considerable difficulties. The Békésy audiogram does not provide any help in the differentiation, that is to say the recording amplitudes may become smaller or remain unchanged. The attempt of Weidauer and Lenarz (1982) to use the fatigue of the stapedius reflex as the criterion of a *noise-induced* sensorineural deafness is logical in the sense that patients with noise-induced deafness should not show any fatigue. Their findings have not yet been confirmed.

Niemeyer (1971) believes that the threshold of discomfort is raised in noise-induced deafness, but not the stapedius reflex threshold, not even in the frequencies with progressed hearing loss. In practice this procedure often remains unproductive, as the determination of the threshold of discomfort is not accurate enough (±12 dB; Forquer 1979) and the stapedius reflex threshold is useless for the diagnosis if there is a middle ear component. Apart from this, Dieroff (1976) thinks that with increasing noise damage the stapedius reflex threshold rises and indeed may be evidence of the involvement of the spiral ganglion.

Slightly asymmetrical hearing impairment is rather to be expected after exposure to pulsed then to continuous noise (Johnsson and Hawkins 1976). Differences, *generally to the disadvantage* of the left ear were described by Sutherland and Gasaway (1978) and also by Chung et al. (1981, 1983). Differing exposure of the two ears had been excluded here. This noise-induced asymmetry involves particularly the frequencies from 2000 to 6000 Hz, it amounts to >10 dB in ca 7% of the cases (Alberti et al. 1979). Nevertheless, the left ear is reported to be the worse one even without any noise stress and independent of age (Glorig and Roberts 1965). Incidentally the former concept that women are more resistant to noise than men has not been confirmed by a statistical analysis of 25,000 workers exposed to noise (Welleschik and Körpert 1980).

With more effective diagnostic facilities *striking* asymmetries have increasingly appeared as a sequel to acoustic neurinomas (Miller et al. 1981). *Central* hearing disturbances existing in addition to the noise-induced deafness, might be diagnosed with the help of directional audiometry (Dieroff 1973).

There are some recent comments on damage to hearing produced by electronically amplified music. Jatho and Hellmann (1972) had found *slight loss of hearing* in 13% of the professionals. The small number, in spite of equal exposure, indicated an individual sensitivity to noise in the persons affected. These observations were in agreement with the results of laboratory tests (Dey 1970, Speaks et al. 1970) and have also been repeatedly confirmed (Strauss and Chüden 1974, Redell and Lebo 1972, Westmore and Everdsen 1981). On the other hand, high frequency dips were seen in 5 of 18 disc jockeys. They were thus not quite so rare but always kept within narrow limits with a maximum hearing loss of 35 dB at 4000 Hz, 6000 Hz or 8000 Hz (Frei 1980). For persons with *non-occupational* exposure to rock music the risk is obviously much smaller – unless they also work in noise during daytime! Nevertheless, the high frequency component in the new electronic amplifiers should be a warning against excessive exposure, all the more since high frequency losses are increasingly being observed in youngsters not otherwise exposed to stress (Koizumi 1980).

In contrast to that, an emission of noise levels of <85 dB (A) have been measured in dental drills and of >80 dB (A) only in a few machines. Hearing damage therefore appears to be excluded (Praml and Sonnabend 1980).

New aspects could also be opened by high tone audiometry. It demonstrates that the frequency band above 12,000 Hz which is initially resistant to noise, becomes more and more levelled off with increasing acoustic trauma (Fig. 9). Moreover, test subjects with otherwise normal frequency thresholds, who show an impaired auditory function in the region of >12,000 Hz are less noise resistant (Osterhammel 1979, Dieroff 1976, 1982).

The attempt of Fritze (1981) as well as Fritze and Gedlicka (1982) to use the temporary *high tone* dip after experimental *low tone* stress as a criterion for the expected noise *resistance* seems to be of too little significance. The theoretical bases of these considerations are the observations by Burdick et al. (1977) and Burdick (1981) that extreme low frequency noises around 63 Hz *A-weighted* are more damaging than for example those around 1000 Hz. Four-hour exposure to

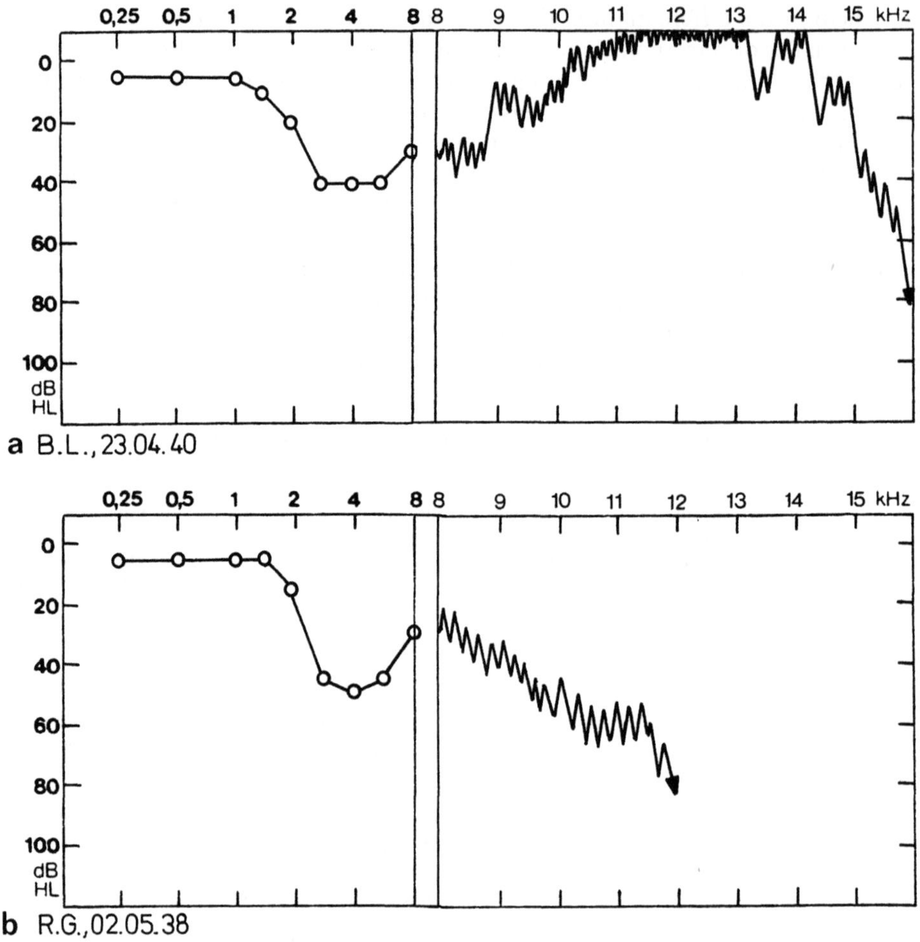

Fig. 9 a, b. Varying behavior of the hearing threshold in the highest frequencies, with similar high tone dip. **a** The hearing function at the frequencies above 8000 Hz is still largely preserved, despite 18 years noise exposure as a weaver. **b** After 22 years exposure as a weaver a clear hearing loss is to be recognized above 8000 Hz. (I am grateful to Prof. Dr. H. G. Dieroff, Jena for these results.) Air conduction only

63 Hz band pass noises had also caused a considerable temporary threshold shift at 1000 to 3000 Hz (Patterson et al. 1977). These results will have to be taken into consideration in the assessment of permanent hearing impairment after exposure to low frequencies.

The experiments of Jerger et al. (1966) represented a transition to vibration stress: the test subjects were exposed to sounds of 119–144 dB in the region of 2–22 Hz. They also showed a TTS in the frequencies from 3000 to 8000 Hz. In occupational, exclusively noise-induced deafness – that is without extreme low frequency stress – Chung (1980) claims to have seen, besides the usual 4000 Hz dip, a second hearing impairment between 500 and 1000 Hz. There now seems to be no more doubt about an additional vibratory effect on the inner ear (Kile and Wurzbach 1980, Hamernik et al. 1981).

Other investigators found lower TTS values and a quicker recovery under simultaneous vibration (Pfander 1978). Possibly the frequency and amplitude of the vibration play a decisive role in this respect, and certainly also the duration of the exposure, on the one hand only in laboratory testing and on the other over many years of employment.

The question remains under discussion as to *how* this additional danger arises for the persons thus exposed: Possibly by the *vibratory stimulation of the sympathetic nervous system* and the resulting vasospastic effect. In any case, the noise-induced damage was particularly severe in those workers who also showed circulatory disturbances in the fingers (Pykkö and Starck 1982). Precisely the opposite effect, however, would have to be expected according to the findings of Handrock and Fischer (1979), which suggest that a sympathectomy in guinea pigs produces a detrimental noise reaction, whereas the experiments of Beickert and Terayama (1965) as well as those of Maass et al. (1977) had shown a positive effect and those of Hultcrantz (1979) no effect at all on the noise-exposed inner ear.

Handrock and his group have produced several articles on the subject of individual noise sensitivity. Smokers are predisposed to noise-induced deafness (Handrock and Matthias 1982), as well as exposed persons with a magnesium deficiency (Handrock et al. 1981, Ising et al. 1982, Joachims et al. 1983). This is quite possible on account of the "very refined diet" or because of *overdosage* of *Vitamin D* in the industrialised countries and leads to a reduction of the magnesium concentration in the perilymph; on its own, this would not cause any functional impairment in the inner ear, but probably under additional influence from noise – or stress (Vitamin D deficiency, cf. also Page 95). Incidentally, *magnesium* deficiency could also be the cause of the mostly slight high tone hearing impairment in the Wernicke-Korsakoff syndrome, especially as it is apparently localised peripherally in the inner ear in contrast to the other central symptoms of this disease (Probst 1983).

There is an obviously clarifying study by Hood et al. (1976) regarding the influence of the eye color on the TTS. With strict statistical precautions a differentiated picture was obtained to the effect that below 110 dB the *adaptation* is dependent on the melanin content of the iris; above this level, there is *fatigue* – independent of its melanin content. Such critical appraisal also applies to the concept that with a melanin pigmented iris the loss of hearing at 4000 Hz in the left ear is greater than in the absence of pigmentation (Carter 1980).

Vitamin A deficiency is said to have no negative effect on the noise resistance (TTS), at least according to the results in guinea pigs (Seinsch et al. 1982). However, some contrary ideas have also been produced, but these are purely speculative (Willemse 1952, Rüedi 1954, Löhle et al. 1982).

As regards the question whether the inner ear reacts to the noise stress with an additional vascular constriction, a definite answer seems to have been found. According to this, the circulation in the guinea pig cochlea remains constant, as shown by the hydrogen clearance in the endolymphatic space and by polarographic microanalysis, even under exposure to 115 dB of wide band noise, over a period of 45 minutes (Maass and Ludwig 1983). The findings were confirmed by Angelborg et al. (1979) as well as Hultcrantz (1979) as they could not detect any vascular reaction caused by noise. Meanwhile these results have again been questioned by the phasecontrast microscopic findings of Axelsson et al. (1983). According to these, long-term stress (100 dB for 10 hours/day over eight weeks) in rats leads to precapillary sphincter contractions in the radial arterioles of the scala vestibuli and to a reduced circulation in the lamina spiralis. These findings, however, involved mainly spontaneously hypertensive animals and much less the normotensive ones (Borg 1979, Axelsson and Vertes 1982). The entire blood supply of the labyrinth, too, is reported to be reduced (Vertes et al. 1980), and noise exposure could even lead to atrophy of the stria vascularis (Clarke and Bohne 1978).

Brown et al. (1982) likewise favor the "vascular genesis" of noise-induced deafness, but they confine this statement to the frequencies below 1.5 kHz.

Ototoxic medication prior to noise exposure may be the cause of disproportionally severe noise damage. In the opposite case, a reciprocal dependence has so far been denied i.e. a previous exposure to noise would not leave any particular sensitivity of the inner ear. Now, Rejtö et al. (1982) suggest that also primarily noise-damaged subjects are particularly endangered by ototoxic agents. Indeed, both noxae attack the sensory cells directly, but in different ways: the exposure to noise leads to a degeneration by unphysiological acoustic overloading and hence to a metabolic exhaustion; the ototoxic substances first of all only accumulate in the organ of Corti, and secondarily – possibly under physiological "stress" – induce cell death.

While in the case of damage exclusively due to noise, loss of hair cells was also observed in the apical turns of the guinea pig cochlea, the combined application of noise and aminoglycoside antibiotics led to an exclusively basal pattern of damage (Dodson and Bannister 1982).

This relatively brief discussion of noise damage in the inner ear must suffice for the present. The standard information may be looked up in the Report on Occupational Diseases (Lehnhardt 1965), in "Noise-induced Deafness" (Dieroff 1975), in "Effect of Noise in Man" (Kryter 1970), in "Occupational Hearing Loss" (Robinson 1971), in "Noise-induced Hearing Loss" (Hamernik et al. 1980), or in "Industrial Noise Pollution and Hearing Impairment" (Sulkowski 1980). The effects of noise on hearing from the physiological point of view were dealt with by Spreng (1982).

Pfander (1975) gave a summarised description of *blast injuries*. The development of new weapon systems has meanwhile produced sound pressure peaks of up to 250 dB SPL (Sound Pressure Level) that is to say, values which by far exceed those of pulsed noise. While pulsed sounds have a duration of <1 ms (ISO R – 1999), blast or detonations produce pressure peaks of <2 ms and explosions such of >2 ms duration. Such powerful discharges of energy are expected to produce predominantly mechanical injuries to the inner ear, even though perhaps only at the microscopic or the ultramicroscopic level, e.g. on the reticular membrane (Meyer and Biedermann 1980). Finally, *extreme noise* stress (140 dB for one minute) may also cause cellular destruction, e.g. in the stria vascularis (Ulehlová 1982). Details regarding the pathology of blast trauma may be read in the textbook article by Spoendlin (1980). In their clinical presentation the non-mechanical, metabolic components of the blast or explosion trauma resemble those resulting from noise exposure.

3.1.2 Explosion and Cranial Trauma

Like blast and explosion the blunt cranial trauma may damage only the upper part of the basal turn (high frequency dip)– also in boxers (Paulsen and Hundhausen 1971) – or the portion near the round window (high tone loss), or it produces – above all in the case of accompanying fractures – functional death of the entire inner ear.

Since the amount of energy acting is difficult to assess the resulting patterns of hearing impairment are bound to be very different i.e. occasionally even flat

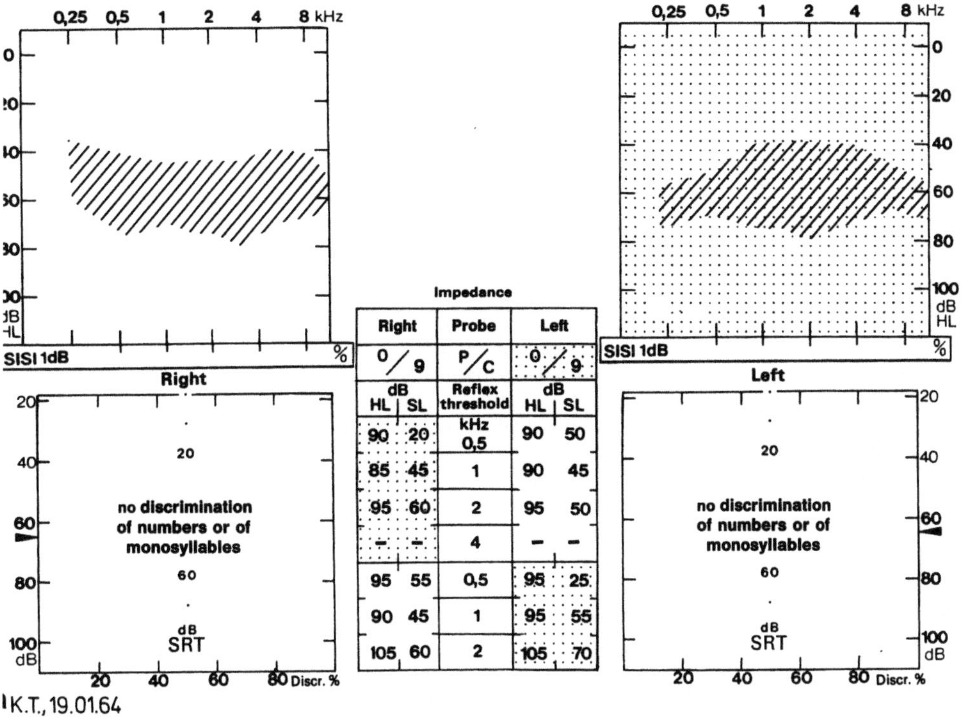

Right		Probe	Left	
0/9		P/C	0/9	
dB HL	SL	Reflex threshold	dB HL	SL
90	20	kHz 0,5	90	50
85	45	1	90	45
95	60	2	95	50
–	–	4	–	–
95	55	0,5	95	25
90	45	1	95	55
105	60	2	105	70

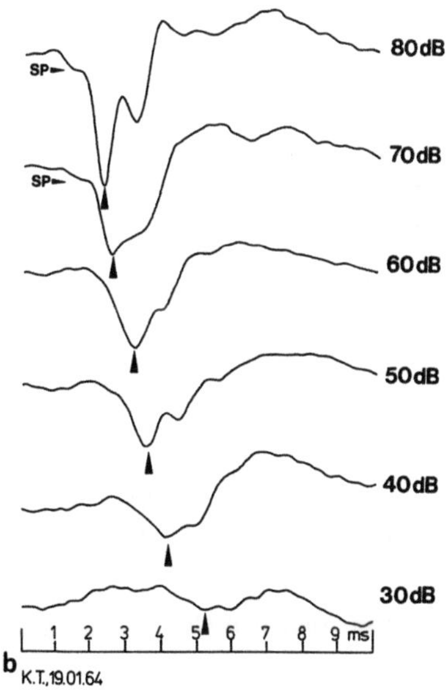

Fig. 10a, b. Example of deafness, *not* inner ear related, after craniocerebral trauma with brain stem contusion. **a** The pure tone hearing still seems to be relatively good, even if the patient's answers were very uncertain (hatched area). Stapedius reflex on both sides largely maintained; no pathological reflex decay. Speech discrimination completely lost. **b** In the ECochG the AP is recordable from 30 or 40 dB onwards, though only for N_1; the SP is clearly recognisable. Brain stem stimulus responses (P_6J_v) are absent

threshold patterns are seen which first of all appear to be nontraumatic (Kerr 1980). They are interpreted by some authors as the manifestation of a traumatic endolymphatic hydrops (Clark and Rees 1977, Rizvi and Gibbin 1979).

Hearing defects following blunt cranial traumata may also exclusively or additionally involve the *central hearing pathway*. These types of deafness which appear "at first sight" to be of inner ear origin can be recognised and localised by special tests (dichotic speech discrimination, stapedius reflex threshold, ECochG, brain stem and cortical ERA, etc) as a lesion somewhere between the auditory nerve and the cortex (Lehnhardt et al. 1981, Fig. 10).

A possibility of distinguishing – by means of audiometric findings – noise-induced from traumatic high frequency damage might be offered by high frequency audiometry. While noise-induced deafness shows a *continuous* deterioration extending to 15,000 Hz, those subjects suffering from an acute traumatic injury are reported to show an *abrupt, complete* hearing loss in the region above the steep fall already recognisable by routine audiometry (Dieroff 1982).

As regards the treatment of acute acoustic trauma, medication with Dextran 40 plus vitamin A and E, Betahistin and Modazepam, has proved ineffective in comparison with NaCl infusions plus placebo tablets (Eibach and Börger 1980). Other authors claim to have achieved significant improvements by ventilation with hyperbaric oxygen (Lamm and Klimpel 1971, Demaertelaere and van Opstal 1981) or with as gas mixture of 95% O_2 plus 5% CO_2 (Ott and von Felten 1981).

Furthermore, the traumatic hearing impairments include those originating from pressure differences and also from electric injury of the ear. These were dealt with in detail in my Report of 1965. In divers and pilots many acute losses of hearing are explained today rather as a window rupture than as a decompression sickness in the original sense (King 1976, Novotny 1980). In the meantime no new points of view have appeared as regards injury by *electric current* or *lightning*.

3.1.3 Rupture of the Windows (Round and Oval)

3.1.3.1 Round Window Membrane Rupture

The integration of this section into the chapter on traumatic inner ear deafness was done with the intention not to count this clinical picture among the atraumatic cryptogenic hearing losses as long as the atraumatic genesis has not been proved – even if the incidence is ever so inconspicuous (Stroud and Calcaterra 1970, Goodhill 1971, Goodhill et al. 1973, Pullen 1972, Fraser and Harborow 1975).

Ruptures of the round window membrane were discribed for the first time by Ulrich in 1926 not, however, as an independent clinical picture, but as a side effect of severe concussion or fracturing of the petrous bone. It is only recently that it has been reported on again (Strohm 1982). Though they are not the topic of the present discussion, it is necessary to mention Ulrich's observations in order to understand why first of all the rupture could only be explained as the sequel of an external insult.

Even in the case of an apparently atraumatic rupture one must look for a force, which acts from within, that is from the perilymphatic space and causes the membrane to be torn. This force seemed not to exist as long as the human aquaeductus cochleae was regarded as extremely narrow. Since, however, no more doubt seems to exist about the fact that this connection between CSF and

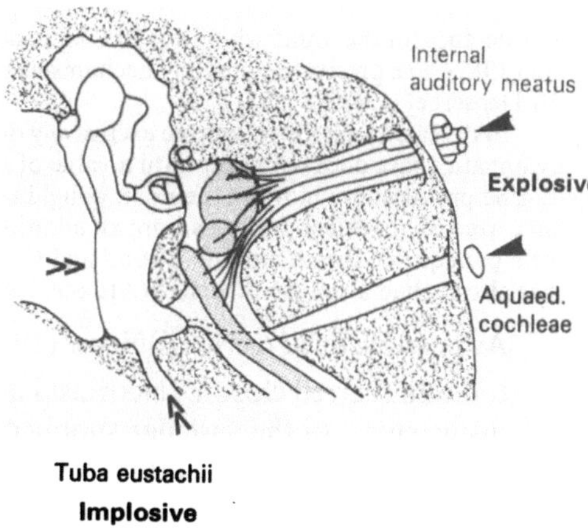

Fig. 11. Semischematic diagram of the connecting pathways between CSF and the inner ear, which are considered to be of etiological importance for the implosive or explosive rupture of the round window membrane. Of particular interest are the close topographical relations between the round window membrane and the aquaeductus cochleae. (After Goodhill 1981)

perilymphatic space in man, too, is wide enough to guarantee a pressure compensation (Palva and Dammert 1969, Schuknecht 1974, Farrior and Endicott 1971, Wlodyka 1978, Sekula and Wlodyka 1982), the most important objection to a "spontaneous" rupture of the round window membrane seems to have been removed (Fig. 11). Apart from the aquaeductus cochleae there exists a connection between the CSF and the perilymph (Kley 1961) via the internal auditory meatus along the auditory nerve and the vessels which usually, however, is scarcely suitable for compensating the pressure differences (Beentjes 1972). In contrast to this, the aquaeductus cochleae is able to facilitate even the opposite compensation, i.e. *from the middle ear* to the perilymph and further in the direction of the CSF space – at least in the cat (Carlborg et al. 1982).

Accordingly the following possibilities are offered for the *mechanism of rupture:*

- implosive by an increase in tympanic pressure
- explosive by an increase in CSF pressure via the aquaeductus cochleae (or also along the auditory nerve? Goodhill 1980, 1981), and possibly also
- explosive as the result of an increased congestion of the inner ear vessels (Carlborg 1981).

For the present, it remains an open question in which way the rupture is caused by the single or combined forces which are necessary for this process, whether by blowing the nose, straining, Valsalva, diving, flying and physical effort or even by acoustic traumata (Lyons et al. 1978). From the morphological aspect, slight force should suffice to tear the "membrane", since the perilymph extends ultramicroscopically as far as the subepithelial space of the tympanic mucous membrane (Arnold and von Ilberg 1972).

In guinea pigs the round window membrane ruptures with an *external* positive pressure of 400 mm water column, a value which indeed exceeds physiological strain (Kleinfeld and Dahl 1979) which, however, is applied by some investigators in measurements of tube function in subjects with defects of the ear drum *and* blocked tubes. An *internal* positive pressure of +350 mm water column is said to develop already by deep lowering of the head. If this coincides with a negative tympanic pressure of <600 mm water column on account of blocked tubes, then a pressure gradient of nearly 1000 mm water column would develop at the round window membrane (Allam 1976, Fukaja and Nomura 1983). Measured as pressure per surface unit the average limit of tolerance for the round window is 29.2 kPa and for the oval window 21.4 kPa (Vogt and Bödefeld 1982). The pressure regulating mechanisms in the perilymphatic space are described in detail by Densert et al. (1978, 1981).

In the cat, an explosive rupture exclusively due to an elevation of pressure in the CSF or perilymphatic space does not occur until a value of 10 to 30 mm Hg is reached. Such pressure could not be produced by blowing the nose, coughing, thoracic or abdominal straining and even by an extreme Trendelenburg's position; an additional weakness of the membrane would therefore be a prerequisite for its rupture (Stroud and Calcaterra 1970, Miriszlai 1981), or the membrane has already had a congenital defect (Althaus 1981).

As possible *local factors* Gülzow (1980) mentions

- too thin scarred closure (Nedzelski and Barber 1976)
- disturbances of the vascular supply of the round window membrane and
- congenital or inflammatory weakness of the round window membrane (Chüden 1979).

Gray and Barton (1981) suspect an unusually large round window as well as an extremely wide aquaeductus cochleae (also Heermann et al. 1976 as well as Grossenbacher 1976), findings which as a part of a malformation (Mondini) may possibly also be recognised by polytomography (Farrior and Endicott 1971, Wolfowitz 1979, Grossenbacher 1976, Gray and Barton 1981). Such wide communications between the CSF – and the perilymphatic space are well known to all surgeons operating on the middle ear, by the gusher of perilymph which sometimes occurs on the occasion of a stapedectomy. It is after all observed in 2% of the operations (n = 1160), but leads in only 0.2% of the patients to severe and persistent loss of hearing (Causse 1980).

An additional danger is said to exist for divers (Freeman 1975, 1978, Molvaer et al. 1978, Pullen et al. 1979, Natali et al. 1980, Gray and Barton 1981). Nevertheless, the inner ear barotrauma cannot be interpreted in every case as a manifestation of a window rupture (Coles 1976, Ristow 1980), but in many cases still as a decompression injury, in the sense of a microembolus caused by bubbles of nitrogen (Farmer 1976, Novotny 1980). A recompression (Pang 1974) or even a simple treatment with vasodilators (Novotny 1980) may then produce an improvement.

Animal experiments on rupture of the round window membrane already go back to the beginning of the 60's; it was on the grounds of these experiments that Simmons and Burton suspected a rupture of the round window membrane in fifteen patients with sudden deterioration of hearing without recognisable trauma (Simmons and Burton 1962, Simmons 1968).

In their experiments on cats Simmons and Burton had observed a disappearance of the CM after opening of the round window membrane; *it was clearer than would have been expected by the histological preparations of the organ of Corti later on.* The CM, however, disappeared only if the perilymph had flown off. Later on, the authors were able to record the complete disappearance of the CM and CAP in two patients also by means of electrocochleography.

If in order to avoid the escape of perilymph, the instrumental perforation of the round window membrane in guinea pigs is made under Ringer's solution the CM and CAP remain present (Lamm et al. 1982). If the perforation did not take place under a fluid level, the potentials improved again after filling the bulla with Ringer's solution. Hence the cause of the hearing loss would be, in the first instance, the lack of perilymph. If this is stopped the electrophysiological values improve, if it is prevented they remain almost constant.

It is probably not only the width of the aquaeductus cochleae which is decisive for the *very variable extent of the hearing losses* after a rupture but also the site of its orifice in the window-near portion of the basal turn or even in a duplication – membrana limitans – of the round window Membrane itself (Franke 1978, Bergmann et al. 1979, Nomura 1982). The unusual bulging of the membrane as described by Grossenbacher (1976) may perhaps be explained by an accumulation of perilymph between the two portions of the membrane or between the round window membrane and a membrane of the round window *niche* (Nomura et al. 1983).

In the case of only a slit-like tear, the perilymph lack is usually replaced by CSF and the membrane will be able to regenerate (McClure and Lycett 1980). In the case of a total absence of the round window membrane (Gülzow 1980) and an aquaeductus cochleae which is relatively wide and possibly even opens into the round window, the CSF will flow directly into the tympanum and will possibly manifest itself here as "serotympanum" or fluid tympanum (Wolfowitz 1979, Fiebach and Plath 1983). The CSF might then "carry along" the perilymph and thus produce an interruption of the perilymph column. This would indeed only be possible if at the same time air reached the scala tympani (Lamm et al. 1984). The sequel would be a momentary break down of the hydrodynamics and hence the sudden loss of the CM in the animal experiment (whereas without perforation of the round window membrane they survive even the death of the animal, though with a markedly reduced amplitude).

These ideas were supported by findings from animal experiments carried out by Robertson (1974). He had opened the scala tympani not in the round window but in the *basal turn* and was able to observe that after an initial drop in the CM – even the secondary potentials appeared again if the perilymph which had leaked away was replaced.

The *pattern of deafness* following rupture of the round window membrane is not uniform as regards the course of the tone threshold, but is uniform in the sense of the recruitment; the loss of hearing is steady or fluctuating. In almost all cases the diagnosis could only be made or confirmed during the operation (Grossenbacher 1976, Stroud and Calcaterra 1970, Frazer and Harborow 1975, Chüden 1979, Boenninghaus and Gülzow 1981) or by transmyringeal endoscopy (Schüssler et al. 1982). About three quarters of the patients complain at the same time of vertigo and half of them about tinnitus (Survey of literature in Strohm 1982). Children are reported to be preferably affected (Arenberg et al. 1974, Grundfast et al. 1978, Knight 1977, Knight and Phillips 1980).

The *indications for operation* in case of a suspected rupture of the round window membrane are based on

- the case history, possibly with obvious or doubtful trauma
- the suddenness of the hearing loss
- a possibly pulsating noise and
- often on the vertigo (Boenninghaus and Gülzow 1981).

Various *operative procedures* are applied: Tonkin and Fagan (1975) excise the margins of the perforation, remove the mucous membrane of the tympanum and place a vein graft on the prepared wound surface. Goodhill et al. (1973) use perichondrium for closing the defect. Others are more cautious on account of the possibility of *spontaneous* healing which was repeatedly observed (Medzelski and Barber 1976, Caruso et al. 1977, Behbehani and Kastenbauer 1978, Kleinfeldt 1978, Meyerhoff 1979). With this recommendation, the question of the operation date is largely settled: the more carefully one proceeds and the more strictly one confines oneself to mere tympanotomy or tympanoscopy in the case of negative findings the sooner is it permitted and advisable, to "operate" early (Goodhill

1971, Wurtele 1976, Jensma 1979, Boenninghaus and Gülzow 1981, Sekula and Wlodyka 1982). *One should avoid in any case a tubal insufflation,* either for diagnostic (Fiebach and Plath 1983), or even "therapeutic" purposes, *on account of the risk of forcing air into the open round window.* The patient must be instructed not to blow his nose, and not to ventilate the middle ear actively from without. This advice requires an early tentative diagnosis already by the first physician who treats the patient – and restraint as regards politzerisation.

The findings of Fukaja and Nomura (1983) obtained in their experiments on guinea pigs, could present basically new aspects on the further development of a round window membrane rupture. The authors recorded the CM, the CAP and the brain stem AEP 10, 20, and 30 days after instrumental perforation of the membrane. After ten days the inner ear impairment only amounted to about 20 dB and had completely recovered after 30 days. A high tone loss only persisted if there had been a simultaneous middle ear effusion. To what extent these findings from guinea pigs can be transferred to man remains to be seen. At all events they are worth noting!

The ultimate clinical results with or without operative treatment and with or without various conservative measures cannot yet be judged. Worth mentioning however, appears to be the recommendation of a treatment with 20% mannitol solution in order to reduce the intracranial pressure (Sekula and Wlodyka 1982); with this medication, six of fourteen patients showed a complete, a further six a partial recovery, and in only two cases no effect was recorded.

The former conception that any manipulation at the *round window* leads to deafness, whereas operations on the *oval* window may be quite feasible and advantageous, is no longer valid (Tonkin and Fagan 1975). Since Schuknecht (1982) introduced even sacculotomy through the round window membrane and after he had carried it out successfully against vertigo and with an appreciable deterioration of hearing in "only" 25% of the cases (n = 51) it appears that from the *noli me tangere* of the round window membrane a first step has been made towards the clarification of many a case of inner ear deafness. What accidental circumstances were involved in the success or failure, of the respective operations has not yet been clarified.

3.1.3.2 Ruptures in the Oval Window

Impairment of hearing as a result of a tear of the *oval* annular ligament in the course of a severe cranial trauma (Fee 1968) requires no renewed discussion. "Spontaneous" implosive or explosive ruptures seem to occur less frequently in the oval window than the round one. A reversed relationship exists if the operative and traumatic ruptures are considered, too. Among the 15 cases reported in the detailed paper by Goodhill et al. (1973) nine were localised in the oval, five in the oval *and* round, and only a single one in the round window. Chronic leaks in the oval annular ligament of the stapes associated with a wide aquaeductus cochleae and raised vestibular perilymph pressure (Farrior and Endicott 1971, cf. Chap. 3.4.1) may be associated with a Mondini malformation, with the risk of a meningitis (Desjardins et al. 1982, Pérez-Garigues et al. 1982, Elverland and Miar 1983).

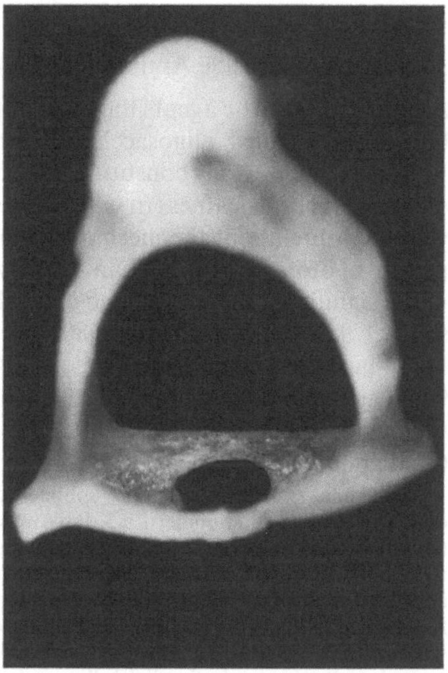

Fig. 12. Stapes with a circular defect in the footplate as part of a Mondini malformation of the labyrinth and the cause of recurrent attacks of meningitis

I am grateful to Prof. H. Feldmann, Münster, for telling me of a similar observation. He treated a six-year-old girl, who had suffered three attacks of meningitis and was now deaf on the left side. No leakage of CSF could be detected, in the X-ray the left cochlea appeared as a vesicle only and the posterior and superior semicircular canals were absent. From a cystic bulging of the mucous membrane between the crura of the stapes, perilymph was leaking and came out in a gusher after removal of the stapes. The vestibule was plugged with connective tissue and after that the fluid came out of the round window, too. Covering of the round window membrane, packing of the tympanum. A small circular defect was found in the footplate of the stapes (Fig. 12) as part of a Mondini malformation of the left ear.

In any case such fistulae in children have to be distinguished from those seen in adults (Guindi 1981). In these, tears in the annular ligament develop less dramatically and the loss of hearing is less severe than in cases of rupture of the round window membrane. Annular ligament defects are also supposed to be a frequent accompaniment of traumatic *rupture of the ear drum,* namely in two-thirds of the cases (Emmett and Shea 1980, Greval et al. 1983), or they occur as a dehiscence after plastic surgery of the stapes (House 1967, Dawes and Watson 1979, Shea 1979). Deafness is then often limited to the lower frequencies (Schmidt 1981; cf. Fig. 45), possibly accompanied by vertigo and tinnitus. An operative repair of tears or dehiscences can usually be achieved without difficulties, but an improvement in hearing cannot always be achieved (Allam 1976, Schmidt 1981). Spontaneous healing is still possible even after months (Tanaka et al. 1983).

A rupture of Reissner's membrane may certainly be regarded as an accidental finding. In one case it occurred in the course of a barotrauma and once without any obvious external cause. In both patients the rupture was situated near the ductus reuniens (Gussen 1981). The clinical appearance of the rupture was that of a "sudden hearing loss."

3.2 Ototoxic Deafness

3.2.1 Aminoglycoside Antibiotics (AA)

Among the ototoxic agents the most important ones are the aminoglycoside antibiotics, also called oligosaccharide or streptomyces antibiotics; according to Rejtö et al. (1982) they constitute 90% of the ototoxic substances. 2% of all cases of sensori-neural deafness (n = 9657) are regarded as toxic in origin (Table 1). The vast literature about the mechanisms of action on the inner ear and the clinical picture of ototoxic deafness can scarcely be surveyed any longer. Detailed surveys of the significant theoretical and clinical aspects are found in the papers of Federspil (1979, 1982), von Ilberg (1980) and Stupp (1970).

It has been known since Caussé (1949) that the AA attack the sensory organ, whereas the spiral ganglion and the nearest neurons remain unaffected for a long time unless they are involved – later on – in the sense of an ascending degeneration (Kellerhals et al. 1967).

In animal experiments the microphone potentials and the action potential disappear very early (Feinmesser and Sohmer 1965, Jankowski et al. 1971) whereas the endochochlear DC potential persists (Logan et al. 1974, Komune and Snow 1981). In these tests the particular sensitivity of the *outer* hair cells was also confirmed electrophysiologically (Rejtö et al. 1982): The recruitment is clearly demonstrable by the action potential (CAP), i.e. in the stimulus-response function, amplitudes are reached which, in the case of great intensities, approximate those of the healthy. Subsequent to kanamycin intoxication, however, the amplitude of the CM remained limited even with loud stimuli (Dallos and Wang 1974). Within the AP, N_1 decreases first whereas N_2 becomes more prominent.

This "dissociated pattern" may be interpreted as the expression of a primary injury to the sensory cells in the basal turn (Ramsden et al. 1980). The spiral ganglion is only affected after complete functional loss of the sensory cells (Koitchev et al. 1982) and also in the central portions of the auditory pathways losses of potential are only seen after extremely high doses, especially as some AA (e.g. neomycin) are not at all detectable in cerebral tissue when administered in normal doses (Desrochers and Schacht 1982).

Schacht (1979) claims to have found in chromatographic studies a particular affinity of the AA for certain lipophosphatides which he considered to be the cause of the ototoxicity. This would perhaps also explain the affinity of the AA for the melanin containing structures in the inner ear, in a similar way as is assumed for quinine and chloroquine (Lyttkens et al. 1979). Lindquist (1973) therefore discussed the possibility that the ototoxicity of the AA like that of chloroquine and quinine arises from storage in the melanin-containing cells; since melanin lies on the surface of the stria vascularis towards the endolymphatic space, disturbances of secretion would be a possible consequence.

Although many details are known from electrophysiological and biochemical findings, the *primary* site of the toxic damage has not yet been definitely localised. Some data suggest an initial alteration of the stria vascularis, above all the potentiating effect of the AA with simultaneous medication of ethacrynic acid which is known to affect the potassium pump of the stria vascularis (Wilson and Juhn 1970, Sellik and Johnstone 1975). A similar loss of potassium and rise of sodium in the endolymph (Mendelsohn and Katzenberg 1972), would have to be produced by an injury of the transport pathways in Reissner's membrane (Watanuki et al. 1968, Kanaka et al. 1970). All these changes would then have a *secondary* effect on the hair cells.

However, in the electrophysiological meaning – as indicated above – the initial persistence of the endocochlear potential in the case of an early decay of the CM and the AP, points to a *primary* damage of the sensory cells. Somehow or other the sensory cell membrane becomes permeable to metabolic toxins (Schacht 1976). The functional loss then proceeds quite abruptly, first of all in the outer and only later in the inner hair cells, starting in each case in the basal turn (Federspil 1972). According to other observations, the degeneration of the inner hair cells advances – in contrast to that of the outer ones – from the apex to the base (von Ilberg 1980, Sato 1983). Presumably the pattern of deterioration is also determined by the dosage.

From pharmacological investigations – also in man (Meyer zum Gottesberge and Stupp 1969) – it is evident that the AA in the serum rapidly pass over into the perilymph, probably because there exists a linear relationship with the serum level which is obtained and because the clearance of the AA from the serum is mainly renal, i.e. does not take place in the case of renal dysfunction. The accumulation in the perilymph proceeds depending on the degree of ototoxicity of the substance – with systemic administration as well as with local application into the middle ear (Stupp et al. 1973, Olitani et al. 1982); the accumulation of kanamycin, for example, is 100 times that in the cerebral tissue (Rejtö 1982). In the individual case the effect is thus predominantly dependent on the *total* dose, and less on the daily dose (Lehnhardt 1970, Jackson 1977, Schönberger 1981, Federspil 1982). Also the subdivision of the daily dose into several single portions has only a limited preventive effect (Federspil and Schätzle 1980). Other authors have again questioned the accumulation of AA in the perilymph, at any rate for neomycin (Descrochers and Schacht 1982).

In the case of disturbed renal excretion the ototoxicity rises to a manifold degree, and with anuria even corresponding to a 20 to 50 fold increase in the daily dosage (Federspil 1982). While patients with healthy kidneys generally did not show any hearing losses even after doses of e.g. 40 to 60 g dihydrostreptomycin (Durska-Zarzewska and Zarzewski 1971), those *with* renal damage, may already suffer from deafness after the intake of only a few grams (Lehnhardt 1970). Corresponding experiences exist regarding medication with gentamicin (Crifo et al. 1980) whereas kanamycin administered over long periods in tuberculosis (in 55.6%, Rempt 1970) and streptomycin after more than 100 mg produced ototoxic impairment of hearing *even in patients with healthy kidneys* (in 82% of the cases, Kitsera and Lyubinets 1982).

The hearing impairment regularly begins in the high frequencies and progresses from there possibly continuously to the low frequencies; the C^5-dip typical of noise is absent. Very early damage is only detectable in the high frequency range, that is above 12 kHz (up to 16 kHz) (Dieroff 1982, Svatko and Kovgalyuk 1979).

The recruitment equivalents are always positive. An allegedly excessive impairment of speech discrimination (Pirsig and Rollin 1968, Rejtö et al. 1982) was probably an expression of the rapid, recruitment-positive failure of hearing. The hearing impairment develops, as a rule, almost identically on the two sides. Unilateral deafness during or soon after medication suggests other causal factors (Fig. 13).

The audiometric picture is probably the same for all ototoxic substances, that is to say it is not dependent on the preparation being used. Only the extent of the deafness differs according to the varying toxicity, for the organ of hearing and/or balance, as also for the kidney (Aran et al. 1982).

The ototoxicity of the newer preparations such as amicacin, sisomycin and netilmycin can be ignored if the necessary precautions are taken (Federspil 1981, Ohtani et al. 1982); even that of Gentamycin C_1 is scarcely important (Fox et al. 1980) always assuming normal function of the kidneys (Hawkins et al. 1969).

In the case of local intratympanic application, basically identical hearing damage may arise, however, the danger is certainly not as great as might be concluded from animal experiments (Stupp 1970, Parker and James 1978, Konishi 1979, Handrock 1982, Renner et al. 1982). Nevertheless, there is no doubt about the fact that e.g. tetracycline, gentamicin and neomycin are able to pass from the middle ear through the round window into the inner ear (Smith and Myers 1979,

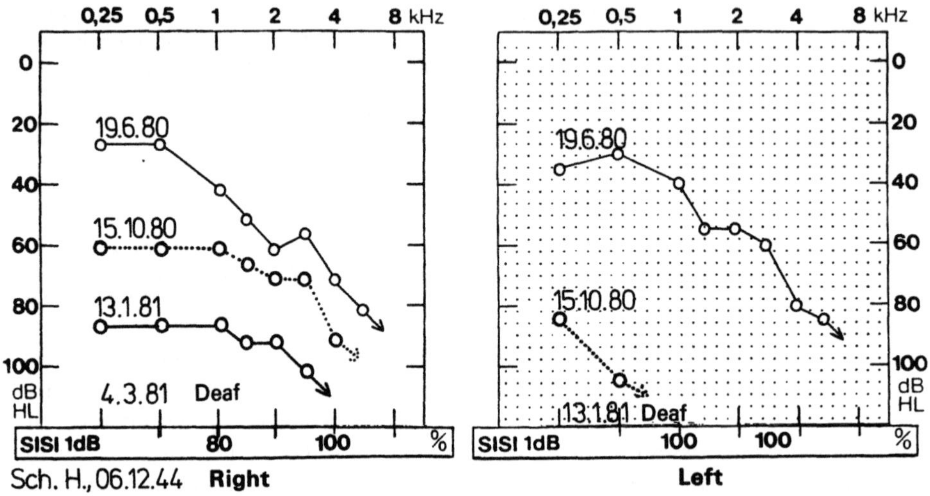

Fig. 13. Progressive hearing loss in post-traumatic renal failure. An osteomyelitic cavity had been treated with gentamicin and nebacetin, among other antibiotics. No details were available about a possible associated systemic treatment with ototoxic substances. After the first audiometric findings further deterioration of hearing could not be stopped although medication was discontinued. BC = AC

Tanaka and Motomura 1981), and to a smaller extent also through the annular ligament of the oval window (Haug et al. 1979, Tanaka and Motomura 1981). The most striking damage to the hair cells has been observed after the use of polymyxin, neomycin and gentamicin (Martin and Martin 1980).

The inflammatory swelling of the tympanic mucous membrane forms a significant protection against the penetration of toxic material into the inner ear; for this reason, particular care is advisable with non-irritated middle ear mucous membranes. However, even in an inflamed middle ear accurate diagnosis is imperative for the use of ear drops containing AA (Matthias and Handrock 1980, Handrock 1981). This equally applies to solvents such as propylene glycol and polyethylene glycol (Stupp 1970, Parker and James 1978, Handrock 1982).

Table 1. List of ototoxic antibiotics (most of them are aminoglycosides) and of neurotoxic polymyxins. (From Federspil 1983)

amikacin	sisomicin
bluensomycin	streptomycin
butikacin	tobramycin
butirosin	yerdamycin
dihydrostreptomycin	fortimicin (pseudodisaccharide)
dibekacin	kasugamycin (disaccharide)
framycetin	spectinomycin (disaccharide)
gentamicin	vancomycin (glycoproteid)
kanamycin	capreomycin (polypeptide)
kanendomycin	viomycin (polypeptide)
lividomycin	minocycline (tetracycline)
neomycin	doxycycline (tetracycline)
netilmicin	erythromycin (macrolide antibiotic)
paromomycin	polymyxin B (basic peptide-antibiotic)
ribostamycin	polymyxin E = colistin

With regard to local application into the middle ear, allowance should also be made for the fact that some antibiotics which are less toxic when applied systemically show a rapid penetration into the inner ear and may cause severe damage after local application, e.g. polymyxin or – though less obviously – tetracycline, chloramphenicol, erythromycin. It is only with penicillin that no damage to hearing is expected (Stupp et al. 1973).

Once the damage has started it usually proceeds for a certain period of time, even if the AA was promptly withdrawn (Federspil 1976) – occasionally even to total deafness (see Fig. 13). This observation was only recently confirmed again by experiments in guinea pigs; even after *premature* stopping of the kanamycin medication the brain stem responses showed a hair cell damage equal to that in the animals where the medication was continued (Nakai et al. 1981).

Hydro- and saline-diuresis or hemodilution exert only little influene on further functional loss – and are nevertheless indicated. Otherwise the *treatment* can only be unspecific and follow that of all the other acute hearing disturbances.

On the other hand, more and more reports are appearing about the reversibility of ototoxic disturbances of hearing (Jackson and Arcieri 1971, Federspil 1982), even in one half of the cases after gentamicin. These reports must be regarded critically and should not stimulate false hopes of spontaneous cure; in general the deafness resulting from AA must be regarded as irreversible (Rejtö et al. 1982)! The possibility of so-called delayed damage, appearing months after withdrawal of the antibiotics, has not been confirmed either clinically or experimentally (Federspil 1978, 1979), always assuming normal renal function (Tiedemann 1978).

The ototoxicity of a second course of treatment is dependent on the time of the first medication and on hearing disturbances possibly resulting from it (Lerner and Matz 1979). There is little danger, if the hearing function is normal before the second course of treatment (Ballantyne 1970) and even less danger the longer the time interval is. Any additional noise-stress is contraindicated as soon as even a suspected hearing loss is judged to be the result of earlier AA medication. As was proved in animal experiments, any noise should of course be avoided during treatment with AA (Kubo and Shida 1973, Quante 1973, Brown et al. 1980).

On account of the poor clearance of AA in premature infants and newborns and hence their greater susceptibility to ototoxic damage (Marcus et al. 1963, Pracic and Salaj 1975, Carlier and Pujol 1980, Eviatar et al. 1981) the possibility of ototoxic genesis should always be investigated in early childhood deafness (allegedly 20–30%, Pellegrini 1966). In premature infants such damage can scarcely be distinguished from that caused by the additional noise of the incubator. Probably there is an interaction of both noxae (Bernard 1981, Potmozakis 1980). On the other hand, a study of 347 newborns has not shown any significant hearing impairment either after gentamicin 5 to 6 mg or after kanamycin 15 mg/kg/day (Finitzko-Hieber et al. 1979) nor has the investigation of incubator noise shown any damaging sound levels (Jacobson and Mencher 1981).

The predisposition to ototoxic damage is assumed to exist above all in the third month of pregnancy (Ganguin and Rempt 1970). At that time the development of the space of Nuel and the tunnel of Corti commences, and this is where Nakai et al. (1983) have seen precipitates in guinea pigs, which they attributed to the administration of kanamycin.

The situation may become extremely obscure, if a familial predisposition to toxic deafness by AA is to be assumed (Podvinec and Stefanovic 1966). For example Tsuiki and Murai (1971) have reported on 16 families in which two or more members showed hearing impairment caused by dihydrostreptomycin – with total doses of only 3–40 g. Even a dosage of only 1 g/day for five days had led to permanent deafness in persons with familial predisposition as for instance in four sisters (Prazić et al. 1964).

According to Tsuiki and Murai (1971) the familial predisposition may not be *specific for streptomycin,* because some families included deaf members who had not been treated with it. The development of deafness in these families might have been caused by various noxae – one of which was streptomycin. The audiograms regularly showed a high tone loss. In such cases we therefore ought to consider the possibility of an hereditary, progressive, sensori-neural deafness, which was only triggered off, aggravated or accelerated by the AA.

An additional ototoxicity is reported to ensue from an elevation of the body temperature. In animal experiments the average hearing loss after kanamycin medication increased by around 20 dB, if the body temperature was maintained at 1° above normal. This observation could be of significance for AA medication in patients with high fever (Henry et al. 1983). It may perhaps also explain the occasional hearing impairment caused by other antibiotics which are scarcely ototoxic, as for example erythromycin (Thompson et al. 1980), or netilmycin (Tjernström et al. 1982).

A *potentiation* of the ototoxicity occurs as a result of the simultaneous administration of *loop diuretics.* Orsulakova and Schacht (1982) believe that the AA – in ototoxic doses – damages the barriers of permeability to, or in, the inner ear and thus encourages the penetration e.g. of ethacrycinic acid. According to Davis et al. (1982), however, the ototoxic interaction is rather determined by the loop diuretics than by the AA i.e. *loop*-diuretics + *non aminoglycoside*-antibiotics (viomycin, capreomycin and polymyxin B) are more ototoxic than *non-loop* diuretics plus *aminoglycoside antibiotics* (Davis et al. 1982). In any case, there is no combined effect as long as both drugs are administered in non-toxic doses (Federspil 1973). However, as soon as one is overdosed or if the AA has an ototoxic effect on account of disturbed renal function, the catastrophe can develop very quickly (Nakai et al. 1977, Brummett et al. 1979, Asakuma and Snow 1980, Tran Ba Huy et al. 1981, Brummett 1983).

Such hearing disturbances are numbered among the dramatic experiences of the ENT specialist, particularly on account of the irreversible hearing losses and the often completely uninfluenceable further deterioration. Thus, we saw a patient who after a heart operation with her circulation in an extremely poor state, with resultant anuria and loop diuretic medication (6 g) certainly owed her survival only to the AA treatment (refobacin 4 g), a survival, however, which was paid for by total deafness. In the otologist's view a doubtful success but for the heart surgeon an unequivocal decision in favor of the operation and the medical treatment.

3.2.2 Loop Diuretics

The ototoxicity of the loop diuretics keeps within narrow limits in so far as any hearing losses which appear after their *exclusive* medication are generally reversible. The type of hearing loss – mostly appearing as a trough or a flat dip around 2000–4000 Hz – and the study of experimental findings, have provided valuable insights into the processes occurring in the inner ear.

Unfortunately information about the pattern of deafness is only sporadically found. Often there are only reports of transitory hearing loss or of fleeting deafness (as in Maher and Schreiner 1965, Matz and Naunton 1968, Hanzelik and Pepperkorn 1969, Ballantyne 1970 and many others). What is missing in particular are the results of adaptation tests, e.g. in the form of the Békésy audiogram or even by means of the ECochG. Indeed such investigations would be attractive since it seems to be certain, that the loop diuretics do not attack the sensory cells, but that their function remains intact.

Among the diuretics mentioned are included ethacrynic acid, frusemide, azosemide, bumetamide, piretanide, ozolinon and mercaptomerine. In the kidney these substances block the active reabsorption of sodium in the ascending limb of Henle's loop and in this way influence the concentration mechanism in the distal section of the tubule. In addition, the reabsorption of ions in the proximal section of the tubule is hindered. The biochemical mechanism consists in the inhibition of the sodium-potassium-ATPase activity, as well as the adenylate cyclase (Kusakari et al. 1978, Bagger-Söbeck et al. 1980, Marco et al. 1981).

In the inner ear, too, the ion-exchange is dependent on the adenylate cyclase and on the ATPase. The loop diuretics may therefore act upon the inner ear according to the same principles as in the kidney (Vosteen 1976, Paloheima and Thalmann 1977, Marks and Schacht 1981) i.e. here, too, the enzyme block leads to a disturbance of the electrolyte transport, the potassium concentration in the endolymph decreases and the sodium rises; at the same time the endocochlear DC potential drops (Silverstein and Yules 1971, Prazma and Thomas 1972, Thalmann et al. 1977, Arnold et al. 1978, Himelfarb et al. 1979) and, in fact, before the shift of ions takes place (Bosher et al. 1973, Bosher 1980).

In animal experiments, the *early drop of the DC-potential* was particularly clear with Ozolinon and was associated with a rise in the chloride activity in the endolymph (Morgenstern et al. 1981). Possibly an inhibition of chloride transport within the endolymph and at the efferent synapses (Klinke et al. 1981) is a (further) component of the ototoxicity. In addition, the glycolysis and the cell respiration, as well as reactions with the sulph-hydril groups and with the magnesium ATPases were found to be disturbed (Thalmann 1981) – above all if associated with a fall in blood pressure and a high CO_2 partial pressure, as side-effects, for example, of the ethacrynic acid (Bosher 1980).

Nevertheless, Thalmann (1982) thinks he has also observed findings contradicting an inhibition of adenylate cyclase by ethacrynic acid in so far as the drop in the DC potential follows so instantaneously on an intraarterial bolus injection of frusemide that the reaction must be limited to the vicinity of the vessels but not involve the adenylate cyclase which is located on the juxtaluminal surface of the stria vascularis.

This would fit in with the idea that frusemide affects the inner ear by an inhibition of the prostaglandin synthesis. Arenberg and Goodfriend (1980) conclude this from their observation that Indomethacin – an inhibitor of prostaglandin synthesis – did not affect the glycerol test, but that the effect of frusemide was weakened or abolished.

How careful one must be in the interpretation even of the effect of ethacrynic acid on the inner ear, is made obvious by experimental results in which no electrophysiological or morphological differences can be discerned after the injection of ethacrynic acid and of sodium chloride into the cochlea (Pollard et al. 1981).

The CM persist for a long time after the administration of loop diuretics, whereas the action potential (CAP) drops rapidly. Also the tuning curve of the single fiber occasionally shows an elevation of the threshold, though only after perfusion of the cochlea (Comis et al. 1981, Klinke et al. 1981). The extinction of the DC potentials already mentioned above precedes the drop in the CAP.

The early drop in the CAP with persistence of the CM suggests that the loop diuretics interfere with a late stage of the stimulus transmission from the still intact sensory cell to the nerve fiber, probably with the release of the transmitter (Klinke et al. 1981).

The reactions mentioned may regress and function may return to normal (Arnold et al. 1978, Brummett et al. 1977). Probably only extremely high doses *and/or* renal dysfunction lead to – permanent – damage *even in the sensory cells* (Quick and Duvall 1970, Nakai 1971, Dilling et al. 1973, Matz 1976, Arnold et al. 1981).

The incidence of deafness is dependent on the flow rate of the infusion and on the dose administered. In the cases of ototoxic side-effects the substance had always been injected intravenously and relatively quickly (Arnold et al. 1981, Arnold 1982) –also in the case of permanent deafness reported by Lloyd-Mostyn and Lloyd (1971). Infusions of e.g. 1000 mg lasix within only 40 min produced hearing losses of up to 70 dB in isolated cases. The reduction of the dose to 600 mg caused the individual hearing losses to recede to a maximum of 20–25 dB, even with terminal renal failure. With prolonged dosage, significant threshold shifts did not appear at all (Maher and Schreiner 1964, Heidland and Wigand 1970, Kohonen et al 1970, Wigand and Heidland 1970). For this reason, a dose of 200 mg/day i.v. or 400 mg (oral) should not be exceeded. Vestibular side-effects are obviously never seen (Schneider and Becker 1966, Wigand and Heidland 1970).

In their mode of action the individual diuretics do not differ basically from one another (Marks and Schacht 1981), but rather in their degree of ototoxicity. For example, bumetamide is said to cause more lasting damage than piretanide and frusemide (Klinke et al. 1981). Even mefrusemide is counted among the so-called "high-ceiling" diuretics (Jung and Schön 1983).

An accumulation in the perilymph as is observed with aminoglycoside antibiotics is not found with the loop diuretics; their rate of excretion from the perilymph, however, is about four times slower than that of the AA (Rybak et al. 1979).

Altogether, the dangerousness of the loop diuretics is less determined by their inherent ototoxicity than by the fact that in case of renal dysfunction the threshold of ototoxicity is depressed to such a low level that even non-toxic aminoglycosides such as capreomycin and polymyxin B or the cytostatic cisplatin may damage the auditory function (Brummett 1980). Such interactions will be rare, but they may have given rise to some reports in the literature, without having been discovered or correspondingly interpreted. The potential ototoxicity in cases of simultaneous administration of loop diuretics and AA was dealt with in the previous chapter.

A quite extraordinary suggestion referring to loop diuretics is to use them in the treatment of inner ear deafness (Nakai et al. 1982). It was made on account of the the observation that, for example, kanamycin even in a non-toxic single dose produces appalling damage to the organ of Corti, if loop diuretics were given beforehand; these are known to lead to a widening of the intercellular spaces in the stria vascularis (v.s.) which is reversible within 1–2 hours after intravenous injection (Brummett et al. 1977, Duvall et al. 1980). If within this period *a therapeutic agent* is administered instead of an ototoxic one an increased penetration into the endolymph – and thus a more favorable therapeutic effect might be expected. This effect would be of use for example in the corticosteroid medication of particular cases of sensori-neural deafness (Igarashi 1982).

3.2.3 Salicylates

After Wittmaack in 1903 and Falbe-Hansen in 1941 had reported on the ototoxic side-effects of salicylates, it was not until 25 years later that the disturbances of the CM, the CAP and the DC potentials were found in animal experiments after correspondingly high doses (Silverstein et al. 1967, Ziemski and Jankowski 1972, Deer and Hunter-Duvar 1982). The ionic equilibrium between endolymph and perilymph was not disturbed, but the enzyme activity in the stria and the outer hair cells was reduced (v. Westernhagen 1968). These reactions are supposed to result from "decoupling" of the oxidative phosphorylation in the mitochondria; this would lead to a deficiency of ATP and hence an energy deficit in the hair cells (Schätzle and Schnieder 1979). No morphological changes could be detected even with the electron microscope (Myers and Bernstein 1965, Deer and Hunter-Duvar 1982).

The clinical correlates are manifested by impaired hearing as well as possible tinnitus and vertigo – without extremely high doses having always been given, e.g. 2–6 g/day (Falbe-Hansen 1941, Badadin 1964, Lucente 1971, Oudot et al. 1979, Reiter et al. 1980). On the other hand, Myers and Bernstein (1965) found a dependency on the plasma salicylate level. The symptoms develop for the most part bilaterally and are reversible within 72 hours – naturally only after withdrawing the drug (Myers and Bernstein 1965). Only exceptionally will the hearing loss after salicylate medication persist (Gignoux et al. 1966). In spite of this, even a unilateral and irreversible hearing disturbance was attributed to salicylate medication (12 g/day for three days) (Jarvis 1966). Also the idea that children might be particularly susceptible is based merely on a single observation after only three aspirin tablets (Kapur 1965).

Interesting characteristics have developed regarding the audiogram. The loss of hearing extends over all frequencies to approximately the same extent, so that the hearing threshold shows a flat curve, if the patient previously had a normal hearing function or shows a parallel shift e.g. in the case of a pre-existing high

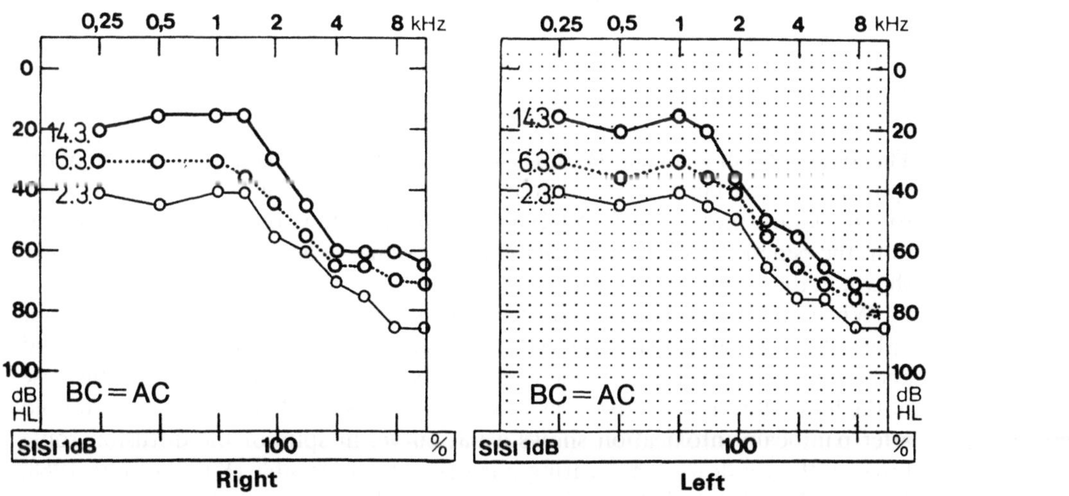

Fig. 14. Transitory impairment of hearing under anti-rheumatic treatment with 3 × 2 tablets of colfarit/day for ten days. No tinnitus or vertigo. After stopping the medication continuous improvement in hearing. The residual high tone loss had probably been existing beforehand. (I am grateful to Dr. G.O. Neumann, Hamburg, for letting me have these records)

tone loss (Fig. 14) (Myers and Bernstein 1965). Pre-existing insignificant losses of hearing, such as a circumscribed c^5 dip of <40 dB, may disappear in the flat course of the pure tone threshold during the intoxication and develop once more in its original form after the auditory function has been restored. The SISI-test indicates a disturbance of function in the inner ear. The uniform involvement of all frequencies has also been demonstrated in experiments on monkeys (Myers and Bernstein 1965).

In addition, in a clinical audiometric study (4 g/day for 4–5 days) a reduction of the "temporal integration" had been demonstrated this means that the hearing threshold climbs more rapidly than normal, with shortening of the presented tones. The continuous tone threshold did not show any recognisable changes. The effect is consistent with the concept of an enzyme inhibition in the inner ear, as a sequel to the salicylate medication (Pedersen 1974).

3.2.4 Atoxyl

The cases of inner ear deafness formerly attributed to arsenic have turned out to be, for the most part, side-effects of the sodium arsenilate Atoxyl, an antihelminthic (Diamant 1958, Moretto 1958). Atoxyl has not achieved any clinical significance in the sense of ototoxicity, but rather as an agent in animal experiments. These date back to Yamakawa (1929) and Miayamoto (1931). During the fifties Nassuphis, and in the seventies Anniko and Wersäll were working with atoxyl. Yamakawa (1929) had already noticed the *apico*-basal pattern of damage – confirmed by Nassuphis – after application of atoxyl, though into the middle ear.

Atoxyl damages the capillary endothelium and inhibits glycolysis earlier and more severely in the kidney than in the stria vascularis of the inner ear. Since the *outer* hair cells are particularly rich in glycogen, above all in the upper turn of the cochlea, it is no wonder that Anniko and Wersäll (1975, Anniko 1976) found maximum damage in the *apical* turn, and here, in the outer hair cells. The inner hair cells which are poor in glycogen remain intact in atoxyl intoxication. There are no clinical reports in the literature about hearing impairment by atoxyl. Von Ilberg (1979) thinks that the *high tone* region was preferentially damaged and that the hearing disturbances were transitory. Both statements are hardly consistent with the experimental findings.

3.2.5 Other Ototoxic Substances

The toxic effect of *local anesthetics* is usually preceded by the disintegration of the epithelial barrier between the middle and the inner ear, that is particularly at the round window membrane (Höft 1969). However even without such a disintegration, the penetration into the inner ear is imaginable as Haug et al. (1978) have shown in the case of tetracyclin.

When applied to the non-irritated tympanum pantocain leads to a drop not only of the CM but also of the CAP (Rahm et al. 1962, Strother et al. 1964, Ward and Honrubia 1969). The primary damage is said to be situated – as in the case of the loop diuretics – in the stria vascularis (v. Ilberg 1980). The tone threshold after pantocain intoxication shows a flat curve, in spite of the diffusion route through the windows. The hearing impairment is reversible (Knothe et al. 1968, 1971, Jankowski et al. 1971), but probably only as long as the damage corresponds to the immediate reaction of the experimental animal within about the first hour. The delayed reaction after days may possibly develop into total deafness (Matthias and Handrock 1980) probably as an expression of an enzyme splitting in the sensory cells (Schätzle and v. Westernhagen 1969). Even if this is of no clinical relevance local anesthetics should not be thoughtlessly applied into the intact tympanum, if only because of the danger of severe vestibular reactions (Ristow 1968).

Also chymotrypsin which had been recommended for use in the middle ear to prevent renewed scar formation appears to be toxic to the inner ear (Flach et al. 1969); the same applies to the autopolymerising tissue adhesive Butyl-2-cyanoacrylate (Fues et al. 1983), which, however, is scarcely being used any more.

An equally ototoxic effect has been found to be exerted by the quaternary ammonium compounds which are being used for skin disinfection; in animal experiments damage to the hair cells resulted, particularly the outer ones, as well as to the capillaries (Aursnes 1982).

The ototoxic effect of some *cytostatics* involved the hair cells of the organ of Corti in animal experiments – in a way quite analogous to the mechanism of action of the AA. Clinical reports mainly refer to hearing losses after perfusion with cyclophosphamide (Conrad and Crosby 1960, Lawrence et al. 1961, Young et al. 1961). Corresponding histological findings have been reported by Schuknecht (1964) and Cummings (1968).

As regards *cisplatin* a sensorineural loss of hearing is said to be the rule, as soon as the total dose exceeds 200 mg (Helson et al. 1978). After doses of 80–120 mg/m^2 hearing losses appeared in only 9% of the cases, and these were so slight that the treatment did not have to be interrupted (Peytral et al. 1981). In most cases some impairment of hearing had already existed, and then deteriorated with cisplatin (Rybak 1981, von Heyden et al. 1984). The distinction between the two components – the pre-existing and the cisplatin-induced – then causes difficulties, even with histological or electron microscopical examination. The five patients described by Wright and Schaefer (1982) had received total doses of 715–1850 mg so that one can certainly not speak of a particular sensitivity of the ear.

In human temporal bone studies (Strauss et al. 1984) and in experiments on guinea pigs cisplatin-induced lesions were detectable especially in the outer hair cells, but scarcely in the stria vascularis. As shown in the AEP of the brain stem, they, nevertheless, tended to improve (Nakai et al. 1982). The histochemical finding was an inhibition of the adenylate-cyclase in the stria vascularis (Bagger-Sjöbäck et al. 1980). In this respect, the mode of action might be similar to that of the loop diuretics (Mees 1983).

In general, single communications about hearing disturbances "caused by" cytostatics are to be regarded with some reservation. In the generally weak patients many noxae may coincide and other possibilities of a deterioration of hearing can scarcely be excluded. Anyhow, the cytostatics are of no great clinical significance in this respect.

The report about hearing losses caused by *misonidazole* has remained unique up to now. This is a 2-nitro-imidazol, which is regarded as a potent agent for the selective increase of the effect of ionizing radiation in poorly oxygenated tumor tissue. Eleven of 21 patients treated per os suffered an inner ear type of hearing loss which, however, kept within limits and was partly reversible and within a month. In these patients there was no evidence of renal disturbance or of pre-existing hearing impairment. The radiation had been excluded as a possible cause of the hearing loss (Waltzman and Cooper 1981). Details of the pathogenetic mechanism of this preparation are not known, and to our knowledge it has not yet been used for scientific experiments.

Among the whole range of "classical" ototoxics it is only quinine that has occasionally aroused some discussion (Koide et al. 1966, Denker et al. 1973). According to this, quinine – like the loop diuretics and the salicylates – causes damage first of all to the stria vascularis and later to the sensory cells. The ototoxicity is explained by the affinity of quinine and chloroquine for melanin (Denker et al. 1973, Lindquist et al. 1973; see also Chap. 3.2.1) – an interpretation, however, that is quite unsatisfactory since the melanin in the epithelial cells of the stria vascularis is apparently not involved in the metabolism of the ductus cochlearis (Beck 1961). The animal experiments of Lawrence (1970) appear more substantiated. By means of capillary microscopy he observed a temporary obstruction of the erythrocytes in the terminal capillaries on the underside of the basilar membrane under the influence of quinine hydrochloride and interpreted this finding as the pathophysiological basis of the temporary deafness. The reports about total deafness in infancy after quinine administration during pregnancy have so far remained isolated cases without any value as evidence.

Cases of impaired hearing after treatment with the *heparin antagonist polybrene* (hexadimethrin bromide) were only seen in hospitals where the preparation had been administered as an anticoagulant to patients on dialysis (Ransome et al. 1966). It has also been used in open heart operations without any hearing disturbances occurring. Polybrene is said to have a contractile effect on the capillaries in the glomeruli; for this reason an analogous effect was assumed for the inner ear (Ballantyne 1966). The effect appears to have been specific for this preparation, for since it has been taken off the market no similar incidents have been seen. The deafness at that time had affected five of fourteen patients with varying severity, was irreversible and for the most part progressive. The tone threshold showed a flat curve or only fell off slightly towards the high frequencies.

Another paper reported on deafness caused by *potassium bromate*, which is used by hairdressers for cold perms (Matsumoto et al. 1980). In most cases it was taken in with suicidal intent; with renal failure, hemolysis and excessive fall in blood pressure the outcome was in most cases fatal. What occurred in the inner ear was not clarified; the authors assumed a reaction similar to that with AA or diuretics, but also considered a "direct damage to the sensory cells" as possible.

The hearing disturbances caused by carbon monoxide, benzene, nitrobenzene, and amino-benzene, lead, fluorine, mercury and carbon disulphide, repeatedly cited in the older literature are nowadays almost forgotten. On the one hand the agents mentioned show their ototoxic action only as part of a real poisoning and on the other hand the industrial health and safety regulations have in the meantime become much stricter. After an *acute* carbon monoxide poisoning the hearing threshold took an almost flat course (Morris 1970). In the case of chronic intoxication the distinction from a noise-induced deafness is often difficult, above all when the persons affected had been exposed accordingly at the same time and high tone loss predominates in the audiogram. The lesions were situated for the most part in the spiral ganglion or in the auditory nerve (Wittmaack 1956), as could also be demonstrated in the suprathreshold audiogram in the few cases so investigated (Lehnhardt 1965).

The sequels to poisoning with organic mercury compounds were recently also described as *retro*cochlear deafness (Minamata's disease) at all events in about half of the cases (Habu et al. 1979).

Hydrocarbon solutions must also be considered as *neuro*-ototoxic (Lehnhardt 1965); the hearing losses shown in the pure-tone and speech audiograms mostly keep within narrow limits but the brain stem latencies may be definitely prolonged (Ödqvist et al. 1982). Anyhow, the sensory organ of the inner ear is less affected than the neural portions of the hearing pathway.

3.3 Infections

Among the hearing impairments in the wake of infectious diseases those connected with spotted fever, typhus and malaria (or quinine medication) or with tuberculosis – unless streptomycin had been applied – are scarcely being observed nowadays (for details see: Lehnhardt 1965). On the other hand, the hearing disturbances caused by *viral* infections are very common. Two different modes of infection are to be assumed for the inner ear (Strauss and Davis 1973). On the one hand the one which leads, through a viremia to an *endo*-lymphatic labyrinthitis, by hematogenous spread via the stria vascularis (e.g. rubella, measles, cytomegaly – and mumps?); on the other hand the meningogenic, peri- or endo-neural infection of the *peri*lymphatic spaces, as with herpes zoster and mumps (Lindsay et al. 1973, Subotić 1976, Murakami 1979, Wilmes and Deinhardt 1983).

Deafness in *herpes zoster oticus* may be of varying extent, from an exclusive high tone loss through involvement of the middle frequencies up to – almost – total deafness. Only exceptionally, however, *total* deafness will result from herpes zoster oticus. The deafness appears to be mainly of the sensorineural type (Lehnhardt 1978), at least according to the conventional audiometric findings. Up to now there do not seem to exist any possibilities of a more detailed differentiation by electrocochleography (Fig. 15).

Lumbar puncture reveals, for the most part, a slight increase of the cell count and of the protein content. The clinical symptoms always involve only one side at least as long as the clinical picture is not characterized by a diffuse varicella-zoster meningo-encephalitis (vide also Chap. 3.6.1).

Mumps shows itself in the ear by a uniform clinical picture, namely a *total unilateral deafness*; there is no residual hearing – appropriate masking provided. The vestibular apparatus may be involved but often it functions normally.

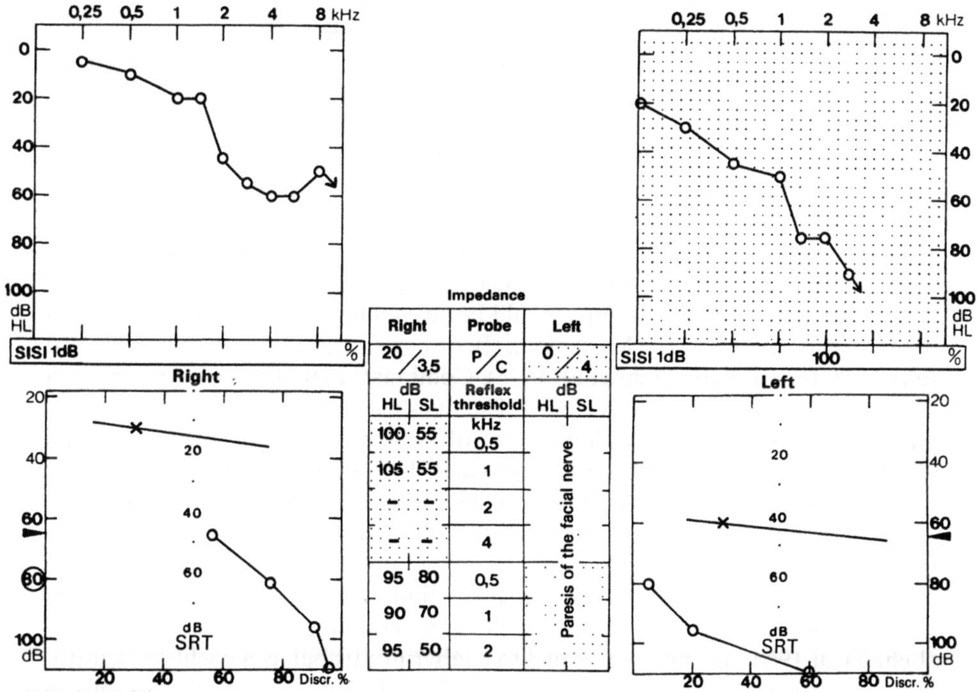

E.H., 26.09.07

Fig. 15. Bilateral high tone deafness. On the left, in addition, an acute deterioration of hearing in the course of a herpes zoster oticus. The SISI reached 100%, however, the stapedius reflex threshold is markedly raised, 100 dB for 500 Hz, 105 dB for 1000 Hz. In the ECochG the CAP was no longer recordable. BC = AC

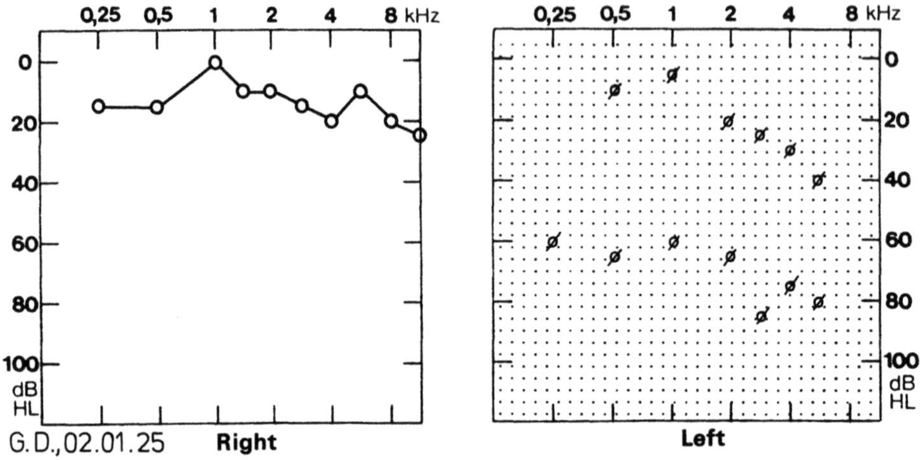

Fig. 16. Complete deafness (*left*) in early childhood, presumably the result of a mumps infection. X-ray Stenver's views the same on both sides. The patient, now 58 years old, hears quite normally on the right even today; i.e. no successive deafness in the second ear. BC = AC. ∅ = BC and AC left without masking

For the most part, mumps-induced deafness develops clinically inapparent. The basic illness need not be specially severe, and often is not at all noticed. In many cases the causal connection is only construed, in other cases positive complement fixation reactions and the anti-hemagglutination test seem to confirm the viral infection retrospectively as the cause of deafness. Up to the seventh day after the onset of the illness mumps virus may be isolated from a throat swab (Brundl et al. 1968).

Therapeutic possibilities – e.g. with immuno-globulin concentrate – do not seem to exist even if the hearing loss was noted *during* the attack of mumps. Prophylactic vaccination against mumps would be advisable. Protection by vaccination with the attenuated vaccine Mumpsvax (Behringwerke A.G. Marburg) is claimed to be 95% for 10 years (Stehr et al. 1975). Combination with measles and rubella vaccine is possible ("Triple vaccine"). The number of such cases of deafness appears to be large from the otologic point of view, but it is apparently too small in relation to all cases of mumps, to convince the non-otologists of the necessity of vaccination. Apart from that, the unilateral loss of hearing is not impressive enough to achieve a broad support for an action of this sort (vide also Chap. 3.6.1).

In accordance with the histological findings of a virugenic neuritis (Wittmaack 1956) we had interpreted the unilateral deafness as neural in origin (Lehnhardt 1962), i.e. not as a sequel to a labyrinthitis but as a cochlear neuritis. The *completeness* of deafness, which is regularly found, and the absence of any restitution supported this assumption (Fig. 16).

This deduction admits more favorable prognostic conclusions as to the *neural or ganglionic* degeneration in so far as one must not in the long run fear a hearing disturbance on the second side like in the case of deafness which accompanies the death of the sensory cells and threatens to successively affect the other ear, too (cf. Chap. 3.10). Nevertheless, the question how these audiometric findings are to be made compatible with the histological findings of Lindsay et al. (1971) or of Schuknecht et al. (1974) is still open; in connection with mumps-induced deafness the authors had found an atrophy of the organ of Corti, the membrana tectoria and the stria vascularis, that is to say not the picture of a neuritis but that of a labyrinthitis. By means of promontory testing it was possible to identify the total deafness after mumps as a *sensory* damage. Also very few remaining CMs inspite of deafness answer the long open question to the effect that the mumps-induced deafness probable is of sensory origin, also from the audiometric point of view (Laszig, Lehnhardt and Battmer 1985).

Deafness following a *meningo-encephalitis* is, for the most part, caused by virugenic infection since bacterial infections are regarded as having a more favorable prognosis. 30–50% of viral meningitides are caused by *mumps* viruses (Marget 1977). As for the rest, they are mainly the various herpes viruses, the measles and varicella zoster virus, the cytomegalovirus, the echo- and Coxsackie viruses and the rubella virus (vide also Chap. 3.5).

The perineural passage is particularly suspected for those cases of viral deafness which go along with a clinically almost inapparent meningeal irritation (e.g. otic herpes). If mumps leads to deafness via a diffuse *meningitis* both ears are generally involved and the loss will be total on both sides. Only Chüden (1978) thinks that he has also seen *uni*lateral deafness after mumps meningitis.

Among the *bacterial* infections, it is *erysipeloid meningitis* (Streptococcus suis) that seems to be particularly dangerous for the inner ear; butchers are especially at risk. An extensive loss on both ears seems to be scheduled and no improvement is to be expected with antibiotic treatment (Schneersen et al. 1980). In one personal observation there was still reasonable residual hearing on both sides.

Deafness following meningitis is said to vary in extent quite frequently, for example after Haemophilus influenzae, and also after meningococcal meningitis (Rosenhall and Kankkunen 1981). No further investigations were carried out to clarify if an endolymphatic hydrops was the basis of these clinical conditions as the authors think, or a disturbance of CSF circulation. In some of these patients the hearing disturbances had only appeared six to twelve months after a free interval. The sound thresholds always showed a flat curve with varying emphasis on the high tone regions and were at times also surprisingly irregular. As post-meningitis deafness – especially in children – may develop after a free interval and be *progressive*, follow-up tests in these patients are strongly recommended (Pappas and Mundy 1982).

It is only very recently, since 1975, that single cases of *fungal labyrinthitis* have been described (Igarashi et al. 1975, McGill 1978, Meyerhoff et al. 1979). It seems to occur only in debilitated patients i.e. after cytostatic, antibiotic or steroid medication or with diabetes mellitus. The infection spreads via the meninges, the tympanum or – more rarely – the blood. The loss of function of the inner ear varies in speed and extent. Cryptococcus, blastomyces, mycospores and candida were identified as pathogens.

In the case of deafness following cryptococcus neoformans infection, described by Harada et al. (1979), the audiometric and histological alterations affected the ganglion cells and the fibers of the auditory nerve and less, in contrast, the inner ear itself. Igarashi et al. (1975) described cryptococcus cysts in the CNS as well as infiltrates in the spiral ganglion and in the inner ear. The impairment affected predominantly the high tones and progressed to total deafness. In one personal observation (Wilhelmina K. 11.02.44) the CAP, too, was absent in the electrocochleogram. A well founded study about hearing loss as a sequel to meningitis was presented by Nadol (1978).

3.3.1 Inner Ear Deafness in Syphilis

The treponema pallidum may persist for a long time, thus also in the labyrinth. Exacerbations lead to sudden (20%), variable (ca 30%), or progressive deafness – often bilateral. It may appear up to sixty years after the primary infection; even congenital syphilis may possibly manifest itself only in later life (Booth 1982).

The tone threshold does not show any characteristic pattern i.e. it may fall off towards the high frequencies or all tones are affected, though to a varying extent. The fluctuation of the hearing loss alone should suggest a specific labyrinthitis (Pillsbury and Shea 1979).

The FTA (fluorescent treponemal antibody) absorption test renders a specifically positive result in 98% of the congenital and in 100% of the acquired disease. If need be the TPHA (Treponema pallidum hemagglutination)-test and the TPI (Treponema pallidum immobilisation)-test are to be carried out in addition. In the congenital form the recurrent interstitial keratitis or a chorioretinitis may lead to the diagnosis; the non-syphilitic Cogan's syndrome then has to be excluded by differential diagnosis (cf. Chap. 3.10). Previous medications may blur the clinical picture (cf. Chap. 3.5).

The congenital form requires, apart from the combined penicillin-corticoid treatment, an additional ACTH medication over several years (Adams et al. 1983). Though deafness will not regress with this treatment an increase in the hearing loss can mostly be avoided (in 22 of 24 cases; Kerr and Adams 1983).

3.4 Heredity

Hereditary deafness – monosymptomatic or as part of a syndrome – is dealt with in comprehensive surveys e.g. by Konigsmark and Gorlin (1976), by Kessler, Tymnik and Braun (1977), by McKusic (1978) and in the dictionary of syndromes by Leiber and Olbrich (1966).

As regards the clinical aspects of inner ear deafness, the *congenital forms* are of secondary importance, because unfortunately they are not (or not yet) accessible to our therapeutical efforts. This applies not only to isolated (and thus) monosymptomatic hereditary deafness but also to those types associated with specific syndromes. It is not necessary, either, to list up in this context the countless syndromes associated among other symptoms, with total deafness or with a hearing defect without progression and apparently without any causal metabolic dependency on another organic or enzyme deficiency.

The incidence in the USA, Great Britain, Japan and Germany is quoted to be one *congenitally* deaf child in every 2000–6000 live births; 10–20% of cases of deafness in children are congenital in origin and 52% of these are genetically determined (Steele 1981). The diagnostic classification is particularly difficult in those cases where the loss of hearing appears to be the only symptom (Kamei et al. 1980). We will here ignore those cases which are of neural genesis and are thus not assumed to originate in the inner ear, as for example the *Norrie-Warburg* syndrome about which reliable audiological findings have meanwhile been presented (Parving and Warburg 1977, Parving et al. 1978, Moreira-Filho and Neustein 1979, Jacklin 1980, Fujita et al. 1980) or the *Cockayne-syndrome* the neural origin of which may, amongst other things, be diagnosed in the CCT by the calcification of the basal ganglia (Konigsmark and Gorlin 1976). The malformations of the external and middle ear will equally be excluded from this discussion.

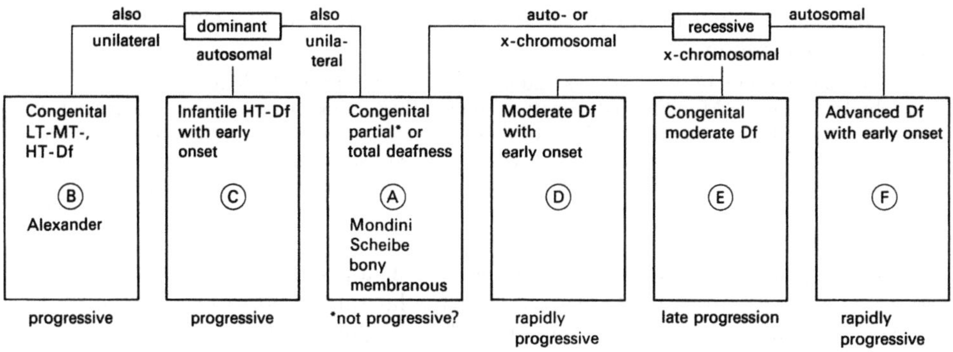

Fig. 17. Attempt of a classification of monosymptomatic hereditary hearing impairments, mainly on the model of Konigsmark and Gorlin (1976). The letters in *circles* will be referred to in the text. Df stands for deafness, LT for low tone, HT for high tone, MT for middle tone

3.4.1 Monosymptomatic Hereditary Hearing Impairments

Congenital hearing impairment or total deafness (A in Fig. 17) may be inherited as a dominant or recessive characteristic. Only exceptionally is it the result of a complete aplasia of the labyrinth (Michel type). The recessive forms are reported to result more often from a *membranous* aplasia (Scheibe type), the dominant forms from a bony dysplasia (Mondini type; Precerutti 1968).

The type of malformation is genetically determined. Aplasia of the labyrinth (Michel type) develops before the fourth week, and the Mondini defect (Illum 1972) at the end of the seventh week. Nowadays the bony malformation can be diagnosed by radio-tomography and indeed at the earliest in the axial views of the petrous bone (Illum 1972), but not so the membranous aplasia.

A clinical picture that may appear as an *apparently isolated* hereditary hearing defect, is the *Klippel-Feil syndrome*. In this case, the bony labyrinth is either not developed or is malformed (Windle-Taylor et al. 1981), in two thirds of the cases only unilaterally. The deformity of the vertebro-occipital junction may remain undetected for a long time, or only be noticed as a "frog neck" (Opitz and Schmidt 1967). The ear is affected exclusively in women; familial incidence has not so far been observed (Eiseman and Sharma 1979). The oto-vertebral symptoms may be accompanied by palatochisis, syndactyly etc, as in the Wildervanck syndrome from which 1% of the congenitally deaf suffer. Similarities exist with the Goldenhar syndrome and with the Duane-Türk syndrome.

With complete aplasia (Michel-type) there is no residual hearing at all; with the Mondini malformation the pattern of hearing is not uniform (Windle-Taylor et al. 1981). As long as the inner ear is malformed but not completely asplastic, hearing impairment or at least some residual hearing may exist; however, there is a tendency towards a progressive hearing loss (Albrecht 1923, 1931).

In the case of a Mondini type deafness it is nowadays possible by means of a very sophisticated polytomographic technique to pick out even the details of the malformation (Mangabeira-Albernaz et al. 1981). In most cases the septum between the two upper turns is missing, less frequently we have the picture of a "cloaca". In the electrocochleogram the threshold of the CAP was found to be possibly more favorable than the x-ray findings might have suggested – perhaps only because the defect is located in the *upper* turns and the ECochG only records the high tone region.

The configuration of the CAP was said to resemble that seen in the Menière patients. Since the children with the Mondini malformation show a fluctuating or progressive impairment of hearing, the authors compared the CAP of these children with those of adults with fluctuating deafness and claim to have found a definite agreement. The stimulus-stimulus response function indicated a recruitment. The endolymph-subarachnoidal shunt operation according to House is said to have led to a stabilisation of the previously fluctuating hearing function or to have stopped the progress of deafness.

This report should certainly be considered as a preliminary communication; however, it is worth while, to search in particular for the above-mentioned findings – not only in infantile deafness but also in adults with fluctuating hearing. All the same, only a short time ago it was reported from the morphological viewpoint (Paparella 1980) that in many Mondini ears the organ of Corti was intact and that this finding gave rise "to interesting speculations regarding further investigations of the hearing function". The endolymphatic duct had been dilated and the longitudinal flow had obviously been functioning.

Into this aspect, namely the inner ear deafness as a sequel to a bony malformation with progressive loss of hearing, a report from Farrior and Endicott (1971) fits very nicely. The authors believe that there may exist a congenital *isolated* widening of the aquaeductus cochleae, that many of these patients are born with normal hearing, but then, however, a combined middle ear/inner ear deafness develops. In contrast to the congenital footplate fixation, it is characterised by the progress of the inner ear component. The disease is mostly not discovered until a gusher of perilymph or CSF appears during plastic surgery of the stapes. There is increased pressure of the perilymph in the inner ear, "*peri*lymphatic hydrops", which is responsible for the decrease in bone conduction and which presses the foot plate of the stapes outwards in such a way that even the air conduction is interfered with. Farrior proposed two different operative procedures for the blockage of the aquaeductus cochleae and is convinced that the progressive deafness is arrested by the procedure and the middle ear component is remedied. Some cases would (additionally) require the closure of the perineural spaces in the internal auditory meatus via a posterior access or the middle cranial fossa. The procedure is described in full detail (Farrior 1966–1968).

The indications and technique are dealt with in the literature, apparently, however, only for extensive Mondini malformations and accordingly advanced deafness (Wolfowitz 1979). The operative procedures were mainly carried out with the aim of preventing recurrent attacks of meningitis [Pérez-Garriguez et al. 1982 (cf. Chap. 3.1.3.2, Fig. 12)].

Partial irregularities of the membranous labyrinth (Alexander type) appear as a high tone deafness (with involvement only of the basal turn) or as a pantonal, mediocochlear or apicocochlear hearing impairment (B in Fig. 17, also Figs. 18 and 19). They are said to always follow a dominant inheritance pattern (Everberg 1960, Märtensson 1960, Konigsmark et al. 1979).

The clinically relevant question concerning the further progress of a case of deafness can, for the most part, only be answered, if there is an opportunity of examining elder members of the family who are also hard of hearing. If deafness has actually been existing since birth, which is often very difficult to recognise, a gradual progress is to be expected in the families which show an autosomal dominant inheritance (C in Fig. 17).

The non-congenital, but earlier or later developing types of deafness as far as they are inherited as a recessive characteristic (auto- or x-chromosomal) (D & F in Fig. 17) tend to develop into total deafness quite early, often even before puberty (Mengel et al. 1967). The later progression begins, the more slowly will it

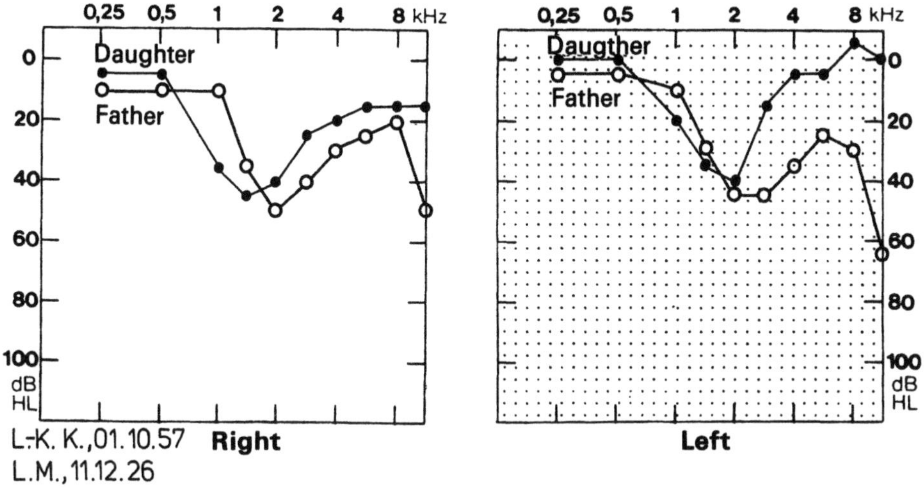

Fig. 18. Middle tone dips in daughter (25 y) and father (56 y). Scarcely any evidence of progress. BC=AC

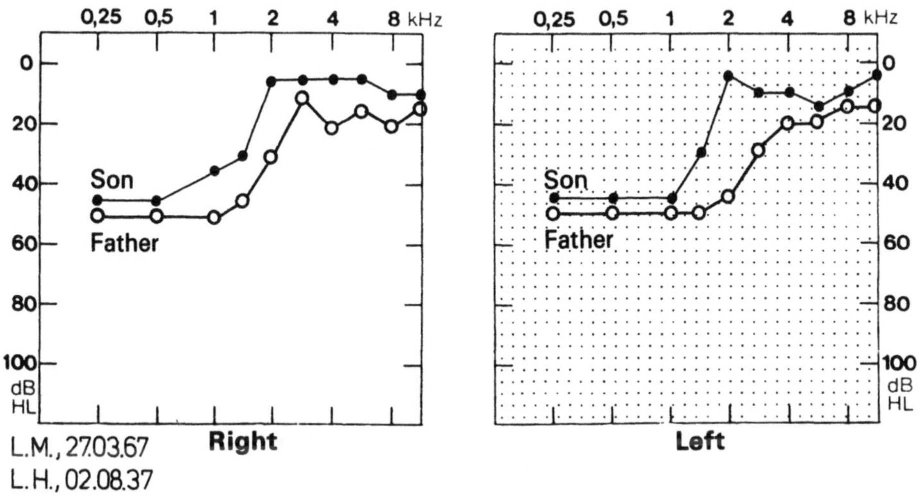

Fig. 19. Low tone deafness in son (15 y) and father (45 y). The hearing losses are identical up to 500 Hz (right) and 1000 Hz (left); progression in middle and high frequencies? SISI in both patients near 100%. Stapedius reflex threshold normal. BC=AC

proceed (Fig. 20). In late-onset deafness, the initial symmetry successively develops into an asymmetry with increasing age (Kanzaki and O-Uchi 1981). From observations in the white mink Flottorp and Foss (1979) conclude that the rapidly progressing deafness in childhood is the result of an inherent circulatory deficiency of the inner ear.

An effort has been made to subdivide these hereditary forms of deafness with a "delayed" onset into primary degenerative (abiotrophic), secondary degenerative and dysgenerative disturbances, as well as into the group "with inadequate reaction" (Jahn and Noyek 1981).

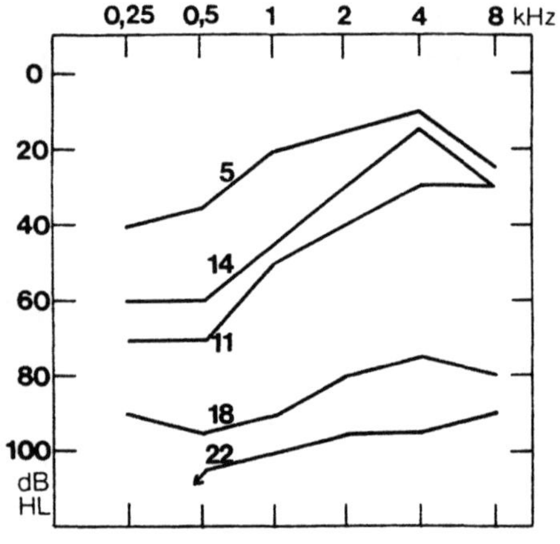

Fig. 20. Tone thresholds from five members of a family with a hereditary, autosomal-dominant rapidly progressive low tone deafness (*B* in Fig. 17). The figures attached to the curves indicate the age of the respective patient. A 38-year-old relative was almost, and a 53-year-old one completely deaf. (From Leon et al. 1981)

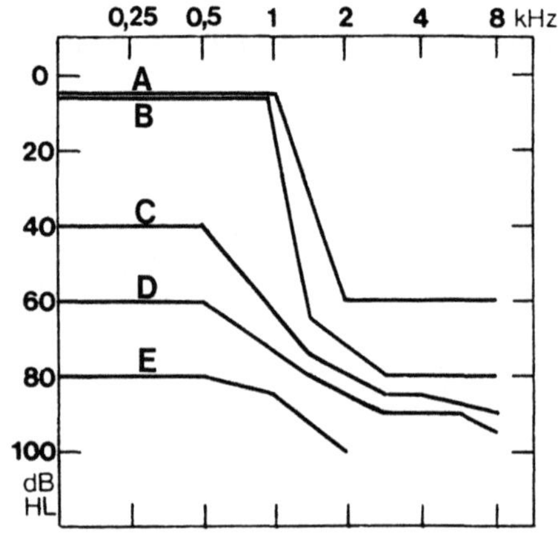

Fig. 21. Five stages (*A–E*) of the high tone hearing deterioration in a family reported on by Huizing et al. (1966)

The last mentioned possibility of a virtually hereditary progressive inner ear deafness should always be considered if *exogenous* "noxae" seem to be the obvious cause, and yet the small doses or their very slight toxicity do not appear to explain the extent of the hearing loss. This may for example apply to the increased familial susceptibility to AA (Tsuiki and Murai 1971) or to patients who after a successful renal transplant show further progression of deafness (Bergstrom et al. 1979).

The prognosis may be more favorable for children, who have a x-chromosomal mode of inheritance because their hearing function may remain constant or only deteriorate later (E in Fig. 17/Konigsmark 1970). Predictions in individual cases are therefore very difficult without accurate knowledge of the mode of inheritance and even then still uncertain (Mohr and Mageroy 1960, Livan 1961).

Huizing et al. (1983) have recently reported once again on several generations of such a family (altogether 104 members of the family) with progressive hereditary sensorineural deafness, after they had repeatedly examined the same patients in the last 20 years. The mode of inheritance was autosomal-*dominant*. The symmetrical hearing impairment started in childhood, *always before the age of 15. Relatives who still showed normal hearing after this time, remained largely unaffected.* The deafness developed with varying speed in the subsequent decades, proceeding from the high frequencies – initially by 7 dB/year. On the other hand, the low tones deteriorated significantly more slowly (only by about 1.5 dB/year). After the age of 40 the progress slowed down still further. No additional findings had been recognised in this family (Fig. 21).

In other families the deafness may progress more quickly, the tone threshold may pursue a flater course and the mode of inheritance may be autosomal-*recessive* (Cremers 1979). Or deafness may only start later showing the picture of a presbyacusis. Examples of this have been found in extensive hearing tests on twins (Gedda and Burno 1974). If there is no familial incidence the distinction between hereditary and endogenous or exogenous probably becomes impossible. This is said to apply to about one third of the cases of inner ear deafness in adults (National Center for Vital Health Statistics 1967, 1968; cited by Konigsmark and Gorlin). In the autosomal-dominant *low tone* loss there might be no progression according to the observations of Nance (1971). The correspondence of the audiograms of these patients was said to be really striking and the hearing disturbance relatively slight (cf. Fig. 19).

For parents and doctor the particularly interesting question is how great the risk of deafness will be for a subsequent child. Nance (1980) tried to answer it on the basis of his virtually unique collection of data (16000 deaf children out of 12000 families!) by a simple rule: If the family anamnesis is negative the risk of having a second child with impaired hearing amounts to about 10%, with a positive anamnesis to about 20%.

Incidentally, remarks about hereditary deafness inevitably form part of the chapter on "deafness in childhood". From the viewpoint of the geneticist this subject has been dealt with in great detail by G. P. Fraser in his report "Profound Childhood Deafness" (1964).

3.4.2 Syndromes Associated with Hereditary Inner Ear Deafness

Among the syndromes with – mostly progressive – inner ear deafness, particular notice should be taken of those in which a causal relationship is suspected between a primary hereditary metabolic or enzymatic deficiency and the ensuing disturbance of inner ear function.

3.4.2.1 Alport's Syndrome

This autosomal dominant or genetically heterogenous illness (Konigsmark and Gorlin 1976) presents itself as a familial incidence of an interstitial nephritis with pathological findings in the eyes, such as cataract and fundus albipunctatus as well as with bilateral progressive inner ear deafness.

The otological interest in Alport's syndrome resulted from the suspicion that there was a causal relationship between the basic renal disease and the progressive hearing loss. Thus, Arenberg (1967) as well as Fujita and Hader (1969) had assumed on the basis of morphological studies a disturbance of nephrogenic metabolism to be responsible for the degeneration of the sense organ. This would have to be some quite specific biochemical mechanism, because not every interstitial nephritis and not every disturbance of renal function leads to a progressive deterioration of hearing. In addition, there were no useful findings suggesting the possibility that the lasting proteinuria and tubular damage caused an excessive loss of metabolically active ions which are indispensible for the function of the inner ear. The nephritis always occurs first or there is no ear involvement at all (Brodehl 1982).

It is difficult to prove whether the occasional *isolated* hearing disturbances without nephropathy in Alport families are really conditioned by the inner ear *and* related with the hereditary disposition; in our investigations they have consistently proved to be of other origin.

The decisive starting point for research into the etiogenetic relationship between the pathological changes in the kidney and in the inner ear was reached when it became possible to demonstrate findings specific to Alport's syndrome in the kidneys; pathognomonic alterations, however, are only detectable by means of electron microscopy (Churg and Sherman 1973, Rumpelt et al. 1974). These changes in the basilar membrane of the glomeruli are so typical of Alport's syndrome which is associated with deafness that every renal biopsy which is done on account of unexplained hematuria and/or proteinuria should also be examined by electron microscopy (Brodehl 1982). In these cases the diagnostic classification of deafness may thus be guided by the renal biopsy, a necessity, which arises particularly from the progressive course of the deafness and possibly also from therapeutic requirements (vide infra).

Making use of these findings in their specific research work Weidauer and Arnold (1976) found corresponding changes in the basal membrane of stria vessels, too. Proceeding from the experiments of Quick et al. (1973) – they were also able to demonstrate in the inner ear a crossed reactivity with antibodies which were directed against the glomerular basal membrane – and thus were able to furnish evidence of an antigen association between the inner ear and the kidney (Arnold et al. 1976, Weidauer et al. 1977).

It does not seem to be out of question that the common immune reactions in both organs are of secondary nature. As for the kidney, they would then have to be understood as an autoantigen reaction to the damaged part of the specific renal tissue. The fact that the basal membrane of the stria vessels – and of the vas prominens – is then also involved in the reaction, is very easy to understand from the experimental results not only of Quick et al. (1973) but also of Arnold et al. (1976), and of Weidauer et al. (1977). This interpretation depending on the antigen specificity, as is expressed for example in the HLA-system, would explain the absence of deafness in about one half of the cases (Turner 1970, Cassidy et al. 1965, Chiricosta et al. 1970, Ferguson and Rance 1972, Hauser 1974). The quoted findings of both groups of investigators, though obtained from animal experiments and not from Alport patients, are of inestimable value for the knowledge of basic relationships between kidney and inner ear.

The hearing impairment in Alport's syndrome is more severe in men than in women (Turner 1970); it often already starts in the first decade and leads in almost one fifth of the cases to total deafness (Purriel et al. 1970), for the most part, however, only after the kidneys have ceased functioning for some time (Gofman and Bátsi 1980). A survey of the auditory function in 54 members of three families was presented by Turner (1970); according to this, the male relatives of affected women are particularly at risk.

In the audiogram a characteristic development of the deafness may be recognised (Fig. 22). Initially the curve is almost flat, that is, all frequencies are affected with a slight emphasis on the middle tones. After this, mainly the high tones are involved to an increasing extent until a diagonal curve results (Kacker and Bajal 1973) which finally develops into total deafness. All supra-threshold tests from the beginning suggest damage to the sensory cells (Spear et al. 1970, Miller et al. 1970). In the Békésy audiogram the amplitudes of the continous tone curve are extremely small – as it seems, regularly already at the onset of the deafness. The ECochG shows a distinct summation potential (SP) (Fig. 23).

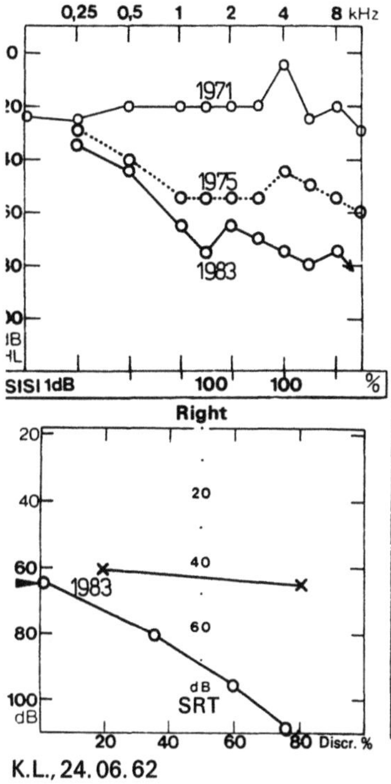

1983
Impedance

Right HL	Right SL	Probe	Left HL	Left SL
−40 / 6		P / C	−20 / 7	
dB HL	dB SL	Reflex threshold kHz	dB HL	dB SL
80	45	0,5	75	35
90	40	1	95	30
85	25	2	95	30
95	35	4	100	25
90	50	0,5	85	50
100	35	1	90	40
100	35	2	85	25

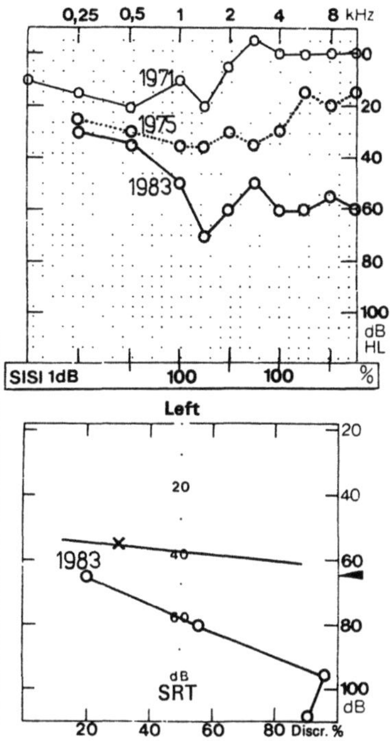

Fig. 22. Alport's syndrome with progressive bilateral inner ear deafness. Already at the age of 13 the broad middle tone trough was apparent, now at the age of 21 it has developed into a high tone loss. According to the SISI and stapedius reflex thresholds, sensory origin. BC = AC

There seems to be a correlation of the audiometric findings with the pattern of decay in the inner ear insofar as an involvement of the middle and the apical turns is already found at an early stage. The death of the sensory cells extends over all the turns, however, in the case described by Johnsson and Arenberg (1981) the *inner* hair cells were more severely affected than the outer ones. The neural elements showed only slight signs of degeneration.

The chances of a successful prophylaxis against further deterioration of hearing have up to now been absolutely nil. From the otological point of view the pediatric fatalism resembles nihilism. The experiences in non-hereditary association of renal dysfunction and inner ear deafness (Mitschke 1977, 1978) might encourage us to force kidney transplantation, possibly also for otological indications – in the hope of achieving an interruption of the otherwise unavoidable further loss of hearing, or even an improvement (Konigsmark and Gorlin 1976, p. 282). Anyhow, this would at the present time be the only possibility of saving the poor patients from total deafness. It should then be clarified in detailed discussion with the nephrologists what stage of renal dysfunction and deafness would have to be reached, in order to be able to account for the indication for renal transplantation – and at what age the operation should take place and whether the patient's own kidneys could or should be allowed to remain, in spite of possible antigenic effects, and whether on account of the possible antigen association, HL-identical kidneys should not be considered. These questions can only be raised here, especially as they have not yet been dealt with in the literature. If, however, any dependence of the cochlear on the nephrogenic process was to be denied all these considerations would be futile.

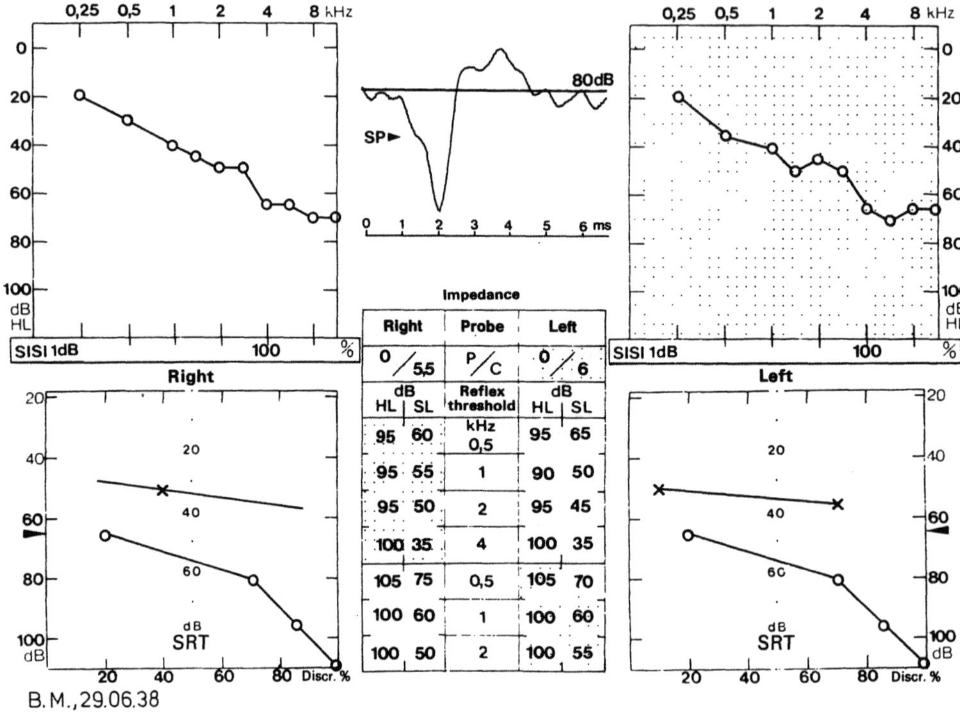

Fig. 23. Symmetrical inner ear deafness with diagonal high tone loss in Alport's syndrome; according to SISI and stapedius reflex threshold of sensory origin. Monosyllable discrimination corresponds with the hearing loss. The action potential (CAP) also includes a clear summation potential (SP_1). BC=AC

3.4.2.2 Alport-like Syndromes

This collective term nowadays includes the hereditary syndromes which

- on the basis of electron-microscopic biopsy findings cannot be classified as Alport's syndrome, *and* those who
- on account of additional symptoms are to be distinguished from Alport's syndrome.

The existence of additional, possibly sporadic disturbances thus does not, on its own, justify the assumption of a separate clinical entity. Even such findings which are interpreted as a phenomenological expression of a pleiotropic gene deficiency coupled with the nephropathy (Brodehl 1982) may be subsumed under the concept of Alport's syndrome, *if the morphological criteria in the kidney are fulfilled.*

On account of this diagnostic classification which has only been possible for a few years, it is difficult to regard as original some of the syndromes surveyed in the literature, especially as no uniform opinion exists regarding the mode of inheritance in Alport's syndrome. These difficulties of delimitation apply e.g. to the Sohar syndrome (1956) with its unclear mode of inheritance and also to the autosomal-recessive Ohlsson syndrome (1963). In both these diseases deafness develops progressively. In the Ohlsson syndrome men are also more severely affected; in both syndromes the involvement of the eyes is shown by a myopia.

The Lemieux-Neemeh syndrome (1967) also seems to be largely identical with Alport's syndrome, but in addition it shows dental anomalies (Charcot-Marie), as well as the autosomal-dominant clinical picture described by Epstein et al. (1972) which, however, – in contrast to Alport's syndrome – predominantly affects women. The rapidly progressing inner ear deafness accompanied by focal nephritis and high blood pressure which was described by Hamet et al. (1973) would be distinguishable from Alport's syndrome by the hypogenitalism; the mode of inheritance is autosomal-recessive.

Clare et al. (1979) described a clinical picture which, on the basis of the renal biopsy, too, was classified as Alport's syndrome, which, in addition, is associated with a thrombocytopenia. Passwell et al. (1981) described another one which, due to the thickening and disintegration of the basal membrane can be counted under Alport's syndrome; also because of the deafness and the ophtalmic findings, otherwise, however, is accompanied by the signs of a Fanconi syndrome i.e. by an excretion of amino-acids and phosphates in the urine, leading to osteomalacia.

The Muckle-Wells syndrome (1962) is characterised by attacks of fever, urticaria, progressive deafness and amyloidosis of the parenchyma of the kidneys and spleen as well as of the vessels of other parenchymatous organs, not, however, in the labyrinth. The deafness develops slowly, but finally reaches a large extent – associated with death from uremia in the third to fifth decade. The mode of inheritance is autosomal-dominant (Sweeney et al. 1979).

The difficulty of classification or differentiation from one another of the majority of similar combinations of nephropathy, inner ear deafness and other variable symptoms, is shown clearly by Goyer et al. (1968) who published the following clinical picture: nephropathy, hyperprolinuria, ichthyosis, and inner ear deafness. Already in 1968 "Swelling of the mesangial basal membrane in the kidney with dense deposits in the matrix" was found by electron microscopy.

Genetic relationships between *proline metabolism* and inner ear deafness have repeatedly been assumed but also been questioned (Konigsmark and Gorlin 1976, p. 356). The inner ear disturbances which are associated with hyperprolinemia and hyperprolinuria therefore need severe scrutiny of their genetic association.

The Herrman-Aquilar-Sacks syndrome is characterized by *progressive* inner ear deafness, starting in the fourth decade – in nine out of thirteen cases (cited from Konigsmark and Gorlin 1976). In the kidneys accumulations of PAS-positive material are found – namely in the tubular cells. In addition, the patients with this autosomal-dominant disease suffer from photo-myoclonic epilepsy and a mild diabetes mellitus.

In the clinical management of inner ear deafness these differential diagnostic considerations are only of secondary importance. The pattern of deafness in all the syndromes mentioned seems to be uniform, i.e. a *relatively flat curve of the hearing thresholds* with the high tone loss becoming increasingly evident. The deafness is always a sensory one, at least as far as the appropriate classification was sought for, or as far as histological findings are available.

Under no circumstances are all hereditary disturbances of renal function accompanied by inner ear deafness. In the congenitally deaf (n = 549) only 2.0% also show a renal damage, and only 2.6% of those with hereditary renal disease (n = 409) are also hard of hearing (Bergström et al. 1979). In half of the cases analysed in this way the family anamnesis was kidney- *and* inner-ear positive.

In other cases one can only suspect – at least without further studies – an accidental genetic coincidence of malformations in the kidneys and in the inner ear, thus in renal caliceal dysmorphism and inner ear deafness (Morse et al. 1980) all the more since there are no disturbances of kidney *function*.

In yet other reports, such as on renal tubular acidosis, the conclusion is really irresistible that there is a causal relationship between deafness and disturbances of renal function.

3.4.2.3 *Renal Tubular Acidosis (RTA)*

Insights into the etiogenesis of some cases of inner ear deafness might be gained from patients in whom renal tubular acidosis (RTA) is associated with inner ear deafness. RTA is not a very unusual clinical picture, but the combination with inner ear deafness is nevertheless uncommon.

The illness results from a deficiency of carbonic anhydrase, an enzyme which is involved in ion transport in the kidneys. Among the three types of this disease only Type I seems to be occasionally combined with deafness. The disturbance is located in the distal tubule; it consists in the inability of the kidney to excrete or exchange adequate amounts of H^+ ions and thus to reduce the pH of the urine below 6 (Schreier 1979).

Type II is an anomaly of bicarbonate reabsorption in the *proximal* section of the tubule, Type III is characterized by a loss of bicarbonate in the distal part. Recently a Type IV has also been described (Brenner et al. 1982).

The number of cases of RTA associated with deafness have so far probably amounted to only 17: 11 collected by Cremers et al. (1980), one by Simon et al. (1979), three by Guibaud et al. (1979) and two by Dunger et al. (1980). The mode of inheritance is autosomal-recessive (Cremers et al. 1980), and in six of eight families there was consanguinity.

The deafness manifests itself in early childhood, possibly starting soon after birth. However, a congenital origin cannot finally be excluded, either (Cohen et al. 1973). The hearing impairment can verge on total deafness or be only moderately developed; a high tone diagonal loss, with a hearing loss of 50 or 60 dB around 1000 Hz (Cremers et al. 1980). There is no information about the audiometric location of the lesions.

A causal relationship between renal and inner ear dysfunction has probably not yet been discussed here, because hearing losses by no means occur in all RTA patients, not even in all those suffering from Type I. Impaired hearing was rather considered an autonomous symptom with a particular autosomal-recessive mode of inheritance (Guibaud et al. 1979).

On the other hand, the carbonic anhydrase (CAH) contained in the distal portion of the renal tubules (and in the gastric mucous membrane) has also been identified histochemically in the stria vascularis (Watanabe 1963). The same evidence was arrived at later by Eggersmann and Bruchmüller (1968).

CAH (carbonic anhydrase) promotes the tubular reabsorption of Na^+ and HCO_3, and it can be inhibited by diamox. A CAH deficiency leads to alkalinity of the urine. In the stria vascularis of the cat, Johnson and Spoendlin (1966) were able to observe a decrease in the vacuoles in the dark cells under the influence of diamox. The authors therefore believe that diamox inhibits the secretory function of the endolymph, whereas CAH encourages the secretion.

Patients with a CAH deficiency as the cause of their renal acidosis may therefore also be suspected suffering from a CAH deficiency as the cause of their impaired hearing. The pathophysiological background of inner ear deafness might then be regarded as a collapse of the endolymphatic cavity – no doubt a speculative, but a possible starting point for further observations and investigations.

3.4.2.4 *Pendred's Syndrome*

This autosomal-recessive functional disturbance of the thyroid gland – associated with inner ear deafness – is relatively frequent: in Scandinavia seen in 1 in 100 000 births (Nilsson et al. 1964). Every one in 10–20 cases of congenital deafness is said to be associated with Pendred's syndrome (Batsakis and Nishiyama 1962, Thieme 1975).

The thyroid is enlarged, sometimes already apparent at the time of birth, otherwise becoming evident in early childhood. The goitre is mostly euthyroid (Barsano and de Groot 1979, Chan et al. 1979) or hypothyroid; it is the incorporation of iodine into the organic form of thyroxin which is disturbed. The positive perchlorate test is said to be evidence of Pendred's syndrome (Morgans and Trotter 1958, Milutinovic et al. 1969, Illum et al. 1972, Hörmann and Held 1980, Maragoni et al. 1983) at least in its intravenous form (Gray et al. 1973), whereas it is regularly negative in endemic cretinism. But the perchlorate test is positive, too, in sporadic cretinism and in Hashimoto's thyroiditis. Also the positive result of the depletion test is said to be pathognomonic for Pendred's syndrome (Gross et al. 1981). The diagnosis is supported by the goitre, the state of metabolism in the thyroid gland, the case history and the autosomal mode of inheritance.

The hearing impairment may already become evident soon after birth. In general it is regarded as congenital, although this has not yet been proved in any case. The assumption that deafness in this case is merely a sequel to intrauterine hypothyroidism, is disproved by the observation that athyroid cretins are mostly not deaf (Barsano and de Groot 1979). For the most part, the deafness is recognised at the start of the third year (Thould and Scowen 1964). In later age, the hearing loss increases only slowly, however, according to personal observations is occasionally also abrupt. The recruitment phenomena are positive (Nilsson et al. 1964, Fraser 1965) – so that there can scarcely be any doubt about the localisation of the deafness in the inner ear. In Pendred's syndrome deformities of the bony cochlea resembling those of the Mondini type have repeatedly been seen in radiography (Hvidberg-Hansen 1968, Illum et al. 1972) – also with perilymph fistula confirmed by surgery (Bergstrom 1980).

The coincidence of a presumably congenital thyroid disease with an early developing inner ear deafness suggests a common enzyme deficiency (v. Harnack et al. 1961) – however, appropriate findings have not been collected.

Up to now it has not been possible to influence the deafness by any treatment. The goitre can be controlled by administration of iodide and thyroid hormone in most, though not in all cases. If necessary, the earliest possible thyroidectomy is then indicated (Hesch; personal communication). Neither the life expectation of the patients are supposed to be reduced nor the intelligence.

3.4.2.5 *Syndromes Resembling Pendred's Syndrome*

In all other hereditary disturbances of thyroid *and* inner ear function, whether with or without increase in the protein-bound iodine (PBI) and epiphyseal disturbances (Refetoff et al. 1967), or whether with delayed growth as well as with proteolytic or lipolytic deficit (Johanson and Blizzard 1971), deafness is already fully developed at birth. It is, however, not progressive and among the congenitally hypothyroid children only one in ten shows deafness to any considerable degree. The tone threshold mostly follows a flat course only falling off a little in the high frequencies (Debruyne et al. 1983).

In the absence of additional symptoms the subordination of an infantile deafness under Pendred's syndrome and its separation from myxedema may be difficult, especially since it was formerly supposed that about one half (Batsakis and Nishiyama 1962) or at least one third of myxedema patients were deaf (de Groot and Stamburry 1975). The differential diagnosis will possibly be facilitated by the additional middle ear component of deafness.

Other investigations, however, have shown, that the impairment of hearing, at least in the *older* myxedematous patients is not greater than in a comparable group of the same age (Schätzle and Haubrich 1967). For that reason, treatment with l-thyroxin did not produce any hearing improvement, either (Parving et al. 1983). In children or young adults the chances of an improvement in hearing by medical treatment should not be considered as quite so unfavorable, since in animal experiments deafness was produceable by myxedema (Meyershoff 1979) – and thus is likely to be influenceable by medicaments. The diverse statements possibly result from a non-uniform definition of the concept of myxedema or from the fact that not the inner ear but the middle ear component had improved.

The detection of a subclinical hypothyroidism in the thyroid in a family with autosomal-dominant inner ear deafness has remained a single observation. There was no goitre, and no additional symptoms could be detected (Lehnhardt 1967).

The hearing impairment started as a middle tone dip during childhood (Fig. 24). With increasing age hearing deteriorated in the high frequencies until in the seventh decade a very advanced deafness was reached. The suprathreshold tests indicated a sensory hearing loss. In all deaf patients X-ray pictures showed a remarkably narrow internal auditory meatus, without this finding being considered as of any causal significance for the deafness (Pagani et al. 1980).

A hearing impairment of the Pendred type was to be excluded here by the absence of a goitre and the late development of the impairment. A causal relationship between the inner ear deafness and the disturbance of thyroid function seemed obvious, was, however, not detectable.

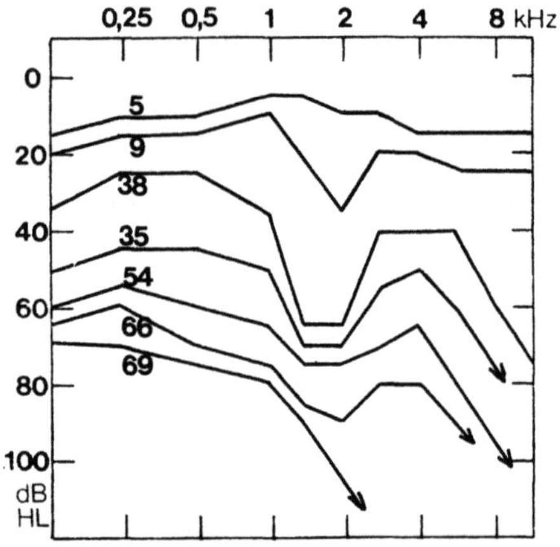

Fig. 24. Familial deafness commencing in childhood with middle tone dip, developing in old age into an extreme high tone loss. Doubtful familial hypothyroidism

3.4.2.6 Disturbances of Parathyroid Hormone Metabolism

Weidauer et al. (1982) described a clinical entity with inner ear deafness, hypocalcemia and vitiligo. The low serum calcium values were explained as a special form of pseudo-hypoparathyroidism. The serum phosphate values were normal and the renal excretion of phosphate was raised. The reaction of the kidneys to parathormone was normal. The reaction in the bones was disturbed. The authors likewise interpreted the hypocalcemia as a hitherto unrecognised special type of pseudo-hypoparathyroidism. The mode of inheritance was autosomal-dominant. Deafness was more severely developed in the father than in the son. The tone threshold showed a flat curve falling off towards the high frequencies. The recruitment was positive. Speech discrimination correlated with the pure tone audiogram in inner ear deafness. No progression had been noticeable.

The authors did not discuss any etiological relationship between the findings of blood chemistry and the inner ear deafness. The combination with vitiligo was said to have resulted from a fortuitous genetic association.

Our own similar observations seem to permit further reflections: Altogether, we have seen five deaf patients with pseudohypoparathyroidism (PHPT). In one case it was a mother and son, in another case a father and son, and in still another case a 58-year-old female without any deaf relatives. The parathormone infusion tests were conclusive, the serum calcium level was reduced and the phosphate raised. The parathormone was increased – at any rate for individual peptide fractions. In one of the boys there was an additional hypogonadism. We have not been able to investigate the blood chemistry of the father[4].

The *tone threshold was running irregularly flat* around 30–40 dB or slightly falling off towards the high frequencies, partly showing clear progression. Genetic investigations had not shed any additional light (Figs. 25 and 26).

There is a disturbance of the cellular parathormone receptors underlying PHPT. In this connection, the receptor protein in the cell membrane or the adenylate cyclase (AC) bound to it may be deficient. The adenylate cyclase complex has the function of initiating the synthesis of cyclic adenosine phosphate (cAMP), which as second messenger regulates the phosphorylation and hence the activity of numerous cell proteins. The specificity of these cell signals lies in the particular structure of the ligand stimulating the receptor e.g. a hormone.

The deficiency can also be caused by a genetically determined, more or less severe lack of a protein (of the guanyl-nucleotide regulating or G-protein) which controls the activity of the AC. The *post*-receptor deficiency represents a third variant.

This interrupts the biologically effective transmission (phosphorylation) of the information from the cAMP synthesized by the AC-stimulation (Fig. 27).

In the first intance (Type Ia) severe genetic deficiencies result in the kidneys and in the skeletal system, i.e. Albright's hereditary osteodystrophy (AHO). To what extent these patients are also deaf has not been explained in the hitherto published surveys and possibly has not been adequately observed.

In the absence of the G-protein (Type I b) this information is not transmitted to the cell by the G-protein in spite of the AC-stimulation. The patients are handicapped to a varying extent.

---

[4] I am grateful to Prof. Dr. Legler, Mannheim, for the loan of the audiograms, to Prof. Dr. Lenard, Mannheim, for the report on the son and also to Prof. Dr. Hesch, Hannover, for the medical examination and advice.

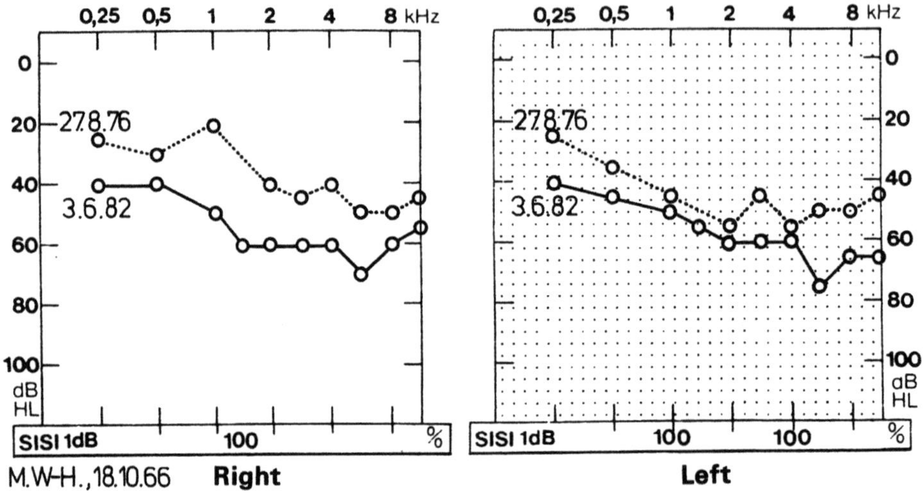

Fig. 25. Deafness apparent since the age of 4. Delayed puberty. Obesity and pseudohypoparathyroidism. Between 10 and 16 obvious deterioration in hearing, also in the speech audiogram. Stapedius reflex threshold bilaterally at 85–95 dB. (For findings in mother see next figure.) BC=AC

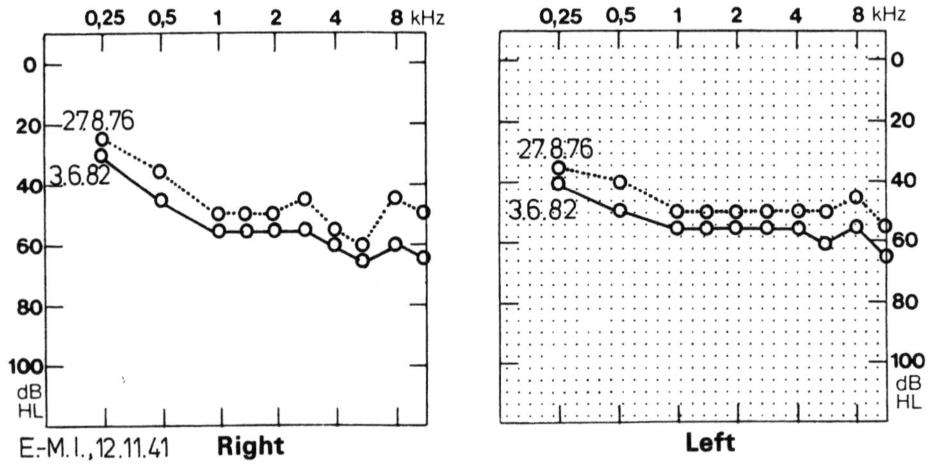

Fig. 26. Deafness existing since childhood. Only son is also hard of hearing (see previous figure). Delayed puberty and obesity up to the age of 15 and now pseudohypoparathyroidism. During the last six years the deafness has only progressed a little. Speech discrimination corresponds to tone threshold. Stapedius reflex threshold bilaterally around 85–95 dB. BC=AC

Type II finally is the least conspicuous one with varying constellations of findings in the kidneys, the skeletal system, the pituitary or the testes. Since there is a post-receptor deficiency, the activity of the AC and the synthesis of the cAMP can proceed unhindered. This defect consists in the disturbance of the cAMP-mediated phosphorylation of the proteins which are able to mediate the distinct cell function. These may be e.g. membrane transport proteins, which are stimulated in their activity by the phosphorylation. In the kidney this leads to a reduction of the phosphate and calcium transport as well as of the excretion in the urine. In the bones the formation

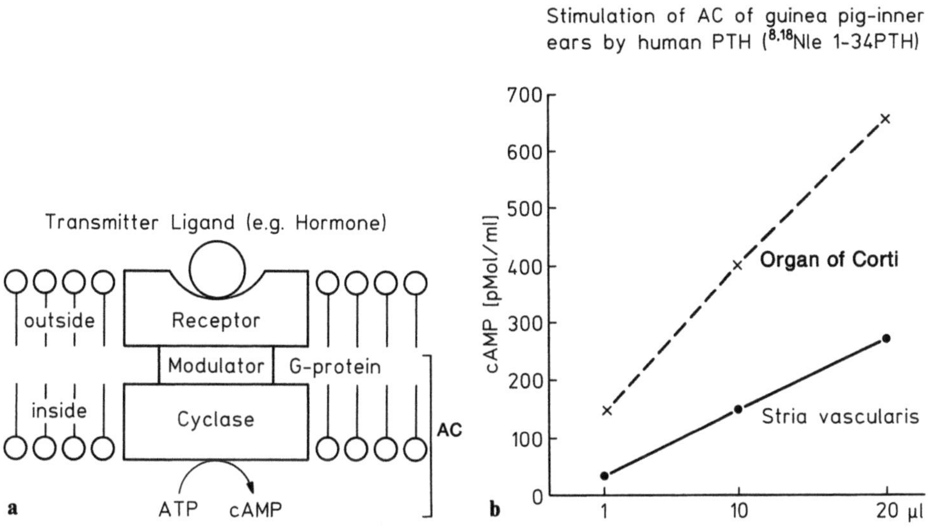

Fig. 27. a Biological sketch of the cell membrane (schematic according to Singer 1974). In the example shown here the parathormone is assumed to be the transmitter, the G-protein the modulator and the adenylate cyclase (AC) the cyclase. **b** With stimulation of the adenylate cyclase in the guinea pig's ear by human parathormone, a dose-dependent synthesis of cAMP is detected, separately for the stria vascularis and the organ of Corti. (According to Hesch and Zenner, cf. Lehnhardt 1984)

Characteristics	Signal	Type		
		Ia	Ib	II
cAMP in urine	Stimulation of AC	0	0	normal
Phosphorus in urine	Post-receptor action of the kidney	0	0	0
Calcium in urine	Post-receptor action of the kidneys and of the bones	↓	↓	↓
G-protein	Activity of AC	↓	normal	
PTH	Stimulation of parathyroid gland by ↓ serum-Ca^{++}	↑	↑	↑

Fig. 28. Graphic representation of the three types of pseudohypoparathyroidism, including their criteria and findings. 0 = absent, ↓ = increased

of osteoblasts is reduced and in the testes the spermatogenesis as well as the testosterone production are disturbed. The disturbances in the kidneys and bones lead to a lowering of the serum calcium level which, on its part, is followed by an increased production of parathormone. *This additional secretion of PTH thus represents the essential feature of pseudo-hypoparathyroidism. Incidentally, it is not the PTH molecule itself which is disturbed but its receptor transmission into the cell* (Fig. 28).

As for the kidneys and the skeleton, it is well-known that the AC is stimulated by PTH, but this is not yet known for the inner ear. As regards the latter, Zenner and Zenner (1979) have demonstrated an activation of the AC by vasopressin and by isoproterenol. In the inner ear of the guinea pig the AC is reported to be an integrated element of the external cell membrane and functionally coupled to the beta-adrenergic receptors. In addition, its acitivity is said to be controlled by the previously mentioned nucleotide-mediating proteins. The authors also discuss possible relations of the activity of this enzyme to synaptic functions, to the transport of ions and to the endolymph secretion. Anyhow, according to Thalmann et al. (1973) the AC, by the production of cAMP, plays a decisive role in the recognition and transmission of regulating signals, also for the cells in the inner ear. However, the location of this enzyme in the inner ear was at that time still unknown. In the meantime Thalmann et al. (1982) have identified the AC on the juxta-luminal surface of the marginal cells in the stria vascularis. Since, in the tubular tissue, structures which are controlled by vasopressin and isoprotenerol also react with PTH, it seems justified to assume a stimulation of the AC by PTH in the same way for the inner ear. If in our patients the parathormone was biologically active whereas the parathormone receptor was deficient, then this defect might also have an effect on the inner ear, above all in the electrolyte transport into the endolymph.

Pseudohypoparathyroidism would thus interfere with the function of the inner ear in the same way as do the loop diuretics. With these, the AC is blocked by an *exogenous* toxin whereas here exists a *genetic* deficiency of the parathormone specific receptor or of the G-protein (Levine et al. 1983). The suspicion that the AC in the inner ear, too, is stimulated by parathormone was in the first place merely an attractive hypothesis for further investigation into the origin of this type of deafness. Meanwhile, at our instigation (Lehnhardt 1984), Hesch and Zenner have succeeded in producing the long awaited proof of this. They were able to demonstrate that the assumed receptor chain for a parathormone-dependent cell stimulation also functioned in the inner ear, i.e. that here, too, parathormone stimulates the adenylate cyclase and hence the production of the cAMP which is so important for cellular metabolism. Figure 27b shows the activation of the cAMP in relation to the dose of PTH applied – indicated separately for the stria vascularis and the organ of Corti or basilar membrane.

In the patients with PHPT *plus* deafness, the genetic deficiency was located in the inner ear, namely in the receptor, whereas the metabolism of the parathormone itself was not disturbed. This raised the question as to whether a true hypoparathyroidism, too, causes similar disturbances of function in the inner ear. We have found no corresponding communications in the literature. Specific observations and investigations will be necessary in order to search for relevant correlations. As regards the insight they give into the molecular biology of the inner ear, these findings are apparently of similar significance as those of Arnold, Weidauer and Seelig (1976) on the pathogenesis of Alport's syndrome. Both clinical pictures show tone thresholds similar to one another without, of course, distinguishing themselves basically from those in other genetic impairments of hearing.

Possibly there also exist direct causal relationships between some osteodysplastic syndromes and the accompanying deafness. Examples of these are Stickler's syndrome (Young et al. 1979, Liberfarb et al. 1981), the osteo-dysplasia and sensori-neural deafness first described by Insley and Astlay (1974) (see also Beighton and Hamersma 1980), or the dysplasia of the femoral head epiphysis plus myopia and sensori-neural deafness (Pfeiffer et al. 1973).

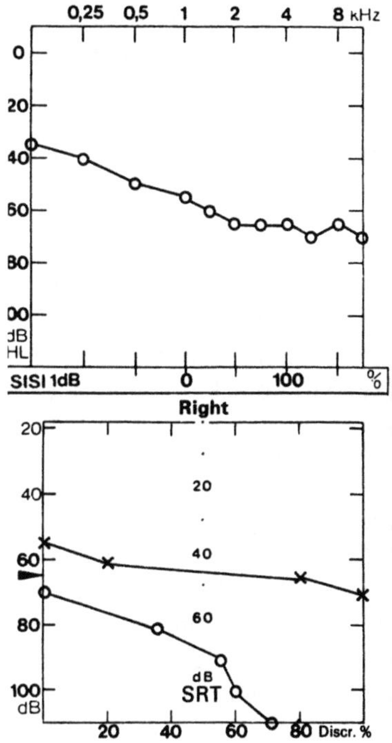

Impedance

Right dB HL	Right dB SL	Probe	Left dB HL	Left dB SL
/		P/C	/	
HL	SL	Reflex threshold kHz	HL	SL
100	60	0,5	100	50
105	55	1	90	35
100	35	2	100	35
115	55	4	100	35
100	50	0,5	100	60
90	35	1	105	55
100	35	2	100	35

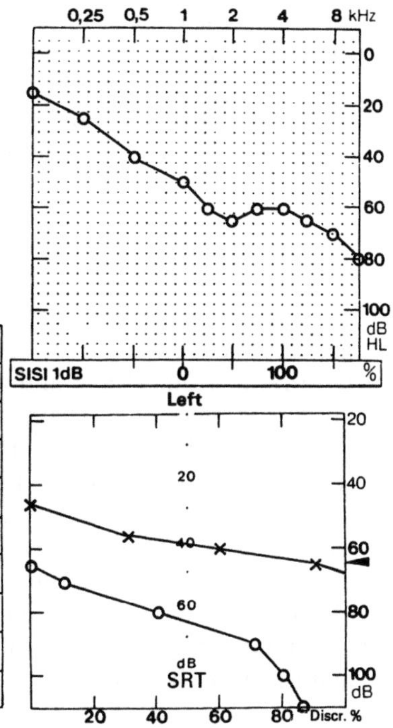

Fig. 29. Impairment of hearing in Refsum's syndrome. Almost symmetrical high tone diagonal loss. No pathological hearing fatigue in the Carhart-test or in the Békésy audiogram. Dichotic speech discrimination at 100 dB right 60%, left 70%. (From Feldmann 1981). BC=AC

3.4.2.7 Refsum's Syndrome

A genetically interesting form of familial deafness is that which forms part of *Refsum's syndrome* (1944, 1946). It is only recently that it has been described in detail in the otological literature (Feldmann 1980, 1981). Other communications were published by neurologists (Goulon et al. 1977, Barolin et al. 1979), ophthalmologists (Refsum 1977), dermatologists (Davis et al. 1977) and internists (Atzpodien et al. 1977, Thümler et al. 1977). The nature of this illness which, if not recognised, may lead to deafness as well as blindness and ataxia has by now been largely clarified. Deafness begins in the second, third or fourth decade (Bergsmann and Djupesland 1968, Feldmann 1981), it exhibits the picture of a sensory hearing defect (Genka et al. 1981), possibly with a neural component, at least as evidenced by the brain stem latencies and the peripheral nerve conduction rate (Feldmann 1981) (Fig. 29). All frequencies are affected, with an increasing tendency towards the high tone region in the sense of a high tone diagonal loss. Speech discrimination correlates with the tone hearing loss, also dichotic, with no hearing fatigue. The etiology of this autosomal-recessive hereditary disease is a disturbance of fat metabolism with pathological accumulation of phytanic acid (for details see: Feldmann 1981). The progression of deafness may therefore be arrested by a specific treatment. This consists in a diet poor in phytol and phytanic acid i.e. in butter and animal fat, but rich in calories, as well as in a large volume plasma exchange transfusion (Gibberd et al. 1979, Gibberd 1980, Lenz et al. 1979, Moser et al. 1980, Refsum 1981).

The diagnosis is derived, apart from the deafness, from a constant increase in the CSF protein concentration and from the accompanying symptoms such as retinitis pigmentosa, ataxia, paresthesia and anosmia; for the most part, vestibular symptoms are absent. It is necessary to make the differential diagnosis from the Usher-syndrome in which, however, deafness is congenital and neurological symptoms besides retinitis pigmentosa are absent. The high phytanic acid level in the plasma is conclusive for Refsum's syndrome.

According to what is indeed a single communication, the CSF – in spite of a normal cell count – is said to contain characteristic vacuolar macrophytes (Scholtz and Barolin 1981), a finding which would indeed be noteworthy from the otological view.

In spite of detailed knowledge about the etiological connection with the fat metabolism, we have still no idea regarding the disturbance of function in the inner ear. We are well aware of the degenerative sequels in the sense organ and in the first neurone (Rake and Saunders 1966, Hallpike 1967) but know nothing about the preceding or continuing changes, that is, the process leading to the functional failure. Deafness in Refsum's syndrome does probably not originate from a direct defect in the biochemical system of the inner ear, but indirectly through its vascular supply. This assumption seems to be supported by the fact that deafness is by no means a regular symptom of Refsum's disease (e.g. Hansen et al. 1979). Not all Refsum patients will thus undergo otological examination. On the other hand, an episodic deterioration of hearing may arise quite acutely (Thümler et al. 1977) and will then force the otologist to make a differential diagnosis from the monosymptomatic vascular sudden hearing loss.

3.4.2.8 Other Storage Diseases

These include *Hurler's*, *Hunter's* and *Scheie's* syndromes. Deafness is only partly due to inner ear dysfunction but originates predominantly in the middle ear.

Thus Scheie (1962) and Kittel (1963) report on an inner ear *component* of deafness in Hurler's syndrome. It is said to be of the *ganglionic* type, though only observed in one single case. In the histological specimen the organ of Corti proved to be normal, however, a broad PAS-positive zone appeared under the stria vascularis; the cytoplasm of the spiral and vestibular ganglia was crammed full of foamy, PAS-positive material (Zechner and Altmann 1968). In contrast to this, Hayes et al. (1980) saw isolated hair-cell defects in two of three cases. In Kelemen's (1966) histological description the middle ear was exclusively affected.

The evaluation of the auditory findings is made difficult by the mental retardation and the frequently early death of the patients. As regards e.g. Scheie's syndrome, there is a complete absence of any results of hearing tests. Only about 20% are reported to be hard of hearing.

The various clinical manifestations of these autosomal or x-chromosomal recessive diseases are based on a disturbance of mucopolysaccharide metabolism. The result is an intracellular storage of unsaturated acid mucopolysaccharides. Normally there are acid mucopolysaccharides in the tectorial membrane of the inner ear but not in the organ of Corti or in the stria vascularis. It therefore seems reasonable to assume an involvement of the inner ear in the disturbed metabolism.

Our knowledge about high tone deafness in mannosidosis (Öckermann 1967, Loeb et al. 1969, Booth et al. 1975, Spranger et al. 1976) is meagre. Up to the age of five these patients are said to remain inapparent (Autio et al. 1973). The pathogenesis of this obviously progressive disease is not clarified.

There are virtually no data of any value, regarding the pattern of deafness in these illnesses. Sometimes middle ear deafness is assumed then sensori-neural deafness and finally *hyper*acusis (Konigsmark and Gorlin 1976). We saw a 21-year-old man with a leucodystrophy which Couchot et al. (1974) counted among the mucopolysaccharidoses. This patient showed the picture of a broad high tone dip; from the SISI (100%) and the normal stapedius reflex threshold it could have been concluded that there was a lesion of the inner ear. The brain stem AEP were normal. Only the responses of the cerebral cortex showed, on the right, a marked prolongation of the latency; findings on the left were normal. Dichotic speech discrimination was likewise markedly reduced on the right.

In this case deafness was therefore *not* arising from the inner ear, but was the result of the central leucodystrophy, an information which is of importance for the etiological classification of the otological findings.

3.4.2.9 Diabetes Mellitus

Among the hereditary disorders of the inner ear associated with diabetes mellitus the most important is *Alström's syndrome* (1959). The mode of inheritance is autosomal-recessive; it leads to retinitis pigmentosa, cataract, nephropathy and to an inner ear hearing loss starting in late childhood and progressing over decades. On the basis of the Békésy audiogram, tone decay test and SISI, the hearing impairment is of sensory origin. The diabetes which only starts in adult life, can thus scarcely be the cause of the deafness, and the renal dysfunction, too, only appears in the third decade (Goldstein and Fialkow 1973).

The time scale is quite different in *Wolfram's* syndrome or the so-called *DIDMOAD* – (*D*iabetes *I*nsipidus, *D*iabetes *M*ellitus, *O*ptic *A*trophy, *D*eafness) – syndrome. Deafness is only associated in about one third of these cases. It affects first of all the high frequencies and later spreads also to the middle and low tone range. The earlier it appears – within the first three decades – the more evident is progression, for the most part over a period of about ten years (Cremers et al. 1977, Ijaiya et al. 1979, Nagi 1979, Likourinas 1980, Morrissey-Walsh and Barry 1980, Bujara et al. 1982).

These and all similar syndromes (Bujara et al. 1982, van den Eyckhaut et al. 1983) are definite rarities and we will therefore forgo any complete description here.

3.4.2.10 Sickle Cell Anemia

The deafness associated with this hereditary hemoglobinopathy affects either the high tones or all frequencies equally and is not serious (Forman-Franco et al. 1982). The faulty development consists in the incorporation of valine instead of glutamic acid into the side-chain of the hemoglobin-molecule – in the USA in 8.5% of the black population. The number of deaf is around

12%; additional lesions in the CNS aggravate the condition (Todd et al. 1973, Friedman et al. 1980). The elevation of the stapedius reflex threshold (Sharp and Orchik 1978) is thus likely to result from central changes in the reflex pathways. Forman-Franco et al. (1982) even think they have found central impairment of speech discrimination in 46% of their patients (n=54); in these, however, the stapedius reflex threshold was not increased.

The hearing losses occur relatively suddenly – with a varying tendency to remissions (Urban 1973, Orchik and Dunn 1977). They are supposed to be the expression of hemolytic crises (Berry 1975), or of ischemic (Morgenstein et al. 1969), or thrombolytic deficiency (Todd et al. 1973). Direct relationships are said to exist between the frequency of the hemolytic crises and the extent of the hearing impairment (Berry 1975).

An obliteration of the spongiosa occurs around the labyrinth with apposition of bone, but without any narrowing of the internal auditory meatus. As regards the cochlea, defects in the organ of Corti and in the stria vascularis have been described (Todd et al. 1973, Serjeant et al. 1975).

Thalassemia major leads to narrowing of the internal auditory meatus by osteo-hypertrophy. It is also known as Cooley anemia, a disturbance of the hemoglobin synthesis at the stage of differentiation from fetal hemoglobin into the adult form (Hb to Hb_A). However, even this is not the direct cause of the bilateral high tone inner ear deafness, either; in the deaf patients the average ferritin level is significantly higher than in those who are not deaf. The sequel to this may be the raised iron values, to which the damage of the high tone elements in the inner ear is attributed (de Virgiliis et al. 1979).

3.4.2.11 Skin Diseases

Most of the numerous syndromes with associated alterations of the skin and the inner ear, are connected with congenital deafness and only a few with *progressive* deafness. These include *Helweg-Larsen*'s syndrome, a dominant hereditary anhydrosis, and *Hammerschlag*'s syndrome, a dominant disturbance of pigmentation. Deafness is progressive in the generalised alopecia described by Crandal et al. (1973) and probably in the atopic dermatitis published by Konigsmark et al. (1968). The details about the pattern of deafness are, however, so meagre that it is impossible to say anything either about the frequency pattern of the hearing disturbance or about the time scale of its progression (cf also Cram et al. 1979, Skinner et al. 1981). Incidentally, these syndromes have so far been observed in only a few families.

In *Waardenburg's syndrome* deafness is also congenital and stationary; it develops to a varying degree (Waardenburg-Klein syndrome: Francois 1979) and may also be completely absent, above all in patients with telecanthus (Type I, Meinecke 1982). The clinical picture is striking by the white hair curl, the broad root of the nose, telecanthus, different colour of irides, vitiligo and patchy hyperpigmentation. In the fundus oculi there is a loss of the pigmented epithelium.

In slight cases the low and middle frequencies are predominantly affected, but in the more severe cases there is only a residual auditory function in the low tone regions or total deafness (Fisch 1959).

The mode of inheritance is autosomal-dominant (Konigsmark and Gorlin 1976). The dysgenetic association of pigment disturbance and deafness is explained by the common origin of pigment cells and the labyrinth from the neural crest (Fisch 1959, Deol 1970).

3.4.2.12 Other Hereditary Syndromes

The great number of hereditary hearing disorders associated with diseases of the eyes has recently been assembled into a table by Gross (1981): This was taken over unchanged if only for its clear arrangement (Table 2). In addition, the combination of a progressive deafness with increasing cataract was recently described, with its autosomal-dominant mode of inheritance evidently a first observation (Nadol and Burgess 1982).

Finally mention should be made of those genetically determined clinical pictures associated with bony appositions which exceptionally also affect the inner ear or the internal auditory meatus. These are the *van Buchem* syndrome with generalised endosteal hyperkeratoses and increase in the alkaline phosphatases as well as *Paget's* syndrome with progressive osteodystrophy or *Albers-Schoenberg's* disease, and many others (Miyamoto et al. 1980). The bony appositions can be partly identified by polytomography, even in the labyrinth. A clear review of the systemic bone diseases which are associated with deafness is found in the article by Booth (1982).

Very difficult to classify is the case of three sisters, all of whom showed *progressive* deafness up to the age of ten. In one case malformations of the cochlea could be excluded, but histological examination revealed a collapse of the endolymphatic sac with an atrophic organ of Corti and a "deformed" stria vascularis, especially in the basal turn. In addition, there was a gastro-intestinal atonia with diverticulitis and ulcerations. One is inclined to suspect the resorption disturbance to be the cause of the inner ear degeneration; up to the present, however, no further clues have been found (Igarashi et al. 1981).

3.5 Deafness in Childhood

A thorough if not exhaustive review of this subject would fill a separate monograph (Beckmann 1962). We will therefore only present the facts which are of importance for the diagnosis of inner ear deafness in children, and even this without any claim to completeness. Many details have already been described in the corresponding chapters such as hereditary and ototoxic hearing impairments, some disturbances caused by viral infection or the search for HLA-associations (cf. Chap. 3.10).

The incidence of congenital or early acquired deafness in Holland was reported to be 0.1% of the total population (Kaaijk 1977); this would result in a total of 60000 in the FRG.

As regards *hereditary* deafness, it is of interest to know its percentage in the incidence of the severe infantile hearing impairments and the distribution among the various genetic disorders. In representative studies (n = 3535, Fraser 1974, Kankkunen 1982) it was altogether about 50% of the congenital, early infantile or infantile cases of deafness which required special care; Kessler et al. (1981) quoted only 30%. The classification is difficult, since the hearing disturbance develops for the most part as an isolated monogenic feature and since the autosomal-recessive forms (80%) are more frequent than the autosomal-dominant ones (20%). There are obviously no possibilities of collecting conclusive findings by means of special audiometric testing in the heterozygous bearers of this characteristic with an apparently normal auditory function (Kessler et al. 1981). 10% of these show autosomal recessive deafness with goitre; one in ten children with genetic deafness thus shows a hearing loss of the Pendred type, and one in fifty is grouped with Usher's syndrome (with retinitis pigmentosa). One half of the dominant inherited cases of deafness are said to develop progressively. Only 0.9% of hereditary deafness is sex-linked (Blumina and Moskovkina 1981, 1981).

Table 2. List of hereditary syndromes with involvement of the ears and eyes. (From Gross 1981)

Name of the syndrome	Symptoms			Mode of inheritance
	Audiologic	Ophthalmic	General	
Alport	End of first decade onset of progressive sound perceptive deafness (symmetrical) mostly in the middle to high frequencies	Lenticonus anterior, subcapsular cataract. fundus albipunctatus, druses on the optic disc	Hemorrhagic nephritis with albuminuria, disturbances of equilibrium, reduced life expectancy in man bearers of characteristics	Autosomal dominant Predilection for males
Alström (1959)	Progressive perceptive deafness from the age of 7	Nystagmus, divergent strabismus, lenticonus posterior. atypical pigment degeneration of the retina (spotty shift of pigment), atrophy of the optic nerve	Obesity, diabetes, hypo-genitalism, hyperuricemia, progressive renal failure reduced life expectancy	Probably autosomal recessive or x-chromosomal
Cockayne (1961)	High grade perceptive deafness	Enophthalmus, reduced reaction of pupils to mydriatics, cataract, retinitis pigmentosa	Disproportionate reduced growth, intracranial calcifica-tion, mental retardation, hepato-spleno-megaly	Autosomal recessive
Diallinas-Amalric (1960)	Perceptive deafness varying in severity	Hypoplasia and heterochromia, of irides central retinopathia pseudo-pigmentosa, no night blindness, normal ERG and EOG, no visual field restriction normal visual acuity	None	Probably autosomal recessive
Familial hypo-genitalism (Weinstein 1970)	Perceptive deafness	Cataract, retinitis pigmentosa with early loss of sight	Obesity, reduced growth, low 17-ketosteroid excretion in urine, closely related to Leber's syndrome	Probably autosomal recessive
Flynn-Aird (1965)	In first year of life onset of progressive bilateral perceptive deafness	Progressive myopia, cataract, atypical retinitis pigmentosa	Muscle hypotonia, ataxia, attacks of reversible aphasia, epileptiform convulsions, sklerodermiform skin alterations, osteoporosis	Autosomal dominant
Forsius-Ericksson (1964)	Perceptive deafness	Microphthalmos, ocular nystagmus. myopia, astigmatism, impaired dark adaptation, dyschromatopsia,	Mental retardation, epilepsy	x-chromosomal

(1976)			mental retardation, progressive tetraparesis	
v. Graefe-Hallgren (1858/1959)	Congenital perceptive deafness	Nystagmus, cataract, retinitis pigmentosa (sometimes without pigment)	Vestibulo-cerebellar ataxia, skeletal deformities, oligophrenia (facultative), schizophrenia-like state	Autosomal recessive
Gregg (1941) (Rubella-embryopathy)	Congenital perceptive deafness	Nystagmus, glaucoma, cataract retinitis pseudo-pigmentosa	Deformed heart, ataxia, convulsions, mental retardation	Not hereditary
Hallervorden-Spatz (1922)	Progressive perceptive deafness	Nystagmus, retinitis pigmentosa, atrophy of the optic nerve	Progressive spasticity, dementia, athetosis, dysphagia, skin pigmentation, muscular atrophy	Autosomal recessive with variable manifestations
Hunter (MPS II) (1917)	Slight to moderate combined deafness in ca. 50% of cases	Corneal opacities, retinitis pigmentosa	Reduced growth, hepato-splenomegaly, gargoylism, skeletal dysplasia. enzyme deficiency (sulphoiduronate sulphatase)	x-chromosomal
Kartagener (1933)	Slight to moderate sound conduction deafness or combined hearing impairment	Myopia, glaucoma, melanosis conjunctivae, coloboma of iris, tortuosity of vessels, retinitis pigmentosa	Bronchiectases, nasal polyps, situs inversus, pansinusitis	Autosomal recessive
Kearns-Sayre (1958)	Combined deafness[a], in most patients perceptive deafness predominantly in high frequencies	Progressive external ophthalmoplegia, retinitis pigmentosa, progressive ptosis	a.v. block, generalised muscular dystrophy, reduced or absent reflexes, progressive ataxia	Autosomal dominant
Laurence-Bardet Bield-Moon (1866/1920/1922)	Perceptive deafness of variable degree (facultative, occasionally progressive)	Ptosis, epicanthus, strabismus, ophthalmoplegia (internal/external), coloboma of iris, retinitis pigmentosa	Obesity, hypogenitalism, polydactyly, mental retardation, heart defects, malformations in urogenital tract	Autosomal recessive
Leber (1969)	Perceptive deafness	Paralysis of eye muscles, nystagmus, keratoconus, cataract, retinitis pigmentosa with congenital amaurosis	Mental retardation, microcephaly, EEG-alterations	Autosomal recessive

[a] In the Kearnes-Sayre syndrome it seems that the deafness only exceptionally affects the middle ear (Weidauer and Lenarz 1984, see p. 2).

Table 2 (continued)

Name of the syndrome	Symptoms			Mode of inheritance
	Audiologic	Ophthalmic	General	
Pfeiffer-Jünemann Polster-Bauer (1973)	Symmetrical, slight to moderate perceptive deafness with high tone loss from 3000–4000 Hz	Nasal supertraction of the disc, retinitis pigmentosa	Epiphyseal dysplasia (femur)	Autosomal recessive
Refsum (1946)	Perceptive deafness in the majority of patients (often asymmetrical), onset in second to third decade with slight progression particularly in the high tone region	Progressive external ophthalmoplegia, pupillary anomalies, retinitis pigmentosa or "inverse" retinitis pigmentosa	Spinocerebellar ataxia, polyneuritis, ichthyosis, a.v. block, phytanic acid-oxidase-deficiency	Autosomal recessive
Reinstein-Chalfin (1971)	Slight to severe perceptive deafness with onset from second decade and slow progression	Inverse retinitis pigmentosa	Hypogenitalism	Probably autosomal recessive
Shy-Gonatas (1967)	Perceptive deafness	Progressive external ophthalmoplegia, corneal dystrophy, atypical retinitis pigmentosa	Neurocerebellar ataxia, dementia	
Werner (1904)	Progressive perceptive deafness with onset in second to fourth decade	Absence of eyelashes, blue sclera, juvenile cataract, perimacular retinal degeneration	Reduced growth, short fingers, small mouth, premature greying and loss of hair, scleropoikilodermia, hypogonadism, osteoporosis, thyroid dysfunction, dysphonia, reduced life expectation	Autosomal recessive
Usher (1913)	Mostly severe, congenital perceptive deafness, bilaterally	Retinitis pigmentosa (without annular scotoma)	Vestibular disturbances	Autosomal recessive
Young-Leon-Barth-Grean (1970)	Moderate to severe bilateral cochlear perceptive deafness	Nystagmus, cataract, retinitis pigmentosa	Migraine (hemiplegic)	Autosomal dominant

A congenital form of infantil deafness with particular clinical significance is the one with malformations of the labyrinth which is associated with a CSF- or perilymph fistula into the middle ear or the Eustachian tube (vide also Chaps. 3.1.3.2 and 3.4.1). These cases are at any time endangered by meningitis, possibly recurring several times. The prerequisites for the diagnosis are the awareness of this possibility and the detection of the leak e.g. by instillation of indigo carmine into the lumbar sac (Sykora et al. 1980, Sterkers et al. 1980).

Among the *not genetically determined* types of infantile deafness almost 20% are acquired *pre*-natally (18% by rubella infection; de Reynier 1979, Kankkunen 1982, rarely as a result of mumps; de Reynier 1964), 25% develop during the perinatal period and the remaining 55% only later.

The occurrence of non-organic, psychogenic hearing disturbances also, and particularly in children has repeatedly been pointed out (cf. esp. Berger 1965). This sort of deafness is always bilateral, less apparent in the speech- and then in the pure tone audiogram and is caused by difficulties at school or at home. Treatment should consist in ignoring the handicap, especially because the little patients are not handicapped in their lessons (Berger 1965, Lehnhardt 1973).

3.5.1 Rubella

Deafness due to *rubella-embryopathy* is thus of great importance – and it is *the* childhood deafness which could largely be prevented. More than one third of those affected by rubella is (nearly) deaf, about 40% have an average bilateral hearing loss of 60–80 dB (Upfold 1970); rarely (in about 4%) only one side is affected (Hardy et al. 1973). Total deafness occurs as a result of infection of the mother during the first month of pregnancy, impaired hearing after infections in the second and third month, often associated with other malformations (Upfold 1970, Rossi et al. 1980).

The audiograms show varying threshold curves (Rossi et al. 1980); sometimes the low frequencies are chiefly impaired, however, not with the typical pattern of an isolated impairment in the low tone range but with a relatively flat curve of the hearing threshold (Fig. 30).

Rubella deafness is said to be often not fully developed at the time of birth but to deteriorate later (Longuebray et al. 1982). This is why some 20% of those children who in their first four years of life are inapparent, by the age of six to eight, still display a hearing disturbance or total deafness sometimes with retinopathy. This, however, is said to apply only to the seropositive cases; in the sero*negative* children such delayed loss of hearing had not been seen (Peckham 1972). Hence, *all* rubella children should be *supervised* up to the age of eight, in order to treat in good time a developing deafness (Menzer and Forrest 1974). There are no concrete ideas about the genesis or the progress of the hearing impairment beginning during early childhood; a faulty diagnosis in the first examination between *one and four years* after birth is excluded by the authors. Barr and Wedenberg (1965) had not seen this. In their opinion rubella deafness – in contrast to the deafness after meningitis or streptomycin – did not increase post partum, not even if a hearing aid was worn.

Rubella vaccination is of outstanding importance, since 24% of all deaf under four years show rubella antibodies as against 9% of those with normal hearing (Peckham 1979, Rossi et al. 1980, Flint 1983).

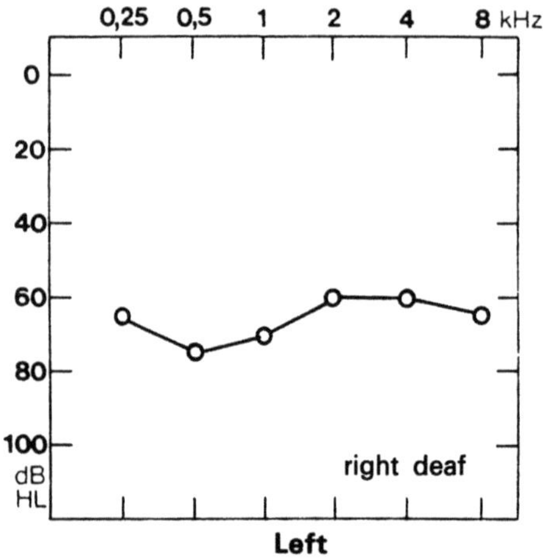

Fig. 30. Rubella deafness in a seven-years-old boy. The right ear only became deaf at the age of four. The slight preponderance of the hearing loss in the low frequencies is said to be characteristic for rubella deafness. (From Hardy et al. 1973.) BC=AC

In addition to this, prenatal rubella infection does more frequently than commonly assumed cause that type of deafness which is combined with macular degeneration (Vick et al. 1979), a condition that generally goes under the *hereditary* Diallinas-Amalric syndrome, or with central changes of the eye-ground but without functional loss (Vick 1981).

Scarcely worth mentioning is the remark made in more recent literature that in 6 out of 13 cases of rubella deafness an abnormal thickness of the cornea was observed (Jensen et al. 1982). In otosclerotics this test is said to be positive in 100% of the cases (Bentzen 1961, 1967).

3.5.2 Cytomegaly

The hearing impairments, caused by the *cytomegalovirus* (CMV) which belongs to the herpes group, is also acquired in utero. Its incidence is estimated to be 9% of newborns with CMV, which for their part represent 0.42% of all newborns. It is just as often unilateral as it is bilateral, mostly severe in extent (Saigal et al. 1982) and it is the sequel to a specific endolabyrinthitis (Myers and Stool 1967, Davis 1977, Stagno et al. 1977) with an affinity of the virus for epithelial structures (Davis 1981). However, not every congenital CMV infection with a positive urine culture is associated with an affection of the inner ear. Here, too, the deafness might progress in the first years of life as with rubella; however, the findings are not very convincing (Dahle et al. 1979).

In comparison to rubella and cytomegaly the remaining viral infections show a much smaller embryopathic effect.

3.5.3 Toxoplasmosis

Toxoplasmosis – likewise acquired in utero – is likely to lead to deafness in 15% (n=101) of congenital infections (Stagno et al. 1977) – often combined with a chorioretinitis. In most cases, the damage remains still subclinical at the time of birth.

A labyrinthitis may develop after experimental inoculation of Toxoplasma Gondii, not only by direct, but also by hematogenous infection. Toxoplasmosis accordingly would be a possible factor in chronic or acute impairment of hearing (Falser 1981), but evidently only a rare one.

As regards the hearing pattern of congenital toxoplasmosis the only thing known is that it varies a lot. Since the report by Kecht (1974) no further communications about this rare cause of deafness in children have been presented.

3.5.4 Erythroblastosis

Deafness from *erythroblastosis* is now rarely encountered thanks to well developed prophylactic or therapeutic measures (Plochl and Tasser 1980, Flint 1983). In 1955, Fisch still reported the incidence of hemolytic hearing impairment to be 5.6%, by 1966 Buch et al. declared it to be only 0.5%. The survey by Kessler et al. (1969) is therefore no longer up to date. Furthermore, the patients described by Pruszewicz et al. (1980) are now 17–30 years old; however, the audiometric findings are interesting in so far as they suggest sensory deafness in 30% of the cases. The hearing damage may therefore also be located in the inner ear, in spite of the *kernicterus* (Kelemen 1956), but is possibly less determined by the bilirubinemia than by the accompanying asphyxia (Buch et al. 1966).

3.5.5 Perinatal Asphyxia

Among the causes of perinatal inner ear deafness the most disastrous one is still, the *asphyxia of the newborn* (Simmons 1980, Taylor 1980). The individual reports do not seem to reflect this fact. According to a recent survey, only one of 26 *new*borns who took at least ten minutes before starting spontaneous breathing suffered from deafness, and this possibly only because this child had not shown any heart beat already during birth (D'Souza et al. 1980). Or only one of 31 *new*borns with severe asphyxia had, as was shown later, suffered damage to the inner ear (Thomsen et al. 1977). Among the *premature* births, however (<1500 g, $n=111$), an inner ear deafness was found in 9% of the cases which the authors attributed mainly to the apneic conditions (Abramovich et al. 1979).

The relative frequency of infantile deafness following perinatal asphyxia matches the observation that almost half of all children with a hearing impairment ($n=10\,778$) show a high tone damage (Barr et al. 1973), that is the finding which one would expect earliest from a hypoxemic condition of the inner ear.

The statistics also show, unfortunately, that the number of children with hearing impairment has remained constant. While middle ear deafness up to the age of 16 is diminishing, the percentage of inner ear deafness is increasing – no pleasant outlook as regards inner ear deafness in children.

3.5.6 Postnatal Deafness

Largely the same aspects apply here as those of deafness in adults. Nevertheless, circumscribed high tone losses or middle tone dips in school children should be more frequently considered to be of genetic rather than of exogenous origin (Claux and Coll 1979, Nance 1980). Thus, Andersson and Wedenberg (1970) often found similar threshold patterns in siblings or in parents. The increase of the stapedius reflex threshold above 1000 Hz is reported to indicate heredity (Klockhoff and Lyttkens 1982), especially as it was found in children whose hearing threshold still ranged within the norm (Fig. 31).

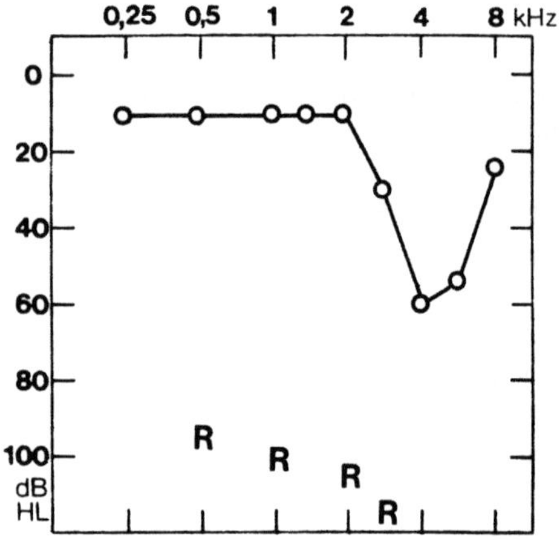

Fig. 31. Infantile high tone dip without any identifiable noise trauma. Stapedius reflex (*R*) increased raised (right). Klockhoff and Lyttkens (1982) interpreted this appearance as the expression of a genetic disposition

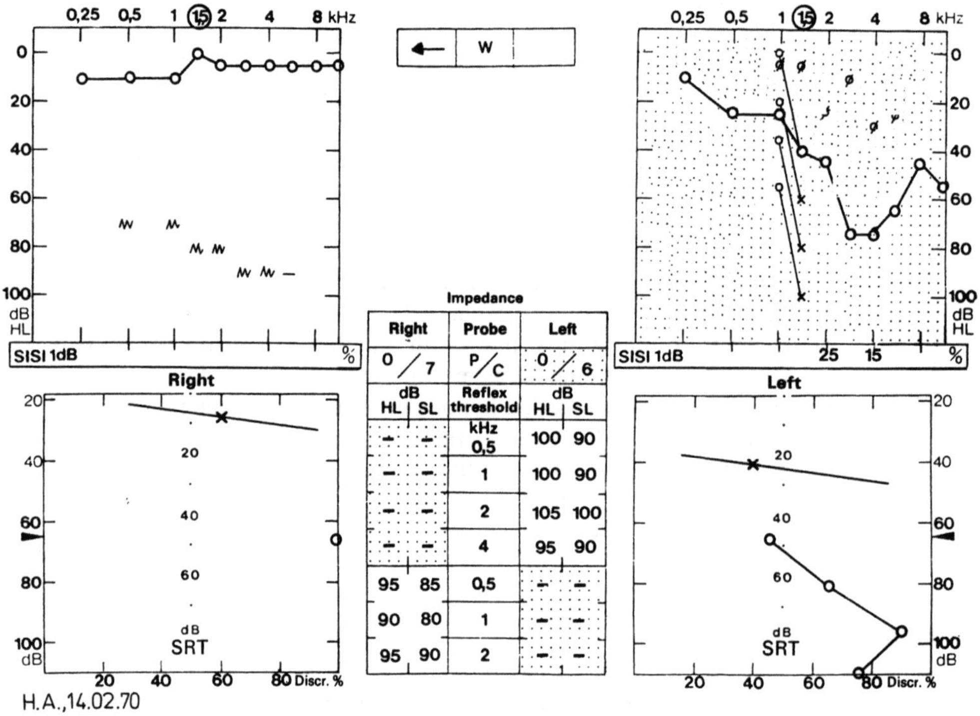

Right	Probe	Left
0 / 7	P / C	0 / 6
dB HL | SL	Reflex threshold	dB HL | SL
– –	kHz 0,5	100 90
– –	1	100 90
– –	2	105 100
– –	4	95 90
95 85	0,5	– –
90 80	1	– –
95 90	2	– –

Fig. 32. Example of a neural (?) high tone deafness in a ten-year-old girl. Recruitment negative, SISI 15 or 25%, respectively. Stapedius reflex not obtainable from the left. As also shown by the prolonged I–V latency of the AEP, not of sensory origin. Acute viral deterioration of hearing or a defect existing since early childhood? Follow-up after three years showed almost identical results. BC=AC. Masking of BC= ⁓, of AC= – (right). BC without masking=∅ (left)

Almost opposite experiences have been published in the USA. There, every fourth school boy (average age 15.2 years) showed a high tone dip which was attributed to the frequent handling of firearms in that rural area, certainly a regional observation which does not yet have general validity (Kramer and Wood 1982). Axelsson et al. (1981) finally combined both ideas in assuming a hereditary sensitivity to relatively slight noise and pop music exposure to be the cause of circumscribed high tone damage in teenage boys. The etiological interpretation of hearing impairments in childhood often remains difficult, in spite of thorough audiometric and pediatric examination because the time scale of its development is for the most part unclear (Fig. 32).

We would recommend Jahnke (1979) for his survey of the differential diagnosis of childhood hearing impairment.

3.6 Vascular and Metabolic Disturbances

3.6.1 Acute Inner Ear (Sensori-Neural) Deafness

There may be many causes of *acute deterioration of hearing*. Only those localised in the inner ear will be discussed here. This delimitation should be understood first of all in the wider sense of deafness *with an identical threshold pattern for bone conduction and air conduction*. Proceeding from this approach it is possible and necessary to define the term "sudden hearing loss" and to distinguish it from apparently similar clinical entities by differential diagnosis.

The term "sudden hearing loss" was created in the fifties with the intention of giving a name to a clinical observation which up to then – in parallel line with the then "isolated vestibular failure" – had been referred to as sudden cryptogenic hearing disturbance, sudden deafness or something similar (Fowler 1950, Beickert 1956, v. Dishoeck and Biermann 1957, Lehnhardt 1958). Vestibular neuronitis or neuronopathy became definite terms for the isolated disequilibrium whereas the isolated hearing disturbance was to be called "*sudden hearing loss*". This implied that in every single case the acute inner ear deafness was regarded "as a challenge and it was tried to interprete it as a symptom of a superordinate disease" (Feldmann 1981 b). It is only in this way that a *symptomatic* acute deterioration of hearing can be distinguished from an isolated idiopathic sudden hearing loss. "Symptomatic sudden hearing loss" would be a contradiction in itself.

For this reason, the diagnosis "sudden hearing loss" (Hörsturz, surdité brusque) should only include those sudden deteriorations of hearing:

- which, on the basis of comprehensive audiometric findings may be assumed to originate in the sensory organ of the inner ear
- the genesis of which is to be interpreted as probably vascular and
- the etiology of which cannot be delimited any further.

Only if these strict definitions were generally taken into consideration – also internationally – various publications could be compared with each other. However, this will not be possible as long as, for example merely on account of the tone threshold and the suddenness of the (observed) deterioration the term "sudden hearing loss" is used uncritically and thus becomes too all-embracing.

3.6.1.1 Symptomatic Acute Deterioration of Hearing

A relatively acute deterioration of hearing in the course of *multiple sclerosis* may, for example, have the appearance of a sudden hearing loss. The disseminated inflammatory foci of demyelination have then affected the myelin sheaths of the auditory pathway – somewhere central of the inner ear. The deterioration of hearing may be quite a solitary and first symptom of the multiple sclerosis; there may even be no tinnitus or vertigo. Mostly it will be felt unilaterally and "noticed suddenly". The distinction from (vascular) sudden hearing loss may be difficult. Perhaps only the evaluation of the many results of a thorough audiometric examination will suggest a non-inner-ear genesis. Spontaneous remissions may possibly appear so soon that later diagnostic efforts fail in finding an explanation. Among the specific audiometric findings the most decisive ones are, in particular, the pathological tone decay of the threshold (> 30 dB) as well as the absence of recruitment, the absence of the stapedius reflex (though only if the focus of demyelination is not central of the reflex pathway), the extremely bad monosyllable discrimination and the disturbed dichotic understanding (Lehnhardt 1975, Plath 1980). Already the enumeration of these findings makes clear which extensive diagnostic measures – if only in audiometry – are necessary today, in order to be able to report competently on the "sudden loss of hearing". As regards the diagnosis of multiple sclerosis, the CSF findings of polyclonal bands and the subsequent neurological course of the disease are decisive (Fig. 33).

An *acoustic neurinoma* or a *cerebellopontine angle tumor* may show a quite similar picture of an acute deterioration of hearing; the suddenness of its development remains, in general, unexplained. It was either a relatively abrupt increase in pressure of whatever nature, a phase of rapid growth or only a sudden awareness of the deafness precipitated for example by masking or ear wax occlusion of the opposite ear. The diagnostic classification of such deterioration of hearing to disturbances in the internal auditory meatus or in the cerebellopontine angle may cause great difficulties as regards audiometry, insofar as the pattern of deafness is not necessarily a neural one – if only for the reason that the deterioration of hearing for example may be due to venous congestion and thus has actually arisen in the inner ear. The vestibular findings *may* in this case facilitate diagnosis, but in general extensive investigations are necessary in order to discover the actual cause of such symptomatic deterioration of hearing – and not to classify as "sudden hearing loss", what will one day prove to be a false diagnosis. The assumption that a tumor may be excluded by infusion treatment "ex juvantibus" is certainly not justified since treatment with low-molecular-weight dextran and possibly diuretics may also bring about a relief of intracranial pressure and thus an improvement in hearing, too.

Other *intracranial tumors, foci of softening* or *hemorrhages* may possibly cause acute deterioration of hearing already before the clinical picture has become so severe and so obvious that the diagnosis is self-explanatory (Fig. 34). In the same way acute hearing deteriorations as the initial symptom of an intracranial aneurysmal hemorrhage (Arnold and Vosteen 1977, Colclasure and Graham 1981), of a basilar thrombosis (Kley and Werner 1980) or of an embolic basilar insufficiency (Meyer zum Gottesberge and Stupp 1972), may appear to be "sud-

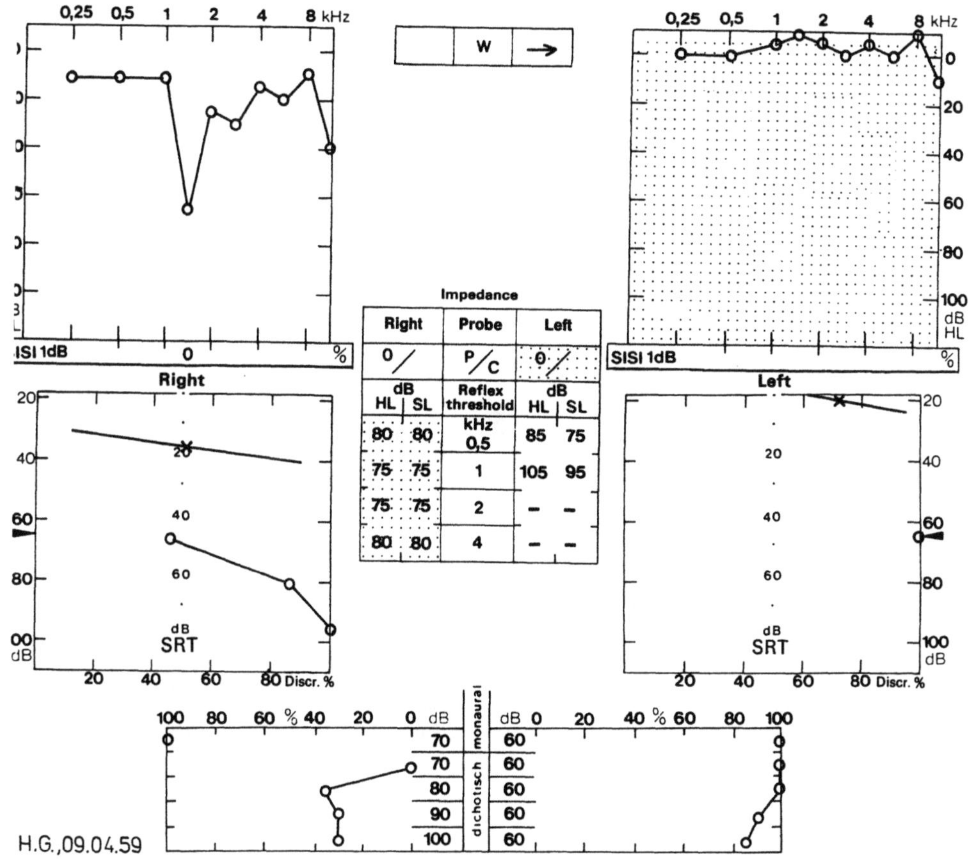

Fig. 33. Steep middle tone dip (Right), treated elsewhere as sudden hearing loss. SISI 0%. Stapedius reflex threshold raised on the right; dichotic speech discrimination definitely restricted on the right. Deafness in multiple sclerosis. Follow-up two years later showed normal findings bilaterally in every respect. BC = AC

den hearing losses" but – as the authors emphasize – should not be interpreted or even treated as such.

Acute – probably inflammatory – deteriorations of hearing in the course of *syphilis* may likewise be misinterpreted as sudden hearing losses. The congenital luetic infections of the inner ear often show an intermittent course and may then appear as "recurrent sudden hearing losses." Their true etiology may possibly only be clarified with the help of the new, extremely sensitive, serological tests: FTA-Abs and TPHA. Syphilitic deafness is uni- or bilateral, and the tone threshold shows an irregular pattern. Its pathological basis is a labyrinthitis and for that reason it exhibits the picture of a sensory disturbance of hearing. The mere possibility of an erroneous classification as a vascular sudden hearing loss makes it necessary to exclude syphilis in every case of acute deterioration of hearing, possibly even by CSF examination.

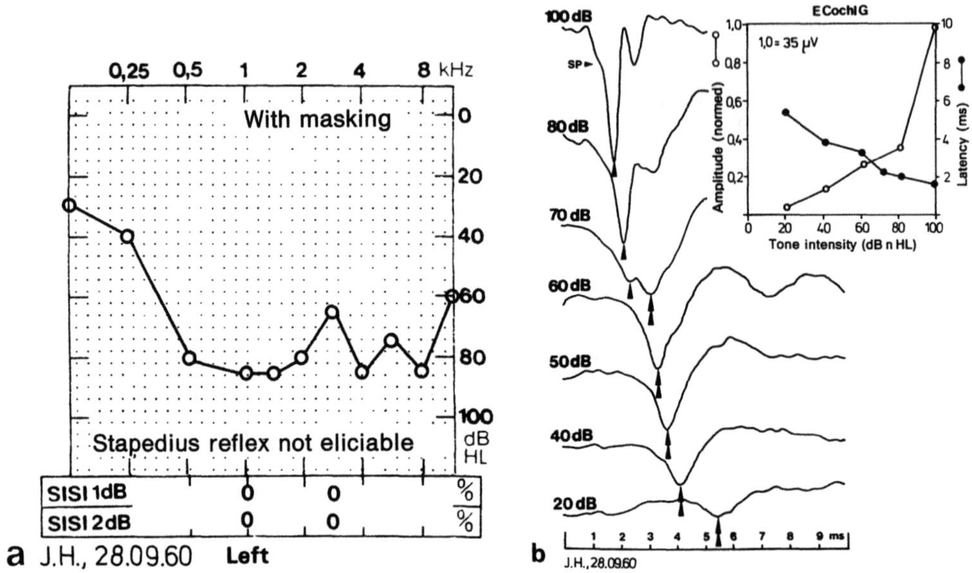

Fig. 34a, b. *Apparent* sudden deafness, actually loss of hearing caused by a brain stem spongioblastoma (piloid astrocytoma). **a** Hearing threshold around 80 dB, SISI 0%, even for 2 dB increments. Stapedius reflex not elicitable. **b** ECochG with input-output function for latency and amplitude. Summation action potential up to 20 dB (HL) detectable (▲ = N_1, ⯭ = N_2), SP = summation potential. The hearing loss therefore could not have originated in the inner ear or in the spiral ganglion (Stimulation rate 29/s, frequency 4000 Hz, Ref. 100 dB = 24 nV; 80–20 dB = 12 nV). P_6J_v not identifiable. BC = AC

A significance not to be underestimated for the correct use of the term "sudden hearing loss" is to be attributed to the recognition of *psychogenic hearing disturbances*. These also "arise" suddenly, without any obvious cause, *mostly bilateral and symmetrical*. If they are unilateral (Hülse 1981) some element of aggravation should be considered. Psychogenic hearing disturbances are more often met with than is generally assumed provided that this possibility has been considered at all, and the audiometric testing is carried out accordingly. In the case of such a suspicion one is surprised by the discrepancy between good discrimination of conversation and the mostly far worse tone threshold. In addition, the speech audiogram will appear relatively too favorable. The stapedius reflex can be elicited without difficulty (even if the hearing threshold was shown to be very poor), and the other supplementary tests may show varying results. The Békésy test with a constant frequency recording very often shows the specific finding of the congruent decrease of the continuous tone and the *pulsed tone threshold* (Lehnhardt 1974). Anyhow, without the above mentioned tests the psychogenesis of an acute hearing loss cannot be excluded (Fig. 35).

Although the psychogenic (or the aggravated) hearing disturbance may not always occur bilaterally, the organic vascular sudden hearing loss is indeed regularly confined to only one ear. The *one-sidedness of the acute deterioration of hearing should therefore be considered as a further criterion of sudden hearing loss* – above all for the distinction from non-organic bilateral hearing disturbances. If

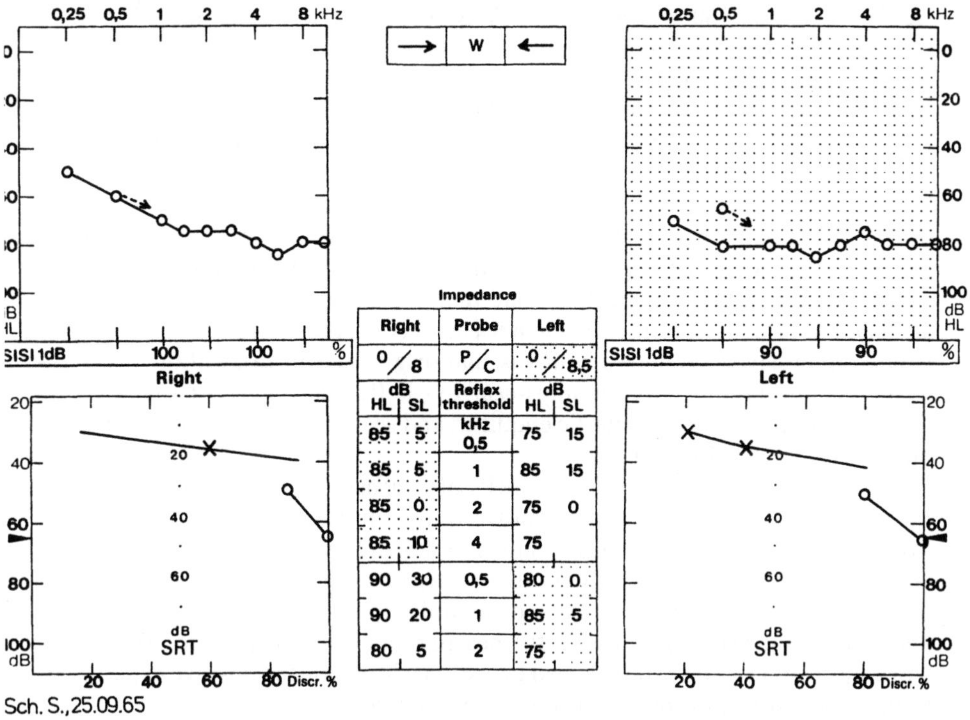

Fig. 35. Non-organic hearing disturbance. Results of speech audiometry much too good as compared with the tone threshold. Even the dichotic speech discrimination was completely preserved. SISI bilaterally = 100%. Stapedius reflex threshold normal. No signs of aggravation. Probably psychogenic disturbance of hearing. ERA: P_6/J_v, *right* from 10 dB, *left* from 0 dB detectable

the psychogenic hearing disturbances are not recognised as such and not distinguished from the organic vascular hearing disturbances the prognosis appears to be remarkably good e.g. 70% *complete* remission (Kleinfeldt 1968). Bilateral acute deteriorations of hearing are mostly described in the literature as hearing loss with an almost horizontal hearing threshold (Lehnhardt 1958, Barr 1960, Berger 1965, Weber 1970). This already suggests that they do not reflect the pattern of a peripheral vascular disturbance in which case one can scarcely expect symmetrical findings. Incidentally, one should always consider that with psychogenic hearing disturbances, the patients are not actually deaf, but only feel as though they were deaf. Hence, the "remission" is not dependent on any medical treatment, but merely on the psychological skills of the doctor, – possibly also on the medicinal framing of this treatment.

Sudden deafness *in children* appears to be a contradiction in itself if it is to be understood as a microvascular dysfunction. Are such vascular reactions conceivable in the juvenile ear, too? At all events, they certainly do not represent a separate clinical entity (Berg and Pallasch 1981). Accordingly, the former communications in the literature appear less convincing, for example if during a class exercise a unilateral hearing loss occurred which disappeared within a few days (Kessler 1968) and if such hearing disturbances showed an almost identical *bilat-*

eral hearing loss of 60–80 dB (Barr 1960, Berger 1965). Since an objective assessment has become possible by means of the ERA and – within limits – by means of the stapedius reflex threshold the number of cases in children described as "sudden hearing loss" should have drastically decreased. However, a critical preliminary assessment can be made already by means of a thorough anamnesis. In each of 19 children who had at first been classified under the diagnosis "sudden hearing loss", Radü (1980) could thereby discover criteria, which permitted another explanation: Trauma, psychogenesis, pre-existing deafness due to hypothyroidism, sequelae to meningitis, perinatal hyperbilirubinemia, familial predisposition to deafness etc. The deafness had therefore by no means always occurred acutely, but often it had only been *noticed* acutely. In the few remaining cases one would rather have to assume a *viral*-vascular origin (vide infra), without necessarily always interpreting it as a mumps-*neuritis* (de Reynier 1964). At any rate, one should make intensive anamnestic enquiries and search very thoroughly for other possible causes (cf. Fig. 32).

Furthermore, the intermittent attacks of deafness in *immuneallergic vasculitides* – e.g. in Cogan's syndrome – may give the impression of a sudden hearing loss and then also on both sides as shown in Fig. 52. As long as the basic disease is not recognised in the individual case, it may be difficult to understand the etiology of the deafness. However, as soon as additional symptoms become obvious, above all in the eyes, the cause of the hearing loss is also explained. To witness a prompt response to corticoids and cytostatics is one of the positive experiences in the diagnostics and treatment of inner ear deafness.

In the other vascular diseases such as *periarteritis nodosa*, in *Wegener's disease* or *panchondritis*, hearing loss may also develop acutely (cf. Chap. 3.10) – on one or both sides; it then possibly involves the middle ear at the same time and accordingly exhibits the picture of a combined deafness (Weidauer and Tenner 1973, Jenkins et al. 1981).

Also the occasionally abrupt loss of hearing seen in periarteritis nodosa (Weidauer and Tenner 1973, Jenkins et al. 1981) or in *Behçet's disease* (Brama and Fainaru 1980) would have to be classified as a *symptomatic* deterioration of hearing, but not as idiopathic "sudden hearing loss" (cf. Chap. 3.10). The same applies to inner ear involvement in *Boeck's disease*, an equally rare combination. We are grateful to Feldmann (1981) for a varied survey of such cases as well as for the first report on a sudden hearing impairment in *phosphate diabetes*, an x-chromosomal hereditary disease leading to a loss of phosphate on account of a renal tubular failure, without deafness being necessarily a part of the clinical picture. As for the present, it remains unexplained whether the – obviously gradual – deterioration of hearing in this individual case was the direct expression of a phosphate deficit in the inner ear, or in which way it developed.

Sudden deafness in acute heroin intoxication represents a rarity (Mulch and Handrock 1979). Since the hearing loss was symmetrical (middle and high tone deafness), it must certainly not be classified as a vascular "sudden hearing loss", particularly as the patient showed general signs of poisoning and was unable to undergo further audiometric testing.

Among the cases of *acute virogenic deafness* there are three forms to be distinguished clinically, namely

- the acute total deafness e.g. in mumps
- the probably ganglionic deafness e.g. in herpes zoster oticus
- the virogenic vascular inner ear damage.

The first two forms mentioned must be distinguished from "sudden hearing loss", whereas the third one is probably identical with the *clinical* picture of "sudden hearing loss" in part of the cases.

Infection with mumps – if it involves the ear – leads nearly always to total deafness and is irreversible; it may be recognised as a viral infection by the case history, complement fixation reaction and anti-hemagglutination test with a fourfold rise in the titer. It affects almost exclusively children, always purely unilateral, unless a mumps meningitis develops and leads to bilateral deafness.

From the clinical view, the picture is described as a virogenic cochlear *neuritis* (Gestaltner 1961, de Reynier 1964, Lehnhardt 1962). However, the histological findings, in the sense of a condition following a viral *labyrinthitis* (Lindsay et al. 1971, Strauss and Davis 1973, Schuknecht et al. 1973, Sando et al. 1977), are not consistent with this definition provided that everyone refers to the same disease.

As regards acute viral deafness Wilmes (1983) discussed the following possibilities:
- a specific immune response of the cells to the effect of an anaphylactic or cytotoxic reaction, or
- a direct viral invasion with the breakdown of protein and DNA-synthesis within a few hours.

The decision as to whether these processes involve the auditory nerve or the inner ear, has been left open by Wilmes.

The second group of acute viral hearing impairments is represented by those caused by herpes zoster oticus. It is often recognised as such by the accompanying symptoms (vertigo, vesicles, facial paresis), but may probably also develop in an isolated – and indeed acute – form. In personal observations it appeared nearly always as a high tone loss, at any rate, never as total deafness; it is unilateral and may regress but hardly ever return to normal. Djupesland et al. (1979), however, saw a normalisation of the hearing function within one year in ten of twelve patients "with objective symptoms of viral infection." Thorough investigation is said to often reveal the involvement of other cranial nerves, too. The authors interpret this picture of *acute reversible hearing loss* as a component of viral meningo-encephalitis, without attributing it specifically to herpes zoster oticus.

A *bilateral acute* hearing disturbance caused by a viral infection is certainly a rarity; as observed by Feldmann (1981) it affected the *low* frequencies symmetrically and had occurred in the course of a rubella infection. However, rubella are also reported to be a possible cause of an acute *unilateral* inner ear deafness with a flat tone threshold (Joachims and Eliachar 1982).

The third group of *viral infections* finally leads directly over to the *vascular* origin of the "sudden hearing loss", insofar as here we are suspecting a virogenic inflammatory vasculopathy with perivascular edema and endothelial proliferation, and therefore also a circulatory disturbance in the inner ear. This secondary vascular etiology of deafness in the course of a virus infection corresponds to the above quoted definition of *"sudden hearing loss"*.

Mitschke (1978) identified a *cytomegalovirus* infection in four cases of sudden unilateral deterioration of hearing and suspects inflammatory cellular proliferation in the vascular endothelium, and hence the picture of a virogenic vascular "sudden hearing loss". The prognosis in these four patients was good, possibly on account of the slight neuropathic activity of the cytomegalovirus (cf. Chap. 3.5.2).

Jaffe (1978) believes that about one third of the cases of "sudden hearing loss" might be of viral origin, on account of the frequently preceding or associated infection of the upper respiratory ways. Rowson et al. (1975), too, observed such infections in one quarter (n = 39) of their patients with sudden hearing loss, Shaia and Sheehy (1976) only in 8% (n = 1220) and Byl (1974,

1977) in 20% (n=32). Apart from influenza, the most frequent viruses were said to be mumps and measles, adeno-virus and mucoplasma pneumoniae (Jaffe 1970, 1978) as well as the Epstein-Barr virus (Gregg and Shaeffer 1964). The *serological* identification of a viral genesis, however, was only occasionally successful and frequently not at all (Wilmes et al. 1979, Fritz et al. 1980, Mercke et al. 1980, Hamann 1981). Anyhow, "raised antibody titres" alone, do not justify the assumption that the sudden hearing loss is of viral origin. Examinations carried out months after the event are of little value unless they are done for the purpose of exclusion. For additional information on the various viral infections see the relevant chapter (3.3.1) as well as the report by Wilmes and Deinhardt (1983).

A *further transitional form of idiopathic vascular sudden hearing loss* is represented by the acute hearing losses which are likewise vascular in origin but which are additionally based on a predisposing disease, for example thrombo-angitis obliterans (Kirikae et al. 1962), leukemia (Schuknecht et al. 1965, Sando and Egami 1977), non-Hodgkin lymphoma (Mahajan 1981), Waldenström's macroglobulinemia (Ronis et al. 1966, Ruben et al. 1969, Feldmann 1981, Misawa 1981), cryoglobulinemia (Barr et al. 1950, Hutchinson et al. 1953, Nomura et al. 1982), polycythemia rubra vera (Jaffe 1967), fat embolism (Jaffe 1970), hepatosplenomegaly with secondary porphyria, an immune vasculitis (Cogan) or a diabetes mellitus (Jaffe 1970, Korvar 1973, Feldmann 1981). In the end they include all the factors which may be equally responsible for *chronic* degenerative inner ear deafness. Anyway, in this respect there are probably no basic differences between the acute and chronic types of the disorder.

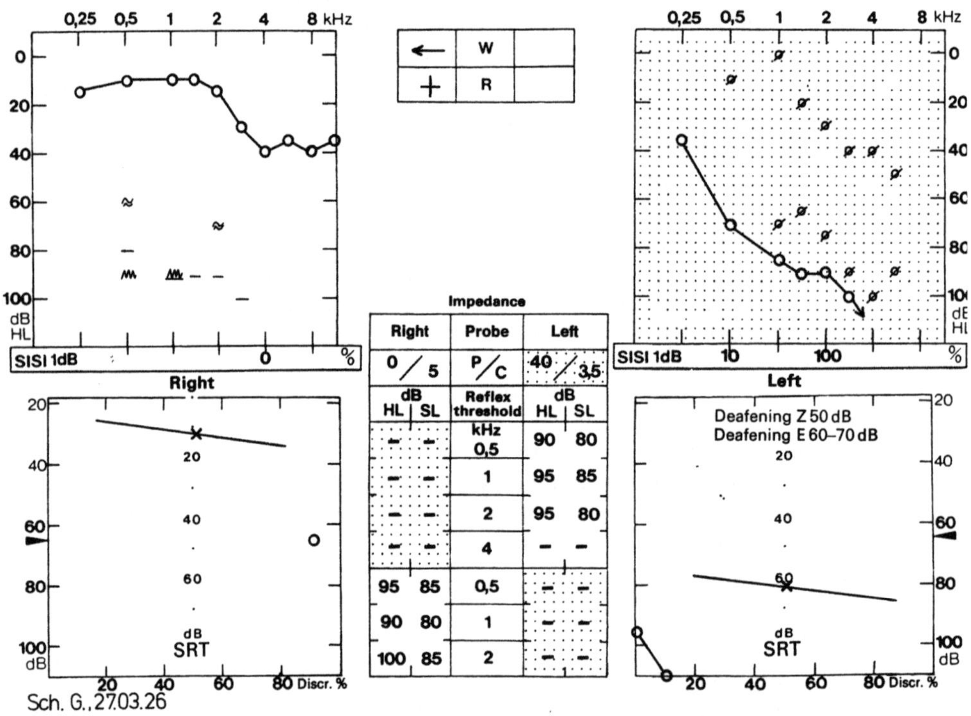

Fig. 36. Acute unilateral deafness immediately following an aortic/coronary bypass operation. No ototoxic treatment. No renal failure, Embolism? BC=AC. For symbols of masking see Fig. 32; masking of SISI = ≈

On the other hand, those hearing defects which occur after coronary by-pass operations and which may be interpreted as of embolic origin are exclusively acute in onset. This applies, however, only to *unilateral* cases, while the bilateral ones must be considered as a sequel to hypoxic states or ototoxic side-effects (Fig. 36). Their incidence is to be estimated at 1‰ whereas the frequency of embolic *cerebral* lesions in the course of cardiopulmonary bypass operations is much higher, namely about 31–53% (Plasse et al. 1980).

Non-excessive exposure to blast or noise immediately preceding some sudden hearing losses should be understood as probably only a *precipitating* factor. This assumption is mainly based on the experience that such apparently acoustically determined hearing disturbances recurr later but then possibly without the external "trigger." The same applies to the sudden deterioration of hearing from merely diving into a swimming pool or during sunbathing (Feldmann 1981). Are they etiologically involved in the occurrence of – unilateral – sudden hearing losses, or are they even their true cause? Could a round window membrane rupture caused by a trivial incident be involved with it? Occasionally such cases will have to be classified as vascular "sudden hearing loss" – and treated accordingly.

The hearing disturbances suddenly occurring during noise exposure originally described by Boenninghaus (1959) and Shapiro (1959) and later referred to as an "acoustic accident" by Becker and Matzker (1961) mostly affect one ear, the audiogram shows a flat curve, and there are no vestibular symptoms. The accused acoustic "trauma" is either the final stage of a chain of injury (Lehnhardt 1965) or the deterioration of hearing has merely occurred fortuitously during a particular situation at work (under the influence of noise; Maurer and Mehmke 1962) but without any causal connection.

3.6.1.2 Idiopathic "Sudden Hearing Loss"

After this detailed differential diagnostic delimitation there remains a substantially dwindled group of *acute, unilateral, sensory, idiopathic* disturbances of hearing for which only two causes can seriously be discussed, namely the viral and the vascular genesis. The *viral* is predominantly favored in the Anglo-Saxon literature (Beal et al. 1967, Schuknecht et al. 1973, Sando et al. 1977). If the virus infection of the inner ear is regarded in the above-mentioned sense as a virogenic vasculopathy with perivascular edema and endothelial proliferation, then the difference between viral and vascular origin decreases quite significantly; the sequel to the pathological processes would also in this case be a circulatory disturbance of the inner ear with the resulting degenerative changes.

Up to now only very few pathological-anatomical findings from the human temporal bone have been presented in favor of the *vascular origin* of sudden deafness (Gussen 1976). Animal experimental studies with the aim of obtaining evidence of the patho-physiological processes within the cochlea during the hearing loss (Handrock 1978), have not contributed any important additional insight, either. However, there seem to be sufficient *clinical* signs supporting the vascular genesis:

- the suddenness of the hearing loss
- the relatively favorable prognosis in respect of spontaneous remission
- the relatively good response to measures stimulating the blood flow
- the tendency to relapse
- the release by psychic stress or hypothermia and
- the frequently identified risk factors in the blood and the blood vessels.

The *nature of the vascular disturbances* in the inner ear during a sudden hearing loss may finally only be guessed at. They are unlikely to differ basically from those which produce a *chronically* inadequate supply of the inner ear (see Chap. 3.6.2).

The attempt to infer, from micro-angiopathic findings in the conjunctiva (Lehnhardt 1958) or in the skin (Oudot and Martin 1979), that there are corresponding changes in the inner ear during the sudden hearing loss, has in the end failed: on the one hand, disturbances of capillary control (Müller 1937) are also found with normal functioning of the inner ear and, on the other hand, they may be absent in patients with sudden hearing loss.

Only exceptionally will there be an organic vascular occlusion or narrowing in the auditory artery, that is thromboses, emboli or sclerotic changes in the vessel walls. A more probable cause are functional ischemias which on their part set off a relaxation of the venous tone and hence a stasis in the capillaries, as well as a subsequent transudation. The extravasation of serum from the capillaries of the stria vascularis probably leads to endolymphatic hydrops as the generally suspected patho-physiological correlate of the sudden hearing loss (Zechner 1980, 1981).

The question as to which factors are considered to *trigger* off the false vasomotor reaction, has not yet been clarified. Most consideration is given to psychological and emotional stress, toxic foci, and allergic influences, as well as basilar impression (Elies 1980) or structural disturbances of the cervical spine about the importance of which, however, there are differing opinions (Terrahe 1979, Elies and Plester 1980, Fritz et al. 1980). The stress factor seems to be too vague to bother further about its definition.

The hearing loss develops within seconds, minutes or hours; many patients are unable to give exact answers to corresponding questions if only because they became aware of the hearing loss when waking up in the morning. It is precisely the observation that hearing losses frequently occur in the early morning hours, i.e. at a time of relative hypotension, which also seems to be an unmistakable hint as to its vascular origin.

If, on the other hand, the loss of hearing develops within hours or days to a variable (fluctuating) or episodically increasing (intermittent) extent, the patient

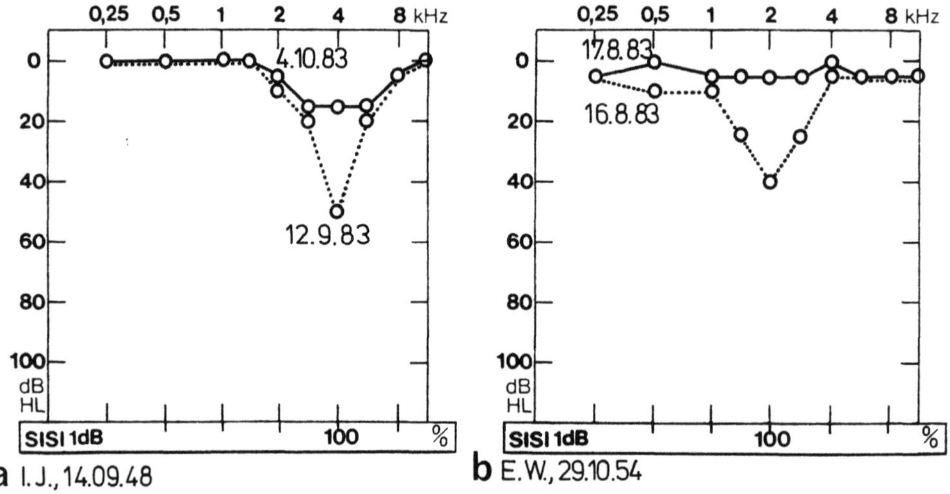

Fig. 37. a *High tone dip* appearing as "sudden hearing loss" (12.9.83) in a dentist who felt deafened by the noise of his turbine drill. Spontaneous recovery. **b** Fleeting *middle tone dip*, in the course of a sudden hearing loss. BC = AC

may then indeed describe this progress of events, however, without us being in a position to draw any conclusions from it, either diagnostic, prognostic or therapeutic ones. Even the frequently alleged feeling of pressure is only a supporting diagnostic piece of evidence.

In addition, the risk factors regarding blood chemistry, blood cells and the vascular wall which are met with almost regularly in the systematic examination of patients with sudden deafness (Wilke et al. 1977, Luetje 1979, Quarante et al. 1980, Khasanov et al. 1982, Friedrich and Wolf 1984), are virtually the same as in chronic inner ear degenerations (see Chap. 3.6.2), an observation which may again be alleged as evidence of the vascular origin of the sudden hearing loss. As a typical example may be mentioned the elevation of five different lipid fractions in 82.5% (n = 42) of the patients with sudden hearing loss (Pruszewicz et al. 1983). Among the vascular risks of sudden hearing loss H. A. Kley (1979) also counts the ovulation inhibitors among which a vasoconstrictor effect is ascribed to progesterone. They are certainly not the only cause of arterial thrombosis and embolism, but are associated with individual susceptibility, nicotine, obesity, diabetes and others (Bausch 1983).

Men are more frequently affected than women and the age distribution corresponds to a broad maximum between the fourth and the sixth decade (Kemper 1977, Wandhöfer 1971). The general incidence is said to be 10–20 cases per 100000 people per year (Byl 1977, Weinaug 1984).

In many aspects, such as diagnostic classification, treatment and prognosis, the initial situation is significant; had the patient's hearing previously been completely sound or had there already been some impairment in the ear now affected or in the opposite ear, or in both to the same or a differing extent? The clarification of these questions often requires very detailed anamnestic questioning or investigations.

In sudden hearing loss no uniform *pattern* of the threshold curve is recognised. Frequently the low frequency range is predominantly affected, otherwise a middle tone dip may occur in the same way as a high tone loss or a pantonal deafness (Fig. 37). Pre-existing hearing impairments may produce threshold curves which only after having been divided into their etiologically different components – possibly also in comparison with the opposite ear – explain the present condition. We have not seen total deafness as the sequel to a sudden hearing loss regarded as vascular. Residual hearing was always detectable, even if only slight in degree (Fig. 38). The suprathreshold audiometric tests regularly indicate a recruitment – indeed, the sudden hearing loss is regarded as the "complete picture" of loudness recruitment with all its equivalents. The Békésy test often reveals a clear reduction of amplitude for the continous tone curve, without this finding being claimed as pathognomonic and indispensible for the diagnosis.

At least the speech audiogram and the stapedius reflex threshold are indispensible, less for the diagnosis than for the differential diagnosis.

However, to deduce the prognosis of sudden hearing loss from the stapedius reflex threshold alone (Gerwin and la Coste 1982), would mean too wide an interpretation of the term "sudden hearing loss"; actually the authors include in this picture not only cochlear, but also retrocochlear and central neural hearing disturbances – indeed everything that may be understood by the term "sensori-*neural*". Such statements are bound to lead to faulty interpretations.

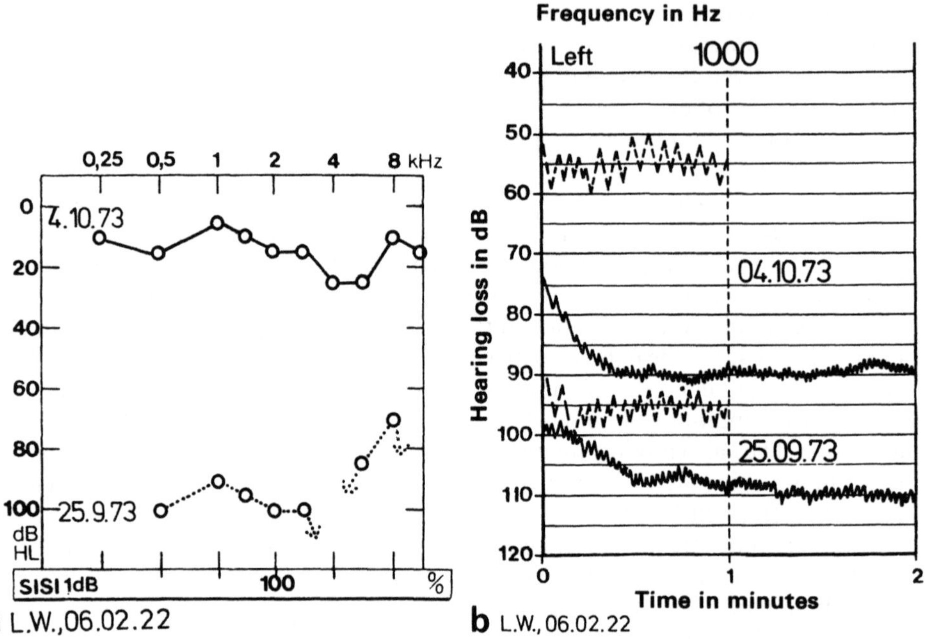

Fig. 38. a *Approaching* total deafness – but with definite residual hearing – developed as a sudden hearing loss (25.9.73). Complete recovery by 4.10.73. BC=AC. **b** In the Békésy audiogram extremely small amplitude with separation of 15 dB on 25.9.73, and actually of 35 dB during recovery (4.10.73)

Only as long as the SP is increased and therefore an endolymphatic hydrops is to be assumed (Eggermont 1976), a restitution of the auditory function is said to be possible. If, however, the SP is no longer present and if hearing has remained poor, it is to be feared that in the meantime the sensory cells have irreversibly degenerated (Nishida 1977, and many others). Less "invasive" – in the presence of a sudden hearing loss! – would be the recording of the brain stem potentials among which the Vth wave is of topodiagnostic significance even at low intensities (<60–80 dB nHL; Lehnhardt 1979), provided that the high tone hearing loss does not exceed the above-mentioned intensity of stimulus. The ERA, however, can only indicate the location in the inner ear, but not the findings specific for the hydrops. Only Yamada et al. (1979) had argued that the extraordinary steepness of the latency curve *immediately above the response threshold* could be interpreted as the criterion of hydrops.

To discuss the question of the *prognosis*, means at the same time to raise that of spontaneous remission. There is no doubt about the fact that sudden hearing loss may regress even without any treatment. The larger the proportion of spontaneous remission, the more difficult becomes the distinction between *post and propter*. Apart from this, there are patients, in whom an improvement or complete recovery from deafness already appears *before* the start of any treatment. Statements about the prognosis of sudden hearing loss therefore cannot be separated from those concerning spontaneous remissions.

The proportion of complete remissions without any treatment is stated to be approximately two-thirds (Mattox and Simmons 1977), that of spontaneous improvement even 89%. For patients under 50 years of age partial or complete remission is to be expected in 96% or 89% of the cases, respectively (Weinaug 1982, 1984). The figures are certainly influenced by the composition of the case material i.e. they will be more favorable in patients treated for the first time, than in previously treated patients referred to large hospitals (cf. Shaia and Sheehy 1976).

The chance of spontaneous remission is less favorable in old age, whereas it is scarcely influenced by the extent of the hearing loss (Mattox and Simmons 1977, Wilson et al. 1980, Koehn and Nickol 1983). For previously damaged ears, the prognosis of a (further) acute deterioration of hearing is generally less favorable, particularly if there is accompanying vertigo (Ristow et al. 1978, Russolo and Poli 1980). For the totally deaf – as far as "sudden hearing loss" may at all be assumed – there is scarcely any chance of recovery – independent of all therapeutic measures (Lehnhardt 1976, Russolo and Poli 1980, Wilson et al. 1980, Friedrich and Wolf 1983, Morgenstern et al. 1983, Eichhorn and Martin 1984).

Middle tone dips or troughs are supposed to have the best prognosis (Wilson et al. 1980), low tone losses a relatively good one, high tone losses and flat curves the worst prognosis (Russolo and Poli 1980). However, improvements in the low frequency range often remain unstable (Eichhorn and Martin 1984), although the low tone losses, in particular, sometimes already appear to be regressing within the first few days. As regards the prognosis, Mattox and Simmons (1977) do not believe they have seen any dependency on accompanying infections, high blood pressure, diabetes mellitus and other systemic illnesses.

If psychogenic (mostly bilateral) and aggravated (mostly unilateral) hearing disturbances are included, because they were not recognized as such, the statistics turn out to be more favorable and include more patients who, after weeks or months, show a "surprising recovery."

On the other hand, a case material with a larger proportion of unilateral *total* deafness or vestibular involvement is likely to show a smaller number of spontaneous (or therapeutic) improvements, precisely because their prognosis is altogether definitely worse (Morgenstern et al. 1983, Friedrich and Wolf 1984). Also the gradual deterioration of hearing in the second ear seems to be prognostically less favorable (Lehnhardt 1958), even though Kumpf and Wandhöfer (1972) thought they were unable to confirm this observation.

The higher the rate of spontaneous remission is, the more difficult is it to assess the value of therapeutic measures. However, if therapeutic measures are at all considered to be successful, this applies mainly to those treatments designed to improve the circulatory conditions in the inner ear: Control of blood pressure and energy metabolism, elimination of possible vasospastic factors and improvement in the flow characteristics of the blood (Kellerhals 1977, Theisen et al. 1980, Zadory et al. 1982) – always related to the *vascular* "sudden hearing loss". As long as the endolymphatic hydrops is regarded as its pathophysiological and anatomical correlate, therapeutic efforts are indicated and indeed indispensable from the medical point of view because the sensory cells are or may be still capable of regeneration. Unfortunately we are not yet in a position to distinguish between sensory cells which show a transitory dysfunction and those which are irreversibly degenerated. The respective possibilities which may be created by the ECochG, have already been mentioned.

A comprehensive discussion of the numerous therapeutic recommendations does not appear reasonable; they range from refusal of any medication (Weinaug 1982) or merely neurovegetative sedation (Sterkers and Renau 1979), through medication with Urografin (Morimitsu et al. 1975, Hirashima 1978, Emmett and Shea 1979, Strohm 1980, Villar et al. 1981, Fiedler 1984), to treatment with fibrinolytics (Donaldson 1979, Altmann et al. 1980, Klemm and Altmann 1983), improvement of fluidility (Luetge 1979, Hörmann et al. 1980), inhibition of platelet aggregation (Zajtchuk et al. 1979, Oudot and Martin 1980, Bosatra et al. 1983), or a thrombolytic therapy (Russolo and Poli 1980). To some extent the intended effects are clearly overlapping. More invasive are the efforts of treatment by intra-arterial ATP infusions (Mörl et al. 1971), by hyperbaric oxygen inhalations (Jakobi et al. 1975, Kühl et al. 1979) or even by ligature of the external carotid artery (Moser and Winkler 1971) just to name a few, picked out at random. For many medications such as Dextran 40, procaine, naftidrofuryl, pyridymethanol, nicotine acid and for stellate ganglion blocks (Strauss and Kunkel 1977) or histamine infusions (Sheehy et al. 1980) no differences were found; on first approximation all these results might be attributed to a spontaneous improvement in hearing. The supposed favorable effect of an early treatment would be conditioned by the selection of spontaneous remissions (Feldmann 1981).

Thorough experiments have been performed with ATP infusions to support this treatment. Since it is an established fact that ATP is broken down relatively slowly (Thalmann, quoted by Jakobi et al. 1979) it is to be expected that the ATP will actually reach the inner ear. In animal experiments it leads directly to an increase in amplitude of the CM which had previously dropped on account of a deficient oxygen inhalation (Jakobi et al. 1979).

As regards experiments with systemic hemodilution or with calcium antagonists (Allen et al. 1983) comprehensive statistics are not yet available. A report on 12 patients mentions a cure rate of 75% (nine patients). The improvements had always occurred immediately after the treatment.

As regards the volume of blood to be withdrawn, the authors (Dauman et al. 1983) recommend 0.5–1.3 liters. At the same time Dextran 60 is infused which had already been shown by Kellerhals (1972) to improve microcirculation in the terminal cochlear vascular system. The hematocrit values are then supposed to amount to 30–35%. Intensive supervision is necessary, though only for one day. In patients with injured coronaries hemodilution is said to be contraindicated.

A remarkable rate of improvement may be expected from short term fibrinolysis with streptokinase, namely in 92% a hearing gain of almost 40 dB (n=28; Klemm and Altmann 1983, Klemm et al. 1983). The average age of these patients, however, was 40 and thus markedly below that of other reports (about 50 years; Mattox and Simmons 1977, Weinaug 1982 and many others).

These measures are expected to reduce the blood viscosity and increase the plasma viscosity and thereby permit a better deformability of the erythrocytes. The regional and particularly the cerebral oxygenation is increased, even in the ischemic areas. The PO_2 in the circulating blood is indeed reduced, but the transport is improved. In order to support the assumption that *high* blood viscosity may have a detrimental effect on the inner ear, the findings of Davis and Nilo (1964) and those of Hildesheimer et al. (1982) were cited, as well as those evidenced by the AP of Rubinstein et al. (1977).

The aim of achieving a better oxygenation of the inner ear also underlies the therapeutic experiments with hyperbaric oxygen (Appaix and Demard 1970,

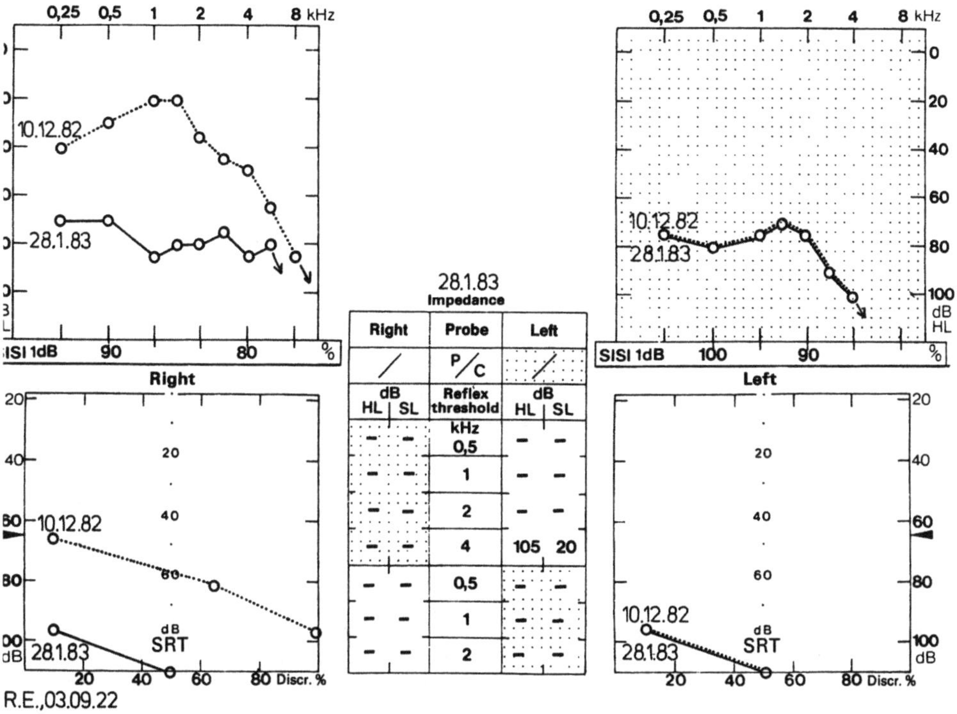

Fig. 39. Example of a hearing deterioration in the second (right) ear which could not be controlled. Twelve years earlier the left ear had become almost completely deaf within months. During the last five years several acute deteriorations of hearing on the right ear, the last one two weeks ago. In spite of comprehensive therapeutic measures, progressive deterioration of hearing *actually while under hospital treatment.* BC = AC

Lamm and Klimpel 1971, Gorlina et al. 1980, Lamm 1980). The results of this treatment are equally differing probably, above all because it is used almost exclusively as a last resort and thus relatively late – a disadvantage which blames all expensive measures.

A warning must be given of uncritical long-term medication with cortico-steroids (Hesch 1982). However, there is hardly any objection to a strictly limited course of treatment, particularly not in the case of gradual deafness of the second ear. Here it might be indicated on the assumption of an auto-immune reaction against the already destroyed inner ear on the side which first became deaf (Lehnhardt 1958, Beickert 1961).

The same applies to the patients who after an acute hearing loss do not show an improvement but a further deterioration of hearing – in spite of manifold diagnostic and therapeutic measures (Fig. 39). However, appropriate caution is of course indicated in these cases, too, as regards premature treatment with corticoids (Mattox 1980) at least as long as inflammatory processes (viral labyrinthitis) or conditions which threaten to cause infections (round window membrane rupture) have not been ruled out (Kanzaki and O-Uchi 1983). Indeed Wilson et al. (1980) by treatment with dexamethasone or methylprednisolone achieved a cure rate twice that in the untreated or in the placebo group, but with 61% it was no higher than the expected spontaneous remission rate. Besides, the report was little convincing in so far as the authors regard the sudden hearing loss as a viral disorder.

As regards nicergolin (Sermion) which like phentolamine (Rogitine) is said to increase the cerebral circulation by means of an alpha-adrenergic receptor blockage (Moretti et al. 1979, Villar et al. 1981), Morgenstern et al. (1982) have tried to demonstrate a completely different mode of action, namely a rise of CO_2 in the inner ear as a *result of the accompanying respiratory depression*. Under the influence of nicergolin a drop in the endocochlear DC potential was detectable which, on the other hand, did not appear when oxygen was administered. In the presentation of this case, however, the authors proceed from the assumption that the functional reaction of the inner ear vessels is the same as that of the cerebral vessels.

According to the experiments of Hultcrantz et al. (1980) it may be regarded as established that administration of CO_2 has a beneficial effect on inner ear function (Snow and Suga 1973); the rate of exchange of the perilymph which is used as a criterion for the cochlear circulation and the metabolic activity of the organ of Corti is definitely raised with CO_2 inhalation, as was shown by the findings of Schnieder (1973). This probably also explains the observation that after previous inhalation of CO_2 and O_2 the noise-induced TTS is less severe (Witter et al. 1980). Frühwald et al. (1979) therefore argue that, at present, the inhalation of $CO_2:O_2$ (10:90) is the only justifiable treatment of vascular sudden hearing loss. Under this treatment the authors found in animal experiments a distinct rise of O_2 in the cochlea, just as with hyperbaric oxygen administration (2 bar absolute). Others had recommended a mixture of 5% CO_2 and 95% O_2 (Shea and Kitabachi 1973, Baghat and Shenoi 1982). For the time being it is still an open question whether the reactions described also apply to the damaged inner ear (Hultcrantz et al. 1980).

The indication for a *stellate ganglion block* in the treatment of sudden hearing loss is still under dispute (Mattox 1980) – independent of the fear of possible accompanying injuries. Dietzel et al. (1971) argue that they have seen a temporary measurable increase in function after the block under experimental as well as under clinical conditions. They intentionally leave the question open as to whether this effect is produced by an increase in oxygen supply. At any rate, the metabolic transfer of oxygen from the vascular system to the respiratory chain is said to be accelerated. Electro-physiological recordings after sympathectomy leave no doubt, either, about the influence of the cervical sympathetic nerve on the inner ear potentials; the mode of action, however, remains unclear (Hultcrantz 1979, Hultcrantz et al. 1979, 1982).

In order to assess the value of this treatment Eichhorn and Martin (1984) gave particular consideration to the *late results*. Among those initially unsuccessfully treated, some eventually still showed a recovery – sometimes after months – (Bailey et al. 1982, Bertram and Luckhaupt 1983). 8.3% of all sudden hearing loss patients later suffered a relapse. In view of the *long-term* development (ca 6 years), the delayed start of treatment, the associated tinnitus and vertigo as well as the long-term medication with vasodilators had *no effect*. Within the period of observation the tone threshold of previous sudden hearing loss patients showed an average deterioration of 1.15 dB/year in the frequencies 0,5, 1, 2, and 3 kHz.

The problem of sudden hearing loss, even though of topical interest, could not be treated exhaustively, the corresponding literature not completely be reproduced. It was rather attempted to report on those discoveries which in recent years have contributed to defining the concept of sudden hearing loss again as accurately as had originally been intended. To the particularly interested reader we recommend the monograph by Neveling (1965) which is still well worth reading, the textbook article by Stange and Neveling (1980) as well as the surveys by Wandhöfer (1979), Feldmann (1981) and Weinaug (1982, 1984).

3.6.2 Chronic Inner Ear Deafness

As a rule, the causal relationship between a *circulatory or metabolic disorder* and inner ear deafness is not very striking. At least it can only rarely be verified without thorough general and blood-chemical examination. Nevertheless, the effort to establish a causal connection with general (internal) clinical pictures is tempting and has repeatedly been made. Yet, in only in a few cases the disorder of the inner ear seems to be interpretable as the direct result of a dysfunction of the thyroid, the kidneys or the circulation. Even Pendred's- or Alport's-hearing impairment do not permit the conclusion that an inner ear deafness may result from every hypofunction of the thyroid or every renal disorder.

However, disturbances of the inner ear will not arise completely independent of generalised circulatory or metabolic disorders. Thus, pathological changes in the vessel wall may also affect the inner ear, without this being an inevitable consequence. Metabolic disorders will rarely act directly on the inner ear, but more frequently do so indirectly via the vascular system. An individual component of various irregularities may remain subclinical. It is *only their multiplicity that becomes a risk for the inner ear.*

Many things which apply to the sudden hearing loss or to the symptomatic sudden deterioration of hearing, also have validity for the chronic degenerative inner ear disturbances. Thus, anyone who misses a particular clue there will probably find it here, or vice versa.

According to what has been said above, the group of inner ear disturbances due to circulatory or metabolic disorders may be subdivided into:

- inner ear dysfunctions directly resulting from disturbed metabolism
- vascular disturbances induced by metabolic disorders and
- direct vascular dysregulations.

For deductive reasons the metabolic disturbances are to be discussed first in order to then lead over to the obviously more important and diverse causes of chronic inner ear deafness, namely those which result from diseases of the vessel wall and of the circulatory regulation. The vascular disturbances due to metabolic disorders occupy an intermediate position.

3.6.2.1 Disturbances of Renal Function

Here the question arises, whether the disturbed renal function – not related to genetic syndromes and independent of the involvement of ototoxic or nephrotoxic substances – may by itself lead to an impairment of hearing. In order to answer this question those cases must be excluded in which the same *noxa* could have damaged not only the kidney but also the inner ear. Or, in other words: What is to be discussed here is the question whether the accumulation of substances usually eliminated with the urine or of metabolites may have a detrimental effect on the function of the inner ear.

This endeavour to find a strict definition already indicates how difficult it will be to find the answer. The statements in the literature vary accordingly. On the one hand, it is said that 33% of all persons suffering from renal disease (Mozzo et al. 1978, Sittoni et al. 1983) are hard of hearing, or 50% (Mitschke 1978, von Ilberg 1980), or even 87.3% (n=71: Yassin 1970). These figures mainly refer to patients with chronic uremia, on regular hemodialysis or to the state after renal transplant. On the other hand, Oda et al. (1974) found deafness only in 18% of the patients after renal transplantation (n=290). And in these, too, the cumulative damage caused by aminoglycoside antibiotics and loop diuretics could scarcely be excluded with absolute certainty. Anyhow, it is indeed convincing that an improvement in hearing was achieved though not during regular dialysis, but after a successful renal transplant, that is by a "complete elimination of those uremic toxins which are difficult to dialyse" (Ferekidis et al. 1980, Mitschke 1980). Nevertheless, the hearing loss and correspondingly also the hearing gain kept within narrow limits (Fig. 40). In the middle tone range the average hearing loss was 15–20 dB, and in the higher frequencies 20–30 dB (Wigand et al. 1972).

It was not possible to identify any correlation between the loss of hearing and the extent of the hyponatremia or other values of blood chemistry (Visencio and Gerber 1979, Ferekidis et al. 1980), although Yassin (1970) regarded the low serum sodium levels as the cause of the impaired hearing and described an improvement in hearing after the sodium levels had returned to normal. According to the pathogenetic possibilities discussed under renal tubular acidosis (see Chap. 3.4.2.3), such an etiological connection is not unlikely.

The average hearing loss "corrected for age", in 58 uremic patients amounted to less than 20 dB even at 8000 Hz, to 15 dB at 4000 Hz, 10 dB at 2000 Hz and 1000 Hz (Wigand and Heidland 1970). These figures suggest that an impairment of hearing should not regularly be expected in uremia patients, even with the inclusion of the standard deviations. As regards the genesis of such hearing losses

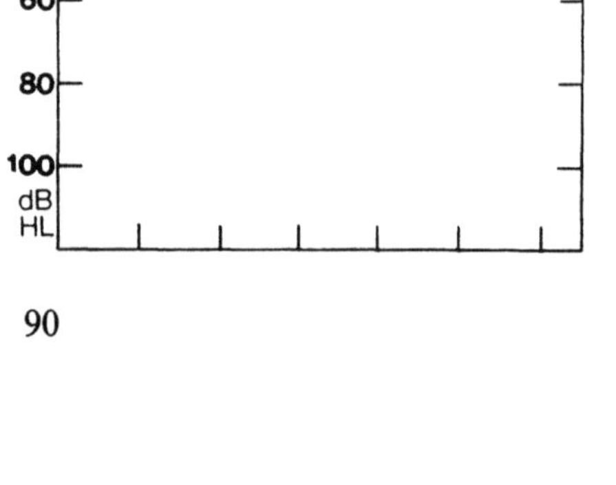

Fig. 40. Tone thresholds before and 19–58 months after renal transplantation (n=14 patients). Mean value and scatter of hearing loss for the individual frequencies are plotted. Altogether, a slight improvement after the transplantation. (From Mitschke 1978)

Wigand et al. (1972) suspect there are transport inhibitors in the blood of uremics e.g. methyl guanidine which at the same time affect the function of the inner ear. Uremic deafness therefore arises through inhibition of the cellular potassium pump; from that follows a rise of the Na^+-concentration in the endolymph and hence an impairment of the ionic balance.

Investigations on nephrectomised guinea pigs led to fundamentally the same results; they revealed an inhibition of the Na^+-K^+-stimulated transport ATPase in the cochlea, too, and thus likewise indicated a disturbance of the cochlear ionic gradient or of the strial function in general (Adler et al. 1980, Mozzo et al. 1978). The concretions seen in the stria vascularis of dialysed patients, however, do not correlate with the extent of the hearing loss; at best they might be regarded as a sign of impending damage to hearing (Bergstrom et al. 1980).

An explanation similar to that of Feldmann (1981) for the *acute* deterioration of hearing is discussed in respect of *fluctuating* deafness or *progressive* loss of hearing during and in spite of repeated peritoneal and hemo-dialysis (Bergstrom et al. 1973, Schmidt and Stange 1976). In one case the tone threshold had shown a flat course around 60 dB (SISI 100%), and twelve days later the patient was deaf on both ears. He had not taken any ototoxic medicines, apparently not even previously. The histological specimen showed a complete collapse of the endolymphatic space with crumpling of the tectorial membrane as well as edema of the stria vascularis and the Hensen cells (Rizvi and Holmes 1980). The authors interpret this finding as a sequel to fluid shifts resulting from osmolar changes. The rapid elimination of the urea is said to leave behind a hyposmolar serum. As a result an osmotic gradient develops as against e.g. the CSF and the brain. This leads to a penetration of fluid into the intercellular and interstitial spaces and thereby possibly to an encephalopathy, the "reverse urea syndrome". A similar mechanism might, on parallel lines, have taken place in the inner ear and led to the ear damage observed.

However, one may try to give a completely different explanation of sudden deteriorations of hearing during or immediately following dialysis, namely a hemorrhage into the labyrinth, particularly if at the same time the clinical picture is characterized by hemorrhages from the nose and into the conjunctiva (Schmidt and Stange 1976). The hemorrhages which for their part were supposed to have been induced by the continuous liquemine (Heparin) medication, would thus only be the indirect result of the kidney disease. In such cases treatment of the hearing loss with low molecular weight Dextran would be *contra-indicated,* since it reduces the viscosity of the blood and thereby might maintain the hemorrhage.

We are grateful to Kligerman et al. (1981) for their valuable contribution towards clearing up the question as to what extent kidney *diseases, without* renal *failure* are responsible for inner ear dysfunction. From this careful investigation the authors conclude that clinically relevant losses of hearing, apart from the hereditary syndromes, do not result from the mere kidney disease. Only renal failure *and* its medical treatment might lead to high tone deafness (54% $n=67$). *Hemodialysis by itself was reported to cause no deterioration of hearing.*

Arnold (1984) discusses the question whether the almost identical percentages of incidence of sensorineural hearing loss in patients with Alport's syndrome (45%) and those with severe renal disorders independent of inherited syndromes indicate a common pathological mechanism in renal diseases followed by inner ear disorders. The answer would require further immunological studies.

3.6.2.2 Diabetes Mellitus

The ophtalmic findings produced by *diabetes* have repeatedly given rise to the assumption that similar changes in the *inner* ear might be the cause of impaired hearing in diabetics.

Actually Kozlov et al. (1979) believed they had seen a direct connection between the duration of the diabetes or the old age diabetes [5] and the findings in

[5] The generally used term "old age diabetes" means diabetes in elderly people, in the sense of a common disease of old age, but not a regular physiological process in old people. The same distinction should be made when using the term "presbyacusis" – q.v.

the vessels and capillaries of the inner ear. In one of every ten diabetics they observed that soon after the onset of the disease deafness had already reached an extent which on the average would have only been expected after twenty years. In previous studies on petrous bone specimen from four insulin patients Makishima and Tanaka (1971) had also found atrophic changes in the spiral ganglion and demyelinisation of the nerve fibers, as well as degeneration in the central auditory pathways; – yet, their patients were not deaf, but were between 56 and 73 years old!

In a study of 14 pairs of human petrous bones, Kovar (1973) thought he had found explanations not only for recruitment deafness but also for ganglio-neural hearing losses. In his opinion, the *acute* losses of hearing in diabetics are caused by hemorrhage into the endolymphatic space or by occlusion of vessels in the stria vascularis, the *chronic* ones by angiopathic changes in the vasa nervorum of the auditory nerve. There were no audiometric records of these patients.

According to other observations the PAS-positive precipitates were located in the thickened capillary walls of the *stria vascularis*; they are reported to have shown a close correlation with the diabetic complications and the duration of the diabetes but to be independent of the patient's age (Jörgensen 1961).

The organ of Corti does not seem to be directly affected, neither in human nor in alloxan-induced diabetes, not even if the changes in the stria vascularis would suggest this (Costa 1967). This assumption was also confirmed by the ability of the ear to recover under successful treatment, at least as regards diabetes in children (Hasanov and Kharsanov 1982). The authors rather consider the spiral ganglion to be the starting point for diabetic hearing impairments; a pathological glycogen concentration was found here in alloxan diabetes. At the same time, however, the free fatty acids in the blood were considerably increased and the glycogen *utilisation* reduced (Khasanov and Popov 1982).

ERA investigations in mice with congenital or alloxan-induced diabetes are said to have shown that there are disturbances predominantly in the central nerve pathways. During medication with gangliosides the prolongation of the latency could be prevented. Cerebral gangliosides are therefore said to be indicated for the maintenance of nerve conduction and synaptic transmission in diabetics (Savastano et al. 1982). In addition to this, an influence on the energy control *in the inner ear*, too, is ascribed to the gangliosides, in such a way that they increase the (Na^+, K^+) ATPase activity and interrupt its inhibition by ethacrynic acid or ouabaine (Molinari 1978, Aporti et al. 1981).

This orientation to *angiopathic* changes in the *neural* and *central* parts of the auditory pathways was not surprising, because in the meantime electro-physiological experiments in streptozotozin-diabetic chinchillas had not shown a reduction of either the CM or the DC potentials (Marshak 1972). Experiments on rats with streptozotozin diabetes as well as on congenitally diabetic mice produced the same results i.e. no diabetic *inner ear* deafness (Strauss et al. 1982). Though Strauß (1981) had found thickening of the inner ear vessel walls probably liable to diabetes these dit not correlate with the animals' audition.

In more recent *audiometric* studies – in contrast to those of the fifties and sixties – it was not possible to demonstrate an average handicap for diabetics (Axelsson et al. 1978, Gibbin and Davis 1981, Strauss 1982) – neither in pure tone nor in speech discrimination.

While the Swedish study (n = 205), as well as Gladney and Shepherd (1970) and Taylor and Irwin (1978) admitted a disease-specific involvement of the inner ear in *individual* diabetics, Strauss et al. (1982) argued that even by the analysis of individual or grouped factors, they were unable to distinguish patients with better or worse audition (n = 660); the authors therefore deny – as do Osterhammel and Christau (1980) on the basis of audiometric comparisons – any causal connection between the diabetic metabolic state and an inner ear deafness. The statistical analysis of a group (n = 51) of diabetic children had led to the same result – even for those with neurological or vascular complications (Sieger et al. 1983).

The few audiometric findings striking as pathologic are supposed to include, apart from a high tone loss, an increased threshold decay and an abnormal fatigue of the stapedius reflex (Strubiński and Malicka 1966, Robin 1981). The diabetes and the retinal microangiopathy are said to have been particularly severe in these patients.

In the Békésy audiogram, an increase in the pulsed tone and continous tone amplitudes by about 3 dB was shown only by *those* diabetics who were also suffering from cardiovascular disturbances (Fiorini et al. 1983) not, however, by those with diabetes *or* cardiovascular diseases. These investigations were performed on diabetics with normal hearing (Roach 1973).

From the results of the various investigations it should be concluded that there is *no* statistically verifiable correlation between the diabetic metabolic state and the hearing function. Diabetes mellitus thus does not directly or regularly lead to an inner ear deafness (Wilson et al. 1982). It rather leads to a thickening of the vessel walls, also in the inner ear (Jörgensen 1961), without a deafness necessarily developing from that alone. However, the angiopathy constitutes a risk factor (Taylor and Irwin 1978), which together with further risks or noxae can produce disturbances of function.

As regards the mode of action of the diabetic vascular changes one should be aware of the fact that the raised HbA_1-concentration in the blood of diabetics impedes the release of O_2 to the tissue, so that the vessel tries to compensate this by dilatation. Nevertheless, with increasing metabolic disturbance the vascular dilatation becomes insufficient, and the tissue hypoxia increases. Additional detrimental effects may be exerted by the diabetic microcirculatory disturbances, an increased thrombocyte aggregation and a reduced deformability of the erythrocytes (Gladney and Shepherd 1970, Hesch 1982).

The discussion of possible disturbances of sugar metabolism as risk factors in the development of inner ear deafness makes it plain that the matter at question is not a direct alteration e.g. of the protein or electrolyte balance in the inner ear, but a mechanism acting indirectly through the vascular system or the microcirculation. In this sense, the resulting metabolic disturbances of the inner ear are once again vascular diseases, namely the sequel to damage of the vascular wall, the endothelium and the microcirculation, as well as the regulation of the cardiovascular system.

3.6.2.3 Disturbances of Fat Metabolism

The influence of disturbances of fat metabolism on the inner ear is to be seen virtually exclusively in their atherogenic effect.

For a long time, the serum cholesterol has served as a parameter of the fat metabolism. In the meantime, however, laboratory diagnostics have become more differentiated i.e. are predominantly based on the lipoproteins. Among these the low density lipoproteins (LDL) are supposed to have a definitely stronger atherogenic effect than the high density lipoproteins (HDL) (Schwandt 1980).

Deaf patients actually did not show higher values either for the serum triglycerides or for the total cholesterol than those of the control group. However, LDL cholesterol and the ratio of LDL cholesterol to HDL cholesterol are said to have been significantly higher in those with hearing impairment (Friedrich and Pilger 1981). The authors therefore recommend the LDL/HDL quotient as "the most sensitive discriminator of a possible risk of arteriosclerosis". In this connection, they *took for granted* that the hearing disturbances had resulted from arteriosclerotic changes.

A completely different approach to the question whether the inner ear is affected by the disturbances of fat metabolism was made by Rosen and Olin (1965). They examined inmates of a psychiatric institution (n = 136) who had been fed exclusively on vegetable fat for five years. It was shown that the hearing of these patients had improved and now corresponded to that of a control group ten years younger. After this group had, for another three years, again been given their customary diet, the hearing once again deteriorated (Rosen et al. 1970).

These findings suggest a general relationship between a "healthy" diet and hearing in advanced age (Marshall 1981). They should not be used, however, for the explanation of "presbyacusis", but only for the interpretation of metabolically determined inner ear deafness (Baba et al. 1980, Carotti et al. 1983).

These findings suggest a general relationship between a "healthy" diet and hearing in advanced age (Marshall 1981). They should not be used, however, for the explanation of "presbyacusis", but only for the interpretation of metabolically determined inner ear deafness (Baba et al. 1980, Carotti et al. 1983). The investigations of Cunningham and Goetzinger (1974) were less significant. They compared twenty patients with hyperlipidemia with 20 healthy subjects aged from 20–50 years, in respect of their *highest* tone hearing at 10–18 kHz. The hearing acuity showed an inverse relationship to the serum lipid values, however this was only barely significant. The question why audiometric measurements were made only in the highest tone region remains unexplained.

In rabbits it has been possible to demonstrate deterioration of hearing if in addition to a renal hypertension, a hypercholesterinemia is produced (Morizono and Paparella 1978) – findings which could not be confirmed in rats with genetic hypertension (Pilsbury 1981). The observations of Bichler and Wieser (1983) might be judged as evidence of a *direct* influence of the fat metabolism. After having fed *chlorphentermine* they observed an accumulation of phospholipid containing lysosomes in the inner hair cells, the dark cells of the stria vascularis, the ganglion cells, some supporting cells and the radial nerve fibers. The authors explain the findings by a local interaction between the drug and the phospholipids; in this way the complex becomes resistant to lipase. The preferential affection of the inner hair cells indicated a particularly active fat metabolism here as well as in the afferent nerve fibers. Electrophysiological testing revealed that the threshold of the CAP and the latency of N_1 were raised; after the withdrawal of chlorphentermine the reactions largely regressed without returning to normal.

3.6.2.4 Disturbances of Liver Function

A direct relationship between inner ear and hepatic dysfunction has scarcely ever been discussed seriously except perhaps for the case of hepatic coma.

Already decades ago, however, a vitamin A deficiency as a sequel to hepatic cirrhosis or to alcoholic liver damage had been regarded as indirectly responsible for impairments of the hearing (Rüedi 1954, Nager 1954 and others).

While formerly this conclusion was purely deductive, from analogy with the retina, vitamin A in the requisite concentration has meanwhile also been detected in the stria vascularis of guinea pigs (Chole et al. 1978, Chole 1980). Vitamin A *deficiency* is said to have caused a loosening of the cuticular membrane of the sensory cells, and later on also signs of degeneration at the afferent nerve endings and in the spiral ganglion (Löhle 1980a, b). On account of the presumed participation of vitamin A in the combined action of osteoclasts and osteoblasts this vitamin is supposed to regulate – "through a calcium-mechanism the permeability of the sensory cell membrane for cations" – as it does in the retina (Kilian and Schacht 1977, Löhle et al. 1982).

Since a vitamin A deficiency seems to be only exceptionally due to inadequate intake, it was attributed to chronic liver disease (Kramp and Schwager 1978, Spitzer and Ventry 1980, Löhle et al. 1982). In animal experiments a drop in the CM by 3.4 dB (!) in comparison to guinea pigs with healthy livers as well as a disturbed adaptation was explained by the impaired liver function (Kramp and Dahle 1978).

The audiometric comparison of the hearing thresholds of subjects with and without hepatic diseases has revealed an additional age-related high tone loss; the loss, however, would have been definitely less had it been compared not with *selected* healthy subjects, but with the normal curve e.g. according to Schmid (1967). The supposed pathological adaptation in 50% of those with alcoholic liver disease persuades just as little as does apostrophizing the preserved stapedius reflex *for* damage in the auditory *nerve* (Löhle et al. 1982). It is therefore also unnecessary to go any closer into the assumption that hearing impairment might be explained by a vitamin A deficiency even in thyroid and kidney disease.

Incidentally, the cause of the supposed vitamin-A-related deafness is not interpreted by Löhle et al. (1982) as a disturbance of function in the stria vascularis or sensory cells, but as pressure atrophy due to bony apposition in the internal auditory meatus or the canal of Rosenthal, that is in the same way as Krmpotić-Nemanić (1971) had suggested for presbyacusis.

Though there seem to exist obvious parallels between eye and ear as regards the role of vitamin A, the hitherto available data are not very conclusive. In children with hearing disturbances of different etiology no significant decrease of the vitamin A (retinol) levels or of the vitamin-A-binding proteins has been observed in the serum (Biesalski et al. 1981).

Also clinically one cannot identify any dependence of inner ear deafness either on vitamin A deficiency or on cirrhotic or alcoholic liver damage. The biochemical effects of reduced liver function are certainly not exhausted in vitamin A deficiency, and disturbances of vitamin A transport are found not only in diseases of the liver but also in those of the thyroid and kidneys (Smith and Goodman 1971, Smith et al. 1973). Nevertheless, deafness is not a regular or even a frequent sequel to disturbed function of the liver, the thyroid or the kidney.

The assumption of a causal connection between a *vitamin D deficiency* and inner ear deafness (Brookes and Morrison 1981, Brookes 1983) likewise requires a critical evaluation; as possible causes of the vitamin D deficiency the authors mention, besides chronic liver diseases, renal dysfunction, inadequate intestinal absorption, anticonvulsives and also a deficient diet.

3.6.2.5 Disturbances of Thyroid Function

Inner ear deafness caused by disturbed iodine metabolism is said to exist in about 30%–45% of the patients with acquired chronic hypothyroidism (de Vos 1963, Haubrich 1975, Dokianakis et al. 1978, Fotin and Ageeva 1981), partly with, but mostly without recruitment (de Vos 1963, Stephens 1970). In two thirds of these cases the middle ear conduction is affected, too (Dokianakis et al. 1978, Jahnke et al. 1979), and also the central conduction pathway can be disturbed as shown by the ERA (Salami et al. 1983). The hearing losses are confined to the high frequency range; obviously there is no characteristic tone threshold pattern. After substitution therapy an improvement in hearing was recorded (Howarth and Lloyd 1956, Dokianakis et al. 1978, Fotin and Ageeva 1981). On the other hand, contrary statements have been made, in the sense that reduced thyroid function is not the cause of occasional high tone deafness (Parving et al. 1983).

The reversibility goes well together with the absence of any morphologically detectable damage in the inner ear, of the ganglion cells or of the auditory nerve. Only histochemical studies in thyroidectomised guinea pigs revealed a storage of mucopolysaccharides in the scalae as well as in the vascular connective tissue around the auditory nerve. Also the concentration of certain enzymes, particularly in the outer hair cells had decreased below normal, a finding which could be regarded as evidence of a disturbance of metabolism, which, however, is likely to be reversible in view of the normal morphology (Schätzle and Haubrich 1967). Kohonen et al. (1971) had indeed also observed a decay of hair cells, however, this was in the apical turns in guinea pigs and could not be correlated with the impairment of the CM.

Thyroid *hypo*function is reported to soften the effects of noise damage, *hyper*function to increase them corresponding to the reduced or increased metabolic rate (Berndt and Wagner 1979). A bilateral hearing loss which developed after treatment of thyrotoxicosis with propylthiouracil, has remained only a single observation. After stopping the medication (and after surgery) the auditory function returned to normal (Smith 1972).

3.6.2.6 Vascular Disturbances

Since a vascular disturbance in the inner ear is so frequently assumed it is necessary first of all to point out the physiological and pathophysiological mechanisms of reaction and regulation. Their knowledge is of fundamental importance for the diagnostic evaluation of the findings obtained and for therapeutic considerations.

On the basis of analogy conclusions, the blood supply of the inner ear had for a long time been classified with the *central* type of regulation (Schnieder 1973, Ritter 1974, 1978). Nowadays we may assume that the artery of the labyrinth does not form part of the cerebral circulation (Maass et al. 1977, Maass 1982), but obeys the rules of the peripheral circulation. Nevertheless, at the same time the distinction between the peripheral and central type of circulation has become less rigid in so far as it is suggested that the cerebral circulation, too, is subject to particular neurogenic, peripheral regulatory influences (Edvinsson and MacKenzie 1977, Paulson and Strandgaard 1978). Within the inner ear there are two functionally separate vascular areas to be distinguished:

- The one *with* adrenergic innervation including the spiral artery of the modiolus, the cochlear plexus and the internal spiral vessels, and
- the one *without* adrenergic innervation, namely the external spiral vessels, the radial arterioles (Maass 1979) as well as the vessels of the spiral ligament and the stria vascularis.

In the adrenergic, *predistal* section – as Hesch (1982) called it – the nervous regulatory mechanisms resemble those of the peripheral arteries of the body i.e. vascular wall-, flow- and blood-factors remain in constant interaction during the development of an arterial circulatory disturbance (Alexander 1977).

The arterial convolutions *in the modiolus* constitute the beginning of the respective units of the vascular system; since they are supplied with muscles, they are probably directly involved in the circulatory regulation.

In the non-adrenergic, *distal* part of the vessels, the terminal anastomosing segmental units of the terminal vascular system are controlled by the *flow-characteristics* of the blood, by local biochemical regulators, by endothelial cells and by pericytes – an organ-specific type of cochlear capillary regulation.

Thus, the vessels with adrenergic innervation are the ones which, together with the spiral vessels underneath the tympanic lip of the osseous spiral lamina, are responsible for the supply of the organ of Corti (Koburg and Maass 1979, Uddman et al. 1982). On the other hand, there also exists the concept according to which the metabolic needs of the organ of Corti are exclusively or to a large extent provided for by the perilymph (Zechner 1974, Arnold and Vosteen 1979). Interruption of the vessels of the modiolus to the capillary loops under the osseous lamina spiralis leads, in spite of an intact stria vascularis and spiral prominence, to a loss of the hair cells, whereas a block in the blood supply of the spiral ligament and the stria vascularis causes a degeneration of the stria vascularis but no loss of the hair cells (Lawrence 1966). In both cases disturbances follow in the respective ischaemic areas (Lawrence 1980). A division of the artery of the labyrinth – for example in the course of surgery of the internal auditory meatus – would cause a degeneration of the entire inner ear except for the ductus and saccus endolymphaticus (Belal 1979).

In the three vascular sections and functions which are to be differentiated vascular disturbances manifest themselves as

- changes in the vessel *wall*
- disturbances of the *vascular innervation*
- endothelial lesions
- disturbances of the microcirculation and
- disturbances of the cardiac output or the blood pressure regulation

Less and less notice is being taken of alterations of the vertebral artery *produced in the cervical spine* – at least, as regards the auditory function (vide also Hesch 1982, Terrahe 1979).

Actually there is little reason to believe that cervicovertebral angiostenoses lead to hearing disturbances. Thus, it is only after ligation of both vertebral and both carotid arteries that the brain stem responses show a radical decay – and that only in four out of ten guinea pigs. The interruption of both vertebral arteries and *one* carotid artery produced only a prolongation of the latency and a reduction of the amplitude of the AEP. These possibilities of reaction or compensation are probably guaranteed by the formation of collaterals, by vasodilator effects and a reactive rise in the blood pressure (Suzuki 1982).

Although the action potential of the auditory nerve (CAP) showed a bilateral decrease in amplitude after ligation of the vertebral and carotid arteries it was not extinguished. Only when the *carotid and subclavian arteries* were ligated *bilaterally* in the mediastinum did the auditory nerves cease to function. However, this occurred in each case only after the fourth vessel had been ligated (Steinert and Mester 1982). These experimental results at the same time illustrate the ability of the inner ear to withstand a deficient *arterial* circulation, above all in comparison with the brain, which responded much sooner to vascular ligation by respiratory arrest. It must be noted as a qualification that these findings were obtained from guinea pigs and therefore cannot automatically be transferred to man. Besides that, narrowings of the vertebral vessels are always associated with stimulation of the accompanying sympathetic plexus.

An extreme decrease in blood pressure and a shock reaction, in the sense of a centralisation of the circulation, seems to be much more unfavorable for the inner ear than arterial ligation. The breakdown of the action potential precisely at the time when the blood pressure sinks below the critical figure of 40 mm Hg (Steinert and Spath 1984) may at least be interpreted to that effect.

The significance of arterio-sclerotic changes in the vascular wall within the circulation area of the labyrinthine artery lies in the arterial "preload" of the inner ear. They become hemodynamically all the more effective as the possibilities of a vicarious perfusion through collaterals are restricted. In such situations additional drops in the cardiac output and the systemic blood pressure may have dreadful consequences for the inner ear.

The O_2 transport from the middle ear into the inner ear through the round window membrane covers merely 10–15% of the consumption in the *basal turn* and even this only with a high O_2 partial pressure in the tympanic cavity (400 mm Hg). It is therefore only of secondary importance (Morgenstern and Kessler 1978) and, in the opposite direction it can be disadvantageous for the inner ear, namely if the PO_2 in the middle ear sinks below 57 mm Hg (Morgenstern 1980).

The *innervation* of the vessel wall by the sympathetic and the parasympathetic influences the cochlear blood flow (Hultcrantz et al. 1975) as well as the O_2 partial pressure in the inner ear in interaction with the systemic blood pressure (Maass et al. 1979).

Nowadays, the *endothelial lesions* are interpreted as of predominantly paraspastic i.e. not primarily organic origin, at all events in the coronary circulation (Maserit et al. 1978). They are followed by an interaction between the adrenergic prostacyclin synthesized in the vessel wall and the thromboxan A_2 released from the thrombocytes; within the resulting vasoconstriction local aggregations of thrombocytes lead to narrowings of the lumina – also in the arteries of the labyrinth (Ritter 1978).

The capillary *microcirculation* is largely regulated by the local products of metabolism as well as by the characteristics of the plasma viscosity and the cellular portion of the blood (for example in cases of polycythemia). As regards the flow characteristics of the blood it is necessary to distinguish between the whole blood viscosity and the plasma viscosity. Their interaction with the blood pressure, the vascular elasticity and the O_2-transport (Ehrly 1981) threatens to have a complex effect as regards a possible inadequate supply of the inner ear. That's why investigations on contraceptives, and their side-effects on the inner ear, do not lack a certain legitimacy (Kley 1978), especially as with local vascular damage, changes in the lipoprotein pattern, disturbances of thrombocyte function *and systemic increase in the blood pressure* they create manifold possibilities for a defective vascular reaction (cf. Chap. 3.6.1.2). The results so far obtained, however, have no substantial significance. It might be a similar summation of adverse factors which explains the greater average high tone loss *in smokers* as compared with nonsmokers (Kothe and Oeken 1983).

Reduced O_2-transport in chronic or acute *anemia* may probably only be regarded as a risk factor in cases of pre-existing additional vascular disease. The same may well be assumed for toxic disturbances of the O_2-exchange e.g. in diabetic coma or with severe burns.

An almost linear correlation exists between high blood pressure and *coronary* heart diseases (Maserit et al. 1978). It is more difficult to answer the question whether this also applies to the vessels of the *inner ear*. In this connection the *constant* hypertension is probably less detrimental than its variability under physical and psychical stress, varying positions of the body or diurnal influences (Krönig and Zschidrich 1979). These variations in the blood pressure are more marked in hypertensives than in those with a normal blood pressure – and can be most effectively assessed if measured by the patients themselves. Particularly unfavorable reductions of organ perfusion threaten during the fall in pressure in *labile hypertension*. *Labile hypo*tension may also have deleterious effects on the peripheral microcirculation, particularly if, on account of a pre-existing vascular disease, it can no longer be compensated by the local regulating mechanisms. Chronic *stable* low blood pressure values are difficult to define as regards their clinical relevance – and hence also their effect on the inner ear. Inadequately treated cardiac insufficiency or irregularities of action, which cause an additional strain on the periphery, may also have an effect on the inner ear, in the sense of *transient ischemic attacks*.

The inner ear is thus dependent on the condition, the reactions and the regulation mechanisms of the entire organism, via the cardiovascular system. The vascular diseases of the inner ear are to be regarded as analogous to the circulatory and vascular reactions of the remaining organs and particularly of the heart. Hesch (1982) has therefore described as *otangina* the clinical picture of deafness in arteriosclerotic, vasospastic, microcirculatory or fluidity disturbances of the inner ear. He thereby also points out the responsibility which rests with the ENT specialist in the diagnosis and treatment of an inner ear deafness. In each individual case comprehensive evaluation of the metabolism and the circulation is necessary, in order to keep the risk of further hearing loss as small as possible – all the more since despite all diagnostic efforts many cases of inner ear deafness still seem very mysterious to us. Despite these concepts borrowed from general heart and circulatory medicine and adapted to the special vascular situation of the inner ear, the clinical criteria of a direct causal relationship often turn out to be meagre, so that the cause of progressive bilateral inner ear deafness remains unclear even after comprehensive diagnostic efforts (Fig. 41 and Table 3).

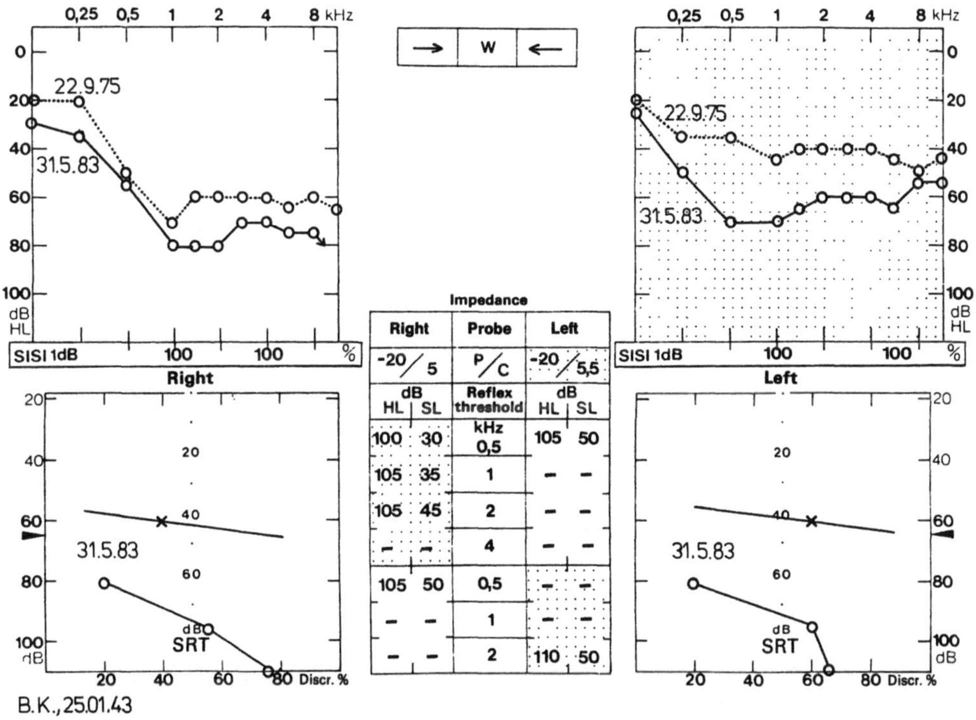

Fig. 41. Etiologically unexplained bilateral inner ear deafness without any familial susceptibility. General medical condition normal, apart from a hypotension. In 1975 the stapedius reflex had still been obtainable at all frequencies (80–105 dB); the speech audiogram, too, had deteriorated since 1975. (The values at that time are not reproduced here). BC = AC

Table 3. Survey of 24 laboratory findings in 205 patients with inner ear deafness In the ordinate the particular tests, in the abscissa the number of pathologic tests results (≦5, 6–9, ≧10) as well as the subdivision into male and female are quoted. The numbers in brackets are the numbers of patients in the respective group. In some fields the hatching is darker, depending on the percentage of the test persons who produced results exceeding the norm, or the number of normal findings obtained; e.g. 0% in the right field above and 100% in the left field below. Viscosity was always extremely pathologic, a result which causes us to doubt the norm-value of the laboratory rather than to think of any causative factor. The left preponderance in the electrocardiogram is rarely missing, corresponding to a hypertensive circulatory state and a hypertonic fundus of the eye – in men with at least only ten pathologic results in only 36% of the cases. They are followed by aortic sclerosis, abuse of nicotine, the disturbance of lipoid metabolism, the microsomal antibodies indicating an immune thyroiditis and the high hematocrit.

Cholesterol, calcium, potassium and sodium in the serum were nearly always normal, as well as T_3, T_4 and alpha- and beta-globulin. In females the same tendencies are recognised, though less pronounced; the sensitivity of the risk factors increases depending on their incidence

	≦5		6–9		≧10	
	m (45)	w (28)	m (66)	w (39)	m (16)	w (11)
Whole blood viscosity	29	33	19	4	7	0
Plasma viscosity	15	17	17	4	13	0
ECG: Left preponderance	78	58	53	59	21	30
Sedimentation (ESR)	72/69	67/63	63/48	22/14	40/20	18/10
Smoking	73	100	44	86	11	55
Hypertensive fundus	81	84	77	87	36	56
Aortic sclerosis	95	88	85	93	75	50
Infarct	97	96	79	100	64	60
Serum-triglyceride	79	94	54	91	43	18
Serum-glucose	83	95	70	76	53	33
Blood urea	87	90	83	81	73	83
Serum cholesterol	100	95	95	94	80	90
Serum-calcium	92	100	94	90	91	89
Serum-potassium	100	100	100	95	93	100
Serum-sodium	100	100	100	100	100	100
Microsomal antibodies	88	81	68	64	82	50
Parathyroid hormone	91	94	88	91	83	83
T_3	97	95	98	87	92	100

Table 3 (continued)

	≦5		6–9		≧10	
	m (45)	w (28)	m (66)	w (39)	m (16)	w (11)
T_4	94	95	98	93	92	100
Hematocrit	89	85	66	82	73	70
Hemoglobin	100	100	89	95	80	82
α_2-globulin	95	100	95	97	86	88
α_1-globulin	100	100	87	94	93	88
β-globulin	100	100	100	97	100	100

Incidentally Rosen and Olin (1965) had found tone perception to be directly dependent on the general atheromatous and coronary arterio-sclerotic conditions, when they compared the tone threshold of the Mabaans with that of an industrialised population. The respective groups also showed corresponding differences in the behaviour of the blood pressure.

Moreover, these statistics were supported by comparisons of two 10–29 year old ethnic groups, one from Finland with a higher and the other one from Jugoslavia with a lower incidence of cardiovascular diseases. The audition of the hypercholesterinemic Finns aged 10–19 was worse than that of the 20–29 year old Jugoslavs without vascular disturbances of the coronaries, however, only regarding the frequencies 14000–18000 Hz (!). On the other hand, the comparison of patients with coronary failure – confirmed by cardiac catheterisation ($n=111$) – with a healthy group aged 30–59 years, showed neither a less favorable average tone threshold nor an increased incidence of inner ear deafness among the cardiac patients – 60% of whom had suffered a cardiac infarct (Brusis et al. 1981).

A comparison of hypertensive persons ($n=90$) with the presbyacusis curves by Schmidt (1967) led to the same result. Again, the patients' audition was not worse than corresponded to the "norm" (Brusis et al. 1982). Only in the case of hypertensive crisis or arteriosclerosis, there would exist greater danger to the inner ear (Carfi et al. 1980).

Deafness occasionally occurs after a coronary or cardiopulmonary bypass operation. If unilateral and acute it is usually regarded as an embolic "sudden hearing loss" (cf. Fig. 36); bilateral prolonged deterioration of hearing is explained by the superimposition of several stress factors, such as cardiopulmonary complications and an aminoglycoside antibiotic or frusemide medication. Systematic follow-up after bypass operations revealed a slight bilateral high tone impairment as compared with the pre-operative findings, however, in most cases only of <10 dB and only in nine of 68 patients of >10 dB (Shapiro et al. 1981).

The effects of arteriosclerotic changes on the inner ear were generally regarded as a significant cause of "presbyacusis"; in particular as there might exist a relationship between the narrowed lumen of the internal auditory artery, the atrophy in the spiral ganglion and the premortal hearing loss. The same coincidence, however, is found with impaired hearing and arteriosclerosis in the circle of Willis, as well as encephalomalacia (Makishima 1978). Accordingly, these findings will have represented advanced arterio- and cerebral-scleroses which naturally do not leave the inner ear unaffected, but are of secondary importance for the clinical aspects of *inner ear* deafness.

For the influence of hematologic diseases on inner ear function cf. Chap. 3.6.1.

In any case, the dependence of the inner ear on the functioning of vascular supply and its regulation cannot be regarded as an isolated and single factor. In most cases several pathological findings are responsible for the acute or chronic deficiency in the supply of the labyrinth. It is precisely the necessary multiplicity of such *risk factors* which makes it difficult in an individual case to produce "evidence" of the vascular origin of the inner ear deafness. With complete exhaustion of the diagnostic means of internal medicine the incidence of relevant, singular or associated cardio-vascular risk factors may amount to about 80% (Lehnhardt and Hesch 1980). The accumulation of such findings, however, demands long term observations and multifactorial statistical evaluations in order to be interpretable as causal relationships. Mere collections of diverse laboratory findings regarded as abnormal are insufficient for a reliable statement, especially if the individual patterns of deafness had only been vaguely defined (Wilke et al. 1977).

In the case of chronic disturbances the *therapeutic consequences* of risk-relevant medical or biochemical findings, mainly come within the *sphere of responsibility* of the *internist*. They should be directed to the prevention of further hearing loss; an improvement is all the more unlikely the more slowly deafness has developed. Prescriptions on part of the otologist should here also be guided by the principle of "nil nocere". Risks of damage do exist if as a result of the medication:

- a systemic fall of the blood pressure occurs and this is followed by a reduction of perfusion of the inner ear
- healthy vascular areas are distended and as a result a steal effect occurs in the inner ear, and if...
- there is a risk of direct vascular damage to be caused by the drug itself e.g. ergotism due to ergotamine preparations, or changes in the vessel walls during prolonged corticosteroid therapy.

For the most part, "vasoactive" or "encephalotropic" substances do not seem to be of benefit. Critical authors therefore advise against such therapeutic attempts on account of the unfavorable relationship of benefit and damage, or approve their application only on the grounds of carefully considered indications (Hesch 1982). The blood pressure conditions should always be taken into consideration. Prior to and also during treatment, the blood pressure should be *checked and recorded* – by the patient himself, if possible.

3.7 Deafness in the Aged

For some years now a fundamental change has been taking place as regards the definition of the term *presbyacusis*. It will probably lead to an even more sparing use of the diagnosis, simply because presbyacusis in its narrower sense will dwindle to a fraction of that which many today still describe as "presbyacusis".

In the fifties and sixties there was a great interest in working out *normal values* for presbyacusis. For this purpose, patient populations of different size were tested after having carefully sorted out all subjects with deafness due to other causes (familial susceptibility, trauma, noise, middle ear infections, otosclerosis etc.). At the same time a distinction was drawn between men and women, and the findings were arranged according to age, in decades or quinquennia. The number of these *old age standards* is large, the data from several of these studies were statistically analysed (Schmidt 1967, Spoor 1967) and have since then, as average threshold curves, frequently

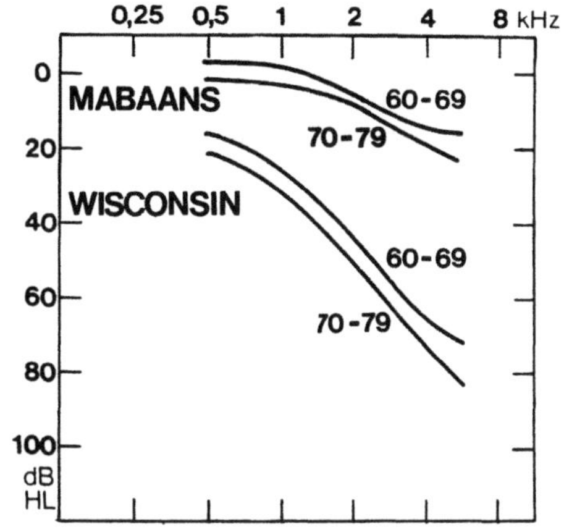

Fig. 42. So-called presbyacusis curves for the seventh and eighth decades, according to the Winsconsin State Fair 1954. In contrast, the hearing losses in the Mabaans in the same decades amounted to only ~5 dB at 2000 Hz, 15 or 18 dB at 4000 Hz and 18 or 25 dB at 6000 Hz. (From Rosen and Olin 1965)

been the basis of the assessment of the "old age component" (Fig. 42). Later on, more such investigations were published, mostly for control and comparison with the data already available (Milne and Lauder 1975, Pearson 1977, Robinson and Sutton 1979, Corso 1980 and others).

After the approximate average extent of "presbyacusis" seemed to be established it was tried to find a clinical audiometric description of the *picture* of deafness due to old age. The respective literature can scarcely be controlled. A survey – not exhaustive, however, – is found in Hülse and Boll (1979), and a very good review of the virtually endless number test results in Marshall (1981). Among the more recent studies those by v. Arentsschild (1972), Hallermann and Plath (1972), Lehnhardt (1978), Hutchinson et al. (1979) and Krüger et al. (1981) may be mentioned.

In recent years special arrangements for the testing of central speech integration were worked out particularly by Jokinen (1973), Granick et al. (1976) and v. Wedel and Opitz (1980). Others investigated the question, as to whether deafness in the aged showed a typical process of hearing-fatigue or adaptation (Jerger 1960, Schindler 1962, Jokinen 1970; Bystrzanowka et al. 1971, Novotny 1975) or whether particular features might be identified in the frequency selectivity (Meurman 1954, Butler and Albrite 1956, König 1957, Gusanti 1967, v. Wedel 1979, Margolis and Goldberg 1980). The findings – certainly on account of the varying objectives, the varying test arrangements, etc. – revealed a striking heterogeneity of the results. All of them had only one feature in common – the age of the patients (Marshall 1981)!

The heterogeneity of the findings was not surprising, since Schuknecht had already in 1955 described four different forms of presbyacusis. For a long time the high tone diagonal loss had been considered to be the typical and exclusive picture of so-called "presbyacusis". However, on the basis of clinical and morphological studies, Schuknecht arrived at the following classification:

- High tone loss as the expression of a hair cell atrophy, particularly in the basal turn: sensory type
- inconstant tone threshold curve as the result of a predominant ganglion cell degeneration – onset in advanced age: neural type
- flat threshold curve as a sign of atrophy of the stria vascularis: metabolic or strial type and
- high tone diagonal loss associated with stiffening of the basilar membrane and the spiral ligament: inner ear conductive type.

The neural type would correspond to the picture of an age-dependent degeneration in the basal portion of the spiral ganglion as described by Fleischer (1956). It would certainly be more reasonable in this connection to speak of a *ganglionic* deafness, especially as it cannot be distinguished from the sensory type by clinical audiometry, whereas negative recruitment would be expected from a neural deafness. Schuknecht emphasized the remarkably bad speech discrimination as the specific criterion of this type of presbyacusis.

The result of Schuknecht's efforts of differentiation is that presbyacusis, with all its variants, is assumed to be located in the *inner ear*, including the spiral ganglion. On the other hand, earlier morphological audiometric findings had indicated an age-dependent disintegration of the *neural* and *central* portions of the auditory pathways including the higher auditory functions.

These findings include:
- disturbance of the binaural summation of two-channel separated speech (Matzker 1956, 1958),
- impairment of dichotic speech discrimination (Hennebert 1955, Feldmann 1956),
- reduction of directional hearing, and hence of the ability to resolve interaural differences in conduction time and intensity (Matzker 1957, Kirikae et al. 1964),
- poor discrimination of redundance reduced, rapid or distorted speech (Bocca 1959).

The two basically different findings in presbyacusis, namely, on the one side the disturbances of inner ear function in their numerous variants and, on the other side, the diversity of the central handicaps, gave rise to doubts about the homogeneity of the term presbyacusis, all the more since the results of suprathreshold audiometric tests were predominantly interpretable to the effect of an inner ear localisation (Lehnhardt 1978, Bernath et al. 1981, Krüger et al. 1981).

Still more frequent and extensive efforts have been made to define separately the individual peripheral and central components (v. Arentsschild 1972, Lowell and Paparella 1977, Lehnhardt 1978, Brinkman 1979, Hülse and Boll 1979, Gilad and Glorig 1979, Krüger 1980, Hülse and Irion 1982, Martin and Martin 1982). It was, however, also tried to differentiate more strictly within the inner ear components. Though the manifestations of central decay were to be classified for the most part as physiological, in old age this does only partly apply to the disturbances of inner ear function.

Schuknechts classification had only pointed out the possibilities as to *pathological* changes with which the inner ear can react and which might be displayed in different ways in audiometric testing. The question as to which of these findings may physiologically develop in old age – and to what extent – must for the time being remain open. The same clinical pictures are sometimes seen in younger patients, too, and, on the contrary, some of the old present considerably more discrete changes. For this reason, those types of deafness which in younger patients would be regarded as of uncertain etiology must not – in the seventh or eighth decade – declared to be presbyacusis for the simple reason that the patient is old.

To delimit the *physiologic* from the pathologic old age component of deafness Kumpf (1970) distinguished a *primary* (sui generis) from a *secondary* presbyacusis (both together then would make up the *average* presbyacusis). These descriptions are not very accurate, if only for the fact that the secondary "presbyacusis" need not be caused by aging (Fleischer 1972).

It is probably more logical to designate as *true* presbyacusis the inner ear component which has developed exclusively as a result of old age – including the neural or central decay equally caused purely by *aging*. The additional peripheral and central disturbances will then require further etiological clarification (cf. Chap. 3.6.2).

As far as this subject is concerned, the central senile losses of hearing or understanding are of less interest. One can scarcely assume, either that central changes are the cause of high tone loss; both the slight peripheral loss of high tones and the impairment of central actions arise independently of each other, but from the same cause, namely progressive aging.

The subjective handicap caused by functional losses at a higher level, however, is intensified by additional high tone losses – actually in the sense of the already existing reduction of peripheral information which, on its part, may be aggravated if, in addition, background noise also blocks the otherwise still functioning low tone region (Schultz-Coulon 1972). This effect is particularly disadvantageous for elderly persons with a high tone deafness since they lack the unvoiced phonemes i.e. the essential sound elements of speech which convey its meaning (Stevenson 1975) and since they are no longer in position to compensate for this by attentiveness, concentration and deduction – though to an individually varying extent (Hallermann and Plath 1971).

But still this handicap is certainly of less importance in those cases of deafness *exclusively* determined by old age than in the other cases of inner ear deafness with an additional circulatory or metabolic component. Plath (1974, 1982) considers deafness in the sense of restricted speech discrimination always to be a sign of *illness*. "Normal aging" does not cause any significant loss of discrimination (Townsend and Bess 1980) and social hearing is preserved (v. Wedel and Tegtmeier 1980). Within these limits, however, speech discrimination may progressively deteriorate with advancing age in spite of constant hearing thresholds (Jerger 1973, Plath 1974) – however, to a significant extent only beyond the age of 80 (Lehnhardt 1977, Krüger et al. 1981).

If there is *also* a hearing loss in the low tone region, an almost flat tone threshold results from senile decay; like all characteristics of the tone threshold it has up to now been interpreted as exclusively related to the inner ear. Since, however, in these – old – patients the Synthetic Sentence Identification Test (SSI) gives a particularly bad result in comparison with the Phonemic Balance Test (PB) it seems that both findings – the additional low tone loss and the deficit in the SSI test – are the expression of *central* aging (Hayes and Jerger 1979).

The probably easiest way to assess the extent of the *actually* age-related inner ear hearing loss is to pick out from a large population of old persons a group of subjects who do not display any striking hearing loss of e.g. >40 dB or even >25 dB in any of the frequencies measured (Menegaux and Pailler 1982). In this way a type of curve *normal for the aged* would result, as shown in Fig. 43. This hearing loss is far less severe than the "standard values", i.e. including the pathological age component of inner ear deafness; it scarcely increases any more – at least from the seventh to the eighth decade (Lehnhardt 1977). The case material underlying these figures is certainly too small, but no comparable figures have been found in the literature.

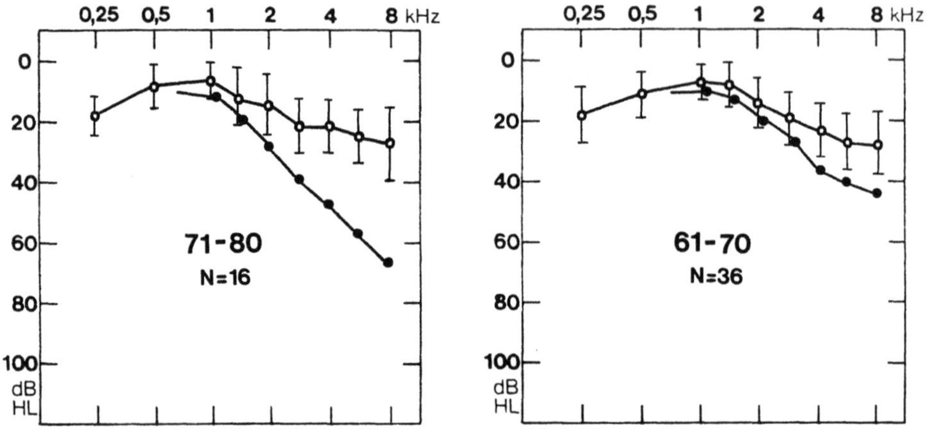

Fig. 43. The upper curves in both diagrams reproduce the average hearing threshold with standard deviations of those with "still good" audition (hearing loss also in the high frequencies <40 dB) among 252 subjects tested, summarized in groups for those aged 61–70 and those aged 71–80 (Lehnhardt 1978). As compared with these, the "standard" curves of the aged by Schmidt (1967 ●—●) are definitely more unfavorable. Probably only the upper curve represents the peripheral loss which is *physiological in old age* wheras the lower one also comprises the *pathological age components* of the hearing loss

The physiological age component is supposed to be represented by the so called saturation phenomenon of the stapedius reflex i.e. the amplitude of the changes in impedance does not increase any further in spite of the rise in the intensity of the stimulus. The authors explain this behaviour by the altered energy integration in the aging ear (Silman and Gelfand 1981) – a process, however, which should not only be related to the inner ear, but may also be neural in origin. Beyond that, the time constant of the reflex is said to show a physiologic increase in old age (Gersdorf 1978).

The other criteria given in the literature for so-called presbyacusis do not refer to the physiological age component of hearing loss but to pathologic disturbances of function in the inner ear within the range of the hitherto customary "norms of the aged". They may be the sequels to various diseases of old age or earlier hearing damage (noise, ototoxics etc.; Hawkins 1973), may be the result of reduced circulation in the inner ear, a general metabolic disturbance, a local enzyme deficiency or a genetically determined premature failure of hearing. It is no wonder therefore that different investigators have obtained different findings.

Thus, e.g the recruitment is said to have been absent or only partially developed; or the mono-syllable discrimination is said to have been too poor as compared with the tone threshold – phonemic regression (Jerger 1973, Bergholtz et al. 1977, Pearlman 1982). The ability to differentiate frequencies is also supposed to diminish with advancing age, particularly in the high tone region and less markedly in the low frequency range (Gryczynski 1981).

Glorig and Davis (1961) described a difference between bone conduction and air conduction in the high tone region and interpreted it as an expression of an age-related stiffening of the basilar membrane or of the spiral ligament. According to Schuknecht, this *gap* ought to be expected in the inner ear sound conduction type. However, it seems more likely that it came about with the technical recording – in the case of different hearing on the two sides by contralateral hearing or – in the case of hearing dips – as a result of the greater content of harmonics in bone conduction as compared with the "purer" air conduction.

Any sex differences in the senile decay of hearing may probably be ignored, as far as they only involve the actual *physiologic* age component; even for the central aging processes they are apparently of no importance (Lowell and Paparella 1977, Paparella 1978).

The *pathologic* age component of inner ear deafness, however, is greater in men than in women. The differences in favor of women are said to be unusually great in black people, even in comparison to white women (Eisdorfer and Wilke 1972). In primitive races this component is definitely smaller than in N. Americans and in Germans (Plester 1962, Rosen et al. 1967, Kapur and Patt 1967). This is presumably accounted for by the more favorable circulatory and metabolic situation in contrast to that in the industrialized population. For this reason, the findings collected from the Mabaans may be equated with our physiological age component of hearing losses (cf. Fig. 42). However, a cardiovascular component of deafness is in no way to be regarded as inevitable in every case in the industrialized nations, either. Thus, Rubinstein et al. (1977) compared 23 healthy persons with 23 cardiovascular patients and in the "invalids" found a hearing loss that was smaller by about 8.5 dB. In the speech audiogram no difference could be demonstrated.

According to our own observations, the audiometric picture of inner ear deafness in old age is largely uniform as far as the suprathreshold tests are concerned (Lehnhardt 1977, Bumm et al. 1980). The respective findings are independent of the tone threshold curve, i.e. of the fact whether it shows a steep high tone fall (sensory, according to Schuknecht) an oblique high tone fall (neural, ganglionic), a flat course (metabolic) or a high tone diagonal fall (inner ear sound conduction). In spite of these varying patterns there are with great regularity findings in the sense of recruitment. SISI almost 100% ΔI (20 dB SL) <1 dB, no tone decay worth mentioning, in the Békésy test no separation of >20 dB, stapedius reflex threshold normal or only slightly raised. Up to the 8th decade even the relationships between the pure tone and speech audiogram correspond to those typical for young patients with inner ear deafness (Möller 1980, Stevenson 1975, Lehnhardt 1978). Even in the dichotic speech test a "surprisingly" good discrimination may often still be seen (Lehnhardt 1977).

What is detectable by the subjective audiometric tests including the stapedius reflex threshold thus appears to be only the disturbance of function in the hair cells. Even if an isolated degeneration of the ganglion cells is found, i.e. not combined with a corresponding destruction of hair cells (Crowe et al. 1934, Saxen 1952, Fleischer 1956, Suga and Lindsay 1976), this "ganglionic" constellation obviously is not reflected separately in the audiometric tests.

In the ECochG specific findings might possibly be expected from the summation potential (SP), but certainly only in inner ear sound conduction deafness according to Schuknecht, namely in so far as the stiffening of the oscillating sections of the inner ear might cause an additional (or a reduced?) asymmetry of the CM. So far the ECochG results have merely shown an atypically broadened, multiple peak CAP – however, in general only in "sensory-neural" deafness i.e. without any specificity for a particular type of inner ear deafness (Bergholtz et al. 1977). The maximum intensity of stimulus was around 75 dB HL, so that the SP could scarcely be recorded.

The decrease in the remote masking effect was regarded as a specific evidence for the *inner ear sound conduction type* with increased rigidity of the cochlear partition – depending on age, as is the case in Menière's hydrops (Cervellera et al. 1978, 1980). This means the rise in the threshold for low tones when masked by high frequency band noise of great intensity (Bilger and Hirsh 1956, Deatherage et al. 1957a, Bilger 1968, Burgeat and Hirsh 1961). This effect is attributed to non-linear distortions of the basilar membrane caused by the obscurity of a non-uniform signal (Deatherage et al. 1957b). The test is said to be regularly negative in an acoustic neurinoma and positive, above all, in hydrops. Up to the present time, no special findings have been presented as to whether the remote masking effect is also specific for Schuknecht's diagonal threshold pattern.

The differentiation of the diverse components comprised by the former collective term of presbyacusis is obstinately pursued here also of the purpose of preventing therapeutic nihilism. As long as every inner ear deafness developing beyond the age of sixty was interpreted as fateful, endogenous or due to old age, any thoughts about treatment seemed useless. We are unable to influence the *physiologic* age component of inner ear deafness and the neural or central decay, regardless of the fact that their effects on speech discrimination are only slight.

Furthermore, we are scarcely able to influence the *pathologic* age component of inner ear deafness; we must, however, endeavour to prevent its further progress. In general this will only be possible in agreement with the internist; for details see Chapter 3.6.2. It should be tried to arrest severe signs of central degeneration by medical treatment (Stutgeron, Encephabol etc). However, vasodilating preparations should only be prescribed with utmost reservation, especially in elderly patients.

Special guidelines apply to the prescription of hearing aids, insofar as infirm patients have difficulties in handling the apparatus and therefore often refuse even bilateral aids (Corso 1977). Mostly one should first of all prescribe *only one* device and wait to see the reaction of the patient; if need be the supply may be accomplished later. On account of its easy handling old patients should preferably receive a CROS-aid mounted in a spectacle-frame, possibly with an open mould (Schultz-Coulon 1983). This, however, is only promising, as long as the monosyllable discrimination at 65 dB is not yet completely lost without the aid. In addition, patients of advanced age often need some auditory training, particularly in the case of a late first fitting (Ventura 1978, Crammond and Gabb 1980).

A special point of view in the prescription of a hearing aid for the "presbyacusis" patient is that which has been mentioned above – namely that in old age the speech discrimination may deteriorate without the tone threshold suggesting this (Jerger 1973, Plath 1974). For checking the apparatus a control of the *tone* threshold is therefore not sufficient, and repeated *speech* audiometric tests are necessary.

3.8 Low Tone Deafness

Isolated low tone deafness deserves particular attention on account of its often fluctuating course and on account of its analogy or identity with Menière's deafness.

The audiometric picture displays a uniformity, insofar as only the low frequencies and, to a varying extent, also the middle frequencies are involved – at least at the beginning. The extension to the high tones takes a long time to appear.

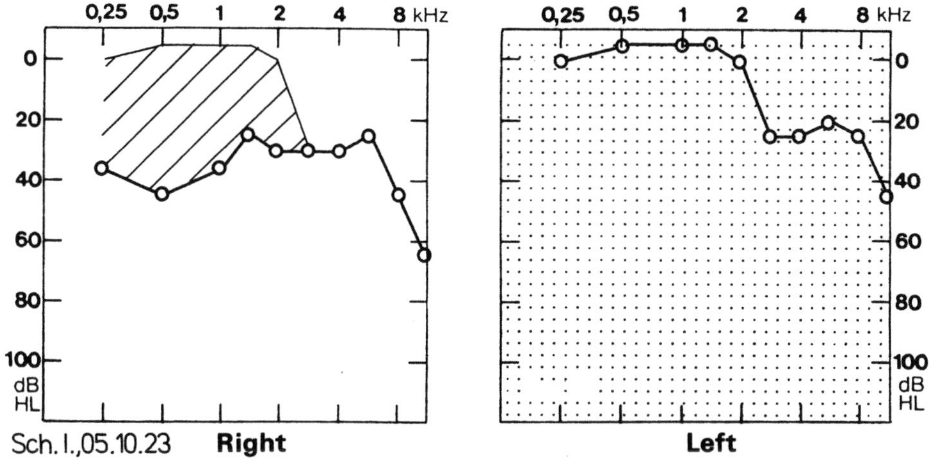

Fig. 44. Acute hearing loss in the low and middle frequencies on the right (*hatched*). Due to a pre-existing slight bilateral high tone loss the hearing threshold now shows an approximately flat curve on the right. BC = AC

If a – bilateral – high tone loss had already existed beforehand the acute low tone deafness may pretend a pantonal hearing loss. The individual components mostly become evident from the comparison with the opposite side (Fig. 44). The fluctuation may persist for a long time, the hearing loss may be consolidated near the norm or around the most unfavorable value of the fluctuation (Megighian 1982).

As regards the etiology, Paparella et al. (1979) suspect a silent or *insidious middle ear inflammation.* In a large-scale study of 560 temporal bone series the authors believe they have demonstrated and statistically confirmed a relationship between signs of inflammation in the window niches (without clinically striking findings in the tympanic membrane) and a hydrops which is chiefly *apical.* In 75 cases they also found subclinical inflammatory changes in the round window membrane as well as the mostly slight hydrops in the apical turn. Any significant decay of hair cells was not shown. This clinically inapparent infection would earlier exert an effect towards the interior than the serous or purulent form which develops towards the exterior.

The explanation given by P. H. Schmidt (1981) is still more "agressive". He had seen a low tone hearing loss in six patients with a *postoperative fistula in the oval window*, and in three patients with a leak from the round window. The operative improvement in hearing by bone conduction appeared likewise in the low tone region. Such a leak may obviously exist without any trauma being identified or, without a chronic perilymphatic hydrops predominating with a wide aquaeductus cochleae. We have also been able to confirm by surgery this cause of acute or fluctuating low tone deafness (Fig. 45). In how far, however, this explanation may be transferred to a larger number of cases of low-tone deafness, or even be assumed to be the rule, remains to be seen. Hitherto the indications for operative revision in such cases have been very carefully considered. In the

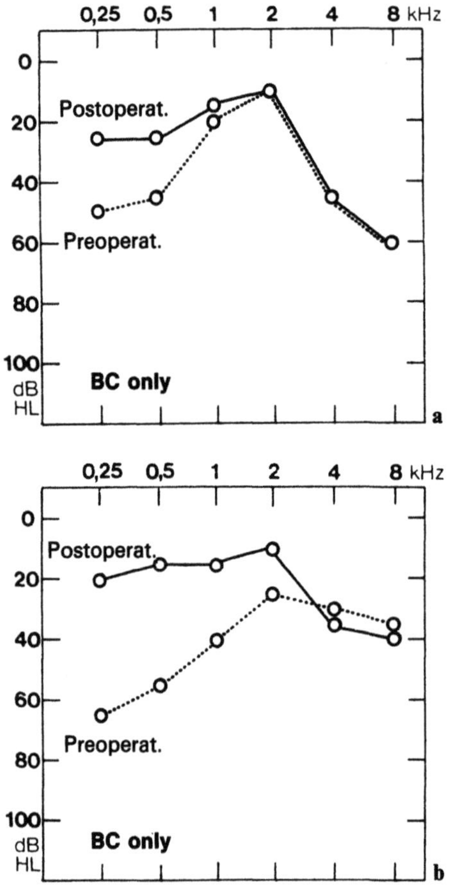

Fig. 45. a Low tone hearing loss after plastic surgery of the stapes with a fistula in the oval window. Closure of the fistula led to an improvement of bone conduction in the low frequencies. **b** Acute loss of hearing in the low frequencies without obvious trauma – personal observation. After closure of a perilymph fistula in the annular ligament of the oval window, bone conduction returned to normal (14.5.84; W., A., * 03.4.41)

case of a constant loss of perilymph through the round window membrane this would indeed be replaced by CSF but with a slight delay (Beentjes 1972). The sequel is a chronic fall in *peri*lymphatic pressure and hence a widening of the *endo*lymphatic sac.

In animal experiments the morphological substrate of a *low tone* related sensory cell damage, that is in the upper turns of the cochlea, was obtained by ligation of the artery of the labyrinth (Kimura and Perlman 1958, Bernstein and Silverstein 1966) or of the anterior inferior cerebellar artery (Afzelius and Aursnes 1979) – however, without endolymphatic hydrops.

In a study including 90 patients with fluctuating hearing disturbances Gosselin and Janick (1975) found in more than one half a slight low tone deafness (average hearing loss of 20 dB at 250 Hz), in more than a quarter a pantonal deafness and in a sixth a high tone hearing loss. Each of these 90 patients was reported to show a *metabolic disturbance*: Hyperlipoproteinemia (33 ×), hypoglycemia (58 ×), hypothyroidism (13 ×). The relevant diet or medical treatment had led to an improvement at least for subjective sensations such as tinnitus or sensation of repletion. However, the study appeared to be too much prejudiced from the audiological point of view to add any new aspects on low tone deafness.

In addition, there are opposing statements from comprehensive careful investigations. Among 204 patients with deafness in the course of Menière's disease (not exclusively low tone deafness) pathologic glucose metabolism was found in nine and thyroid hypofunction in four. In twelve of them the FTA-Abs Test proved to be positive; in each of them an acoustic neurinoma had been ruled out (Meyerhoff et al. 1981). Thus, a general metabolic disturbance may by no means be assumed in every low tone or pantonal deafness.

The *hereditary type* of low tone deafness with an autosomal dominant mode of inheritance (cf. Chap. 3.4.1) is congenital or it starts during early childhood, advances rapidly and already by the third decade has developed into nearly total deafness (Leon et al. 1981; cf. Fig. 20). Another form likewise starts during childhood, but shows only slight (Parving et al. 1978) or no progression (Vanderbilt group 1968). Yet others start only at the age of 20 or 30, progress slowly, but are *not fluctuating* (Konigsmark et al. 1971). These hereditary forms cannot be distinguished to any significant degree from the nongenetic ones either by the tone threshold or by the results of the suprathreshold tests. ECochG findings as well as histological ones are obviously not yet available (Konigsmark and Gorlin 1976), so that nothing more precise is known about the type of the hereditary hearing failure.

All ideas about low tone deafness – with the exception of the hereditary forms(?) – proceed from the assumption that it results from an endolymphatic hydrops – indeed, it is regarded as the prototype of a hydropic reaction. The fluctuation and the frequent reversibility suggest that the function of the affected hair cells has not yet been extinguished but only transitorily impaired. Nevertheless, the recruitment phenomenon shows the same pattern as for example in the irreversible hair cell degeneration caused by noise or ototoxics. In animal experiments an endolymphatic hydrops could be produced by changes in the perilymph components or by destruction of the saccus endolymphaticus (Kimura et al. 1962, Schuknecht et al. 1962, Kimura 1967, Beal 1968, Zechner 1973, 1976, 1980, Schuknecht and Richter 1980).

Tonndorf (1968, 1976) tried to find a physical explanation of the question why in hydropic impairment of hearing the low frequencies are predominantly affected (Fig. 46). He was able to show in models of the cochlea that during *acute* episodes of hydrops, the difference in pressure between endo- and peri-lymph is decisive whereas under *chronic* conditions it is the *mass loading* by increased volume of the ductus cochlearis. With pressure differences, the rigidity gradient decreases towards the apex of the cochlea which results in a low tone loss. Mass loads, on the other hand, lead to a deafness involving all frequencies, that is to a flat curve. Probably both conditions continually merge into each other.

Also the recruitment in low tone deafness may be derived from the *physical* characteristics of the endolymphatic hydrops; this must be done above all, if the failure in the outer hair cells is too slight to explain the recruitment in the same way as e.g. in degenerative hair cell damage.

As a sequel to the hydrops one may assume an interruption in the contact of the stereocilia with the tectorial membrane (Kimura et al. 1976). This may be caused by swelling of the tectorial membrane (Tumarkin 1957), by an increased bulging of the basilar membrane (Boenninghaus et al. 1967), or e.g. by a loss of rigidity of the stereocilia (Tonndorf 1976). In order to explain the balancing of loudness as a sequel to such changes Tonndorf (1981) referred to the phenomenon of *center-clippings*. The decoupling resulted in a central gap which would become smaller and finally ineffective with increasing amplitude, a behaviour which would correspond to the recruitment. Feldmann (personal communication) objected to this explanation, arguing that the decoupling of the tectorial membrane and the cilia of the hair cells would rather lead to a *peak clipping*.

The question arises whether it is at all justified to regard the development of the hydrops and its auditory phenomena as exclusively mechanical. Possibly this applies only to the endolymphatic hydrops resulting from continual loss of perilymph. In the case of "insidious inflammatory" hydrops permanent damage to the sensory cells will probably develop soon. In experiments

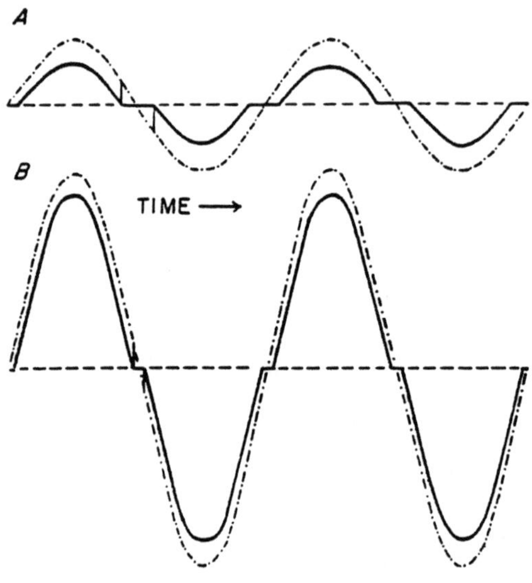

Fig. 46 A, B. Tonndorf's conception of the physics of recruitment in endolymphatic hydrops, with hair cells still capable of recovery. **A** Dotted line shows the wave form of the healthy ear, the continuous line the *center-clipped* wave form. Amplitude distinctly reduced. **B** Like **A** but with three times the amplitude. The plateau at the zero crossing becomes increasingly smaller: center clipping. (From Tonndorf 1980)

the cause of the hydrops is the disturbed resorption of endolymph in the saccus endolymphaticus. However, this will probably not just consist in an interference with water absorption by the saccus endolymphaticus (Arnold and Vosteen 1979). It may rather be assumed that after obliteration of the ductus endolymphaticus the hydrops develops by an accumulation of osmotically active substances in the endolymphatic space. In any case Morgenstern et al. (1982) were able to provide evidence for the assumption that it is not only water which is resorbed in the epithelium of the saccus endolymphaticus, but that there exists an *active* transport mechanism which fails after the occlusion of the ductus endolymphaticus.

In audiometry, low tone deafness is always to be classified as inner ear related; in unilateral deafness, the recruitment is always positive, the SISI test reaches 100%, however, only if – as is typical for the low tones – the loss of hearing amounts to ≧50 dB, and the noise audiogram, too, corresponds to an inner ear lesion (although Langenbeck had not seen this). In fluctuating low tone deafness the stapedius reflex threshold occasionally shows a slight elevation in the frequency range affected; in general, however, it also reflects the picture of recruitment (Fig. 47).

Since in low tone deafness we are concerned with the audiometric registration not only of the recruitment but also of the hydrops, psychoacoustic tuning curves might be of value here. They ought to display a broadening because the basilar membrane is stretched by the hydrops and because the frequency selectivity, as explained above, is already determined by the micromechanics (Morgenstern et al. 1983). However, really specific findings of any value have not yet been presented.

In the ECochG, low tone deafness shows the summation potential (SP) which is described. It is superimposed at ≧80 dB on the action potential and widens this (Schmidt 1976, Gibson et al. 1977, Hirasagi et al. 1979, Moffat 1979, Mangabeira-Albernaz et al. 1981, Coats and Alford 1981). The finding is supposed to have proved specific for low tone deafness or that which begins in the low tone region (Fig. 48). This would provide a criterion easy to recognise because measurements would only have to be performed at *one* great intensity and because the recording of the CAP together with the summation potential requires the smallest expenditure of time and technique in the ECochG. A quantitative assessment of the SP, however, is scarcely possible (cf. Chap. 2.2). The endocochlear *DC-potential* which can only be registered in animal experiments

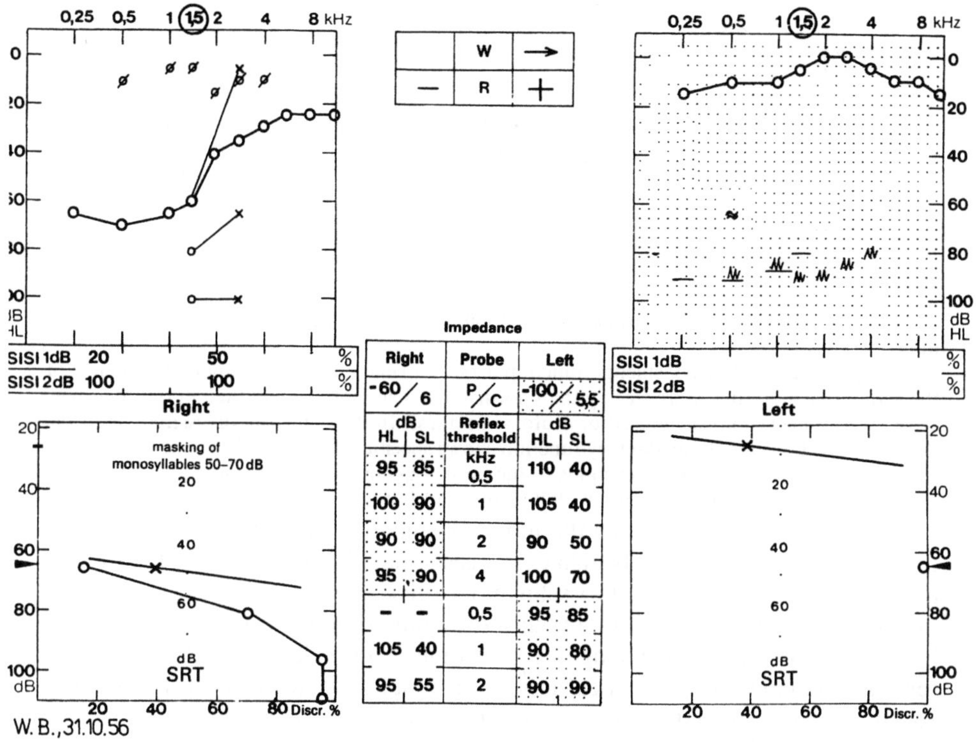

Impedance

Right		Probe	Left	
-60/6		P/C	-100/5,5	
dB HL	dB SL	Reflex threshold kHz	dB HL	dB SL
95	85	0,5	110	40
100	90	1	105	40
90	90	2	90	50
95	90	4	100	70
–	–	0,5	95	85
105	40	1	90	80
95	55	2	90	90

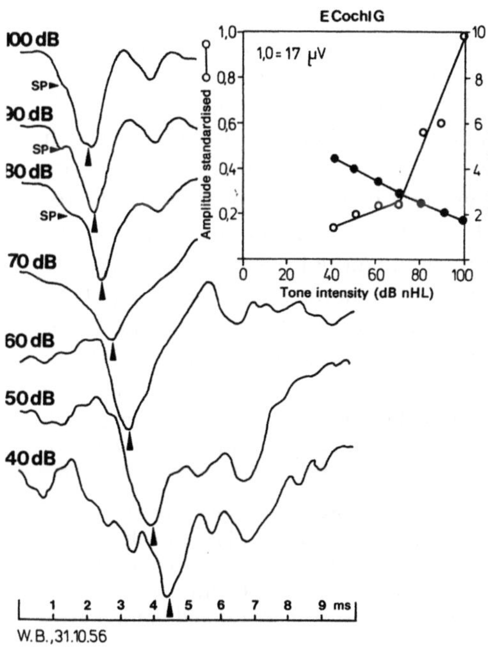

Fig. 47. a Low tone deafness (right) fluctuating and progressive for the last twelve years. Fowler positive. SISI in the low frequencies only at 2 dB 100%. Stapedius reflex threshold slightly increased. BC = AC. For symbols of masking see Figs. 32 and 36. **b** ECochG (right) 4000 Hz alternating click 20/s follow-up-rate. The CAP is recordable from 40 dB, strikingly steep input-output function. N_2 not here, characteristic for low tone deafness. The amplitude function illustrates the characteristic kink at 70 dB

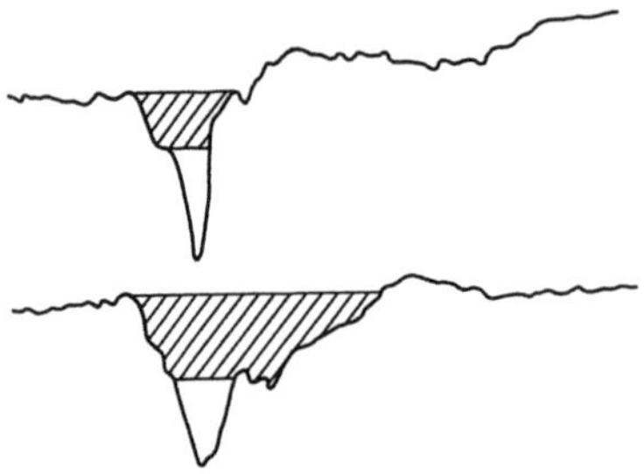

Fig. 48. *Above*: Normal response made up by the action potential (CAP) and the summation potential (SP). *Below*: "Spread out" response due to disproportionate SP-component, allegedly the characteristic picture in endolymphatic hydrops. (From Morrison et al. 1980)

had not changed during the experimental development of the hydrops (Morgenstern and Miyamoto 1979).

In hydrops, the electrocochleographic input-output function for amplitude and latency of the action potential runs more steeply than normal and also more steeply than in the "degenerative" recruitment of noise-induced or ototoxic deafness. In the same way the regression of the double-logarithmic amplitude-latency function shows specific findings for low tone deafness, at least at the early stage i.e. it corresponds to the norm – again in contrast to the hair cell degeneration in high tone deafness (Schmidt 1976, Hoke and Lütkenhöner 1981).

The *fluctuation* seems to be the most conspicuous characteristic of low tone deafness. There may certainly also exist occasional high tone hearing losses with a variable hearing threshold (Gosselin and Yanick 1976), but they are far less frequent and the "fluctuation" there has a different etiology, as for example in the hearing loss associated with Cogan's syndrome. Above all, this fluctuation is observed in unilateral low tone deafness. Occasionally it extends to both sides to a varying extent, so that now one side and then again the other is worse off (Lehnhardt and Hesch 1980).

Low tone deafness may improve and again deteriorate within days or even hours, without any identifiable cause. The attempt to provoke with medicine the remaining possibility of an improvement in hearing, is represented by the glycerol test (Klockhoff and Lindblom 1966). The improvement in hearing after glycerol is judged by some authors as a *conditio sine qua non* for the diagnosis of low tone deafness from hydrops (Morgenstern 1983). Others will only regard it as a positive result if the response to glycerol shows a gain in hearing as compared with the *best* threshold within the last six months (Sauer and Kaemmerle 1981). Those criticising the test argue that they can do without it since the *spontaneous* fluctuation of itself is a more reliable index for the hydrops being the cause of the deafness (Norre and Jessurun 1980). In order to create more favorable preconditions for the action of glycerol, Arenberg et al. (1974) recommended giving the patient a high sodium diet, prior to the test. However, one should be cautious about this recommendation, since it may lead to a *deterioration* in hearing (Bodo et al. 1983). Negative results are all the more likely the flatter the course of the tone threshold (Soldatov and Khrapp 1979) however, only if the initial hearing loss was small, because in these cases a complete return to normal values cannot be expected with glycerol.

Urea is supposed to have a regulatory effect on the hydrops, in the same way as glycerol, i.e. via an increase in the serum osmolarity. Ethanol or mannitol, both of which equally increase the serum osmolarity would have no favorable effect because they diffuse too rapidly into the inner ear (Juhn et al. 1979, Angelborg et al. 1979). However, according to other observations, both ethanol and mannitol also stimulate blood circulation in the inner ear and brain (Larsen et al. 1981, 1982).

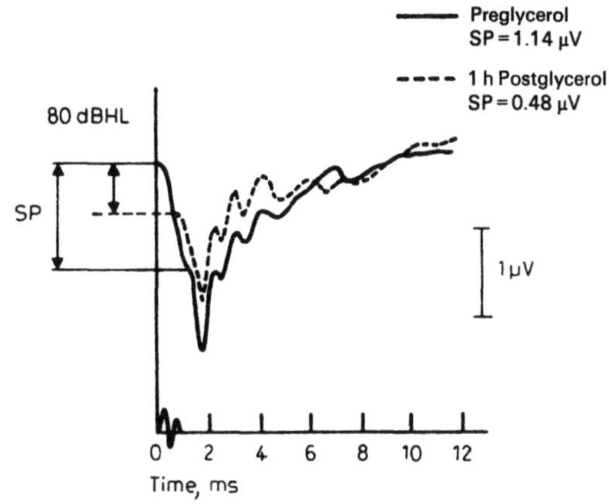

Fig. 49. Decrease of the SP after administration of glycerol (from Menière's Disorders by Extratympanic ECochG 1983). The picture illustrates at the same time the difficulty to assess the SP, especially as in this example along with the fading away of the SP the CAP spreads out and becomes smaller in amplitude

Although the statements in the literature about the Klockhoff test are so contradictory, it remains an established fact that glycerol (2–3 hours after administration of 1.5 g/kg bodyweight) has an effect on the metabolism of the inner ear, predominantly of the stria vascularis (Juhn 1977, Duvall et al. 1980). Glycerol seems not only to reduce the hydrops, but also to exert a favorable influence on the micro-circulation as is shown by the rise in the endolymphatic oxygen pressure in guinea pigs (Prazma 1981). The improvement in hearing may be demonstrated objectively by the SP in the ECochG: under glycerol its amplitude becomes *smaller* (Fig. 49) (Coats and Alford 1981). The glycerol test is therefore suitable for the diagnosis of hydrops; however, it is advisable to critically evaluate the results which may possibly have been influenced by subjective impressions (Thomsen and Vesterhauge 1979). An uncritical use of the test in every vague suspicion of a hydrops may bring it into disrepute quite unreasonably.

What is of value in the differential diagnosis is the observation that low tone and pantonal deafness are obviously never found as the direct sequel to damage by noise or blast and not even after ototoxic medication; only Chung and Gannon (1980) thought that in one case they could attribute a low tone deafness, and thus a hydrops, to occupational noise exposure. In general, however, a flat tone threshold in a hearing disturbance which appeared *during* noise exposure – possibly with additional cervicovertebral strain (Boenninghaus 1959) – is considered to indicate that the noise could not have been the sole cause of deafness (acoustic accident, Becker and Matzker 1961).

Low tone deafness also appears to be the only tone threshold pattern that does *not* suggest an acoustic neurinoma or a cerebellopontine angle lesion, although it is precisely the irregularity of the frequency pattern which is typical for these disorders. As regards the flat tone threshold this does no longer apply.

Low tone deafness in Menière's disease [6] has no characteristics which would not be found in the same clinical picture without vertigo – with or without fluctuation (Lehnhardt 1976). Whether the x-ray findings regarded as pathogeneti-

[6] It was decided not to include Menière's disease in the monograph since the subject would then become too widely extended and, in addition, it would have required the differential diagnosis of vertigo. Tinnitus was therefore also deliberately omitted.

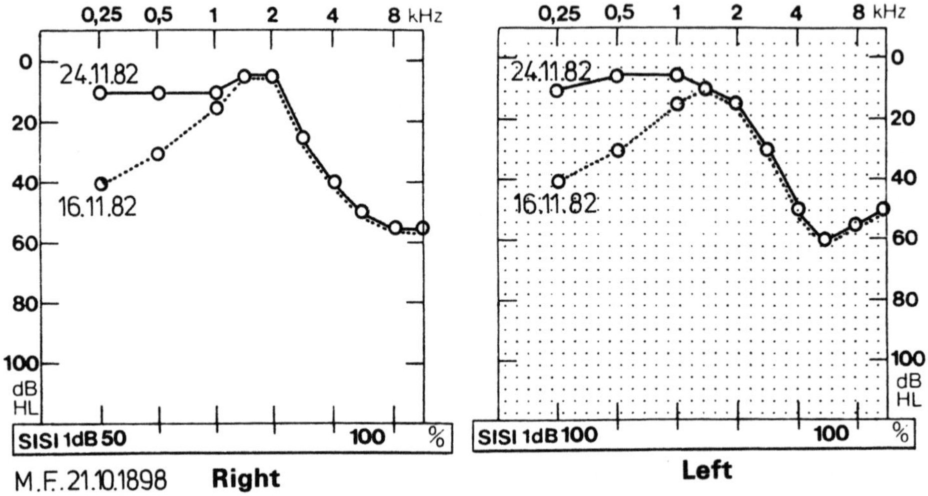

Fig. 50. Nearly symmetrical, acute, bilateral low tone deafness which regressed again within a few days. Pre-existing bilateral high tone loss. BC = AC

cally significant for Menière's disease, particularly the shortness and narrowness of the aquaeductus cochleae (Stahle and Wilbrand 1983), do also apply to isolated low tone deafness, must for the present remain undecided.

On account of its irregular pattern, fluctuating low tone deafness often represents such a difficult finding for the otologist that he is inclined to attribute it etiologically to emotional factors, in the sense of a psychosomatic dysfunction (Lehnhardt and Hesch 1980), as was only recently again assumed for Menière's disease on the basis of a broad classification (n = 457) of causal factors (Oosterveld 1981). Psychosomatic hearing impairment would only at an early stage have to be interpreted as a functional but in the end as an organic lesion in contrast to the exclusively functional psychogenic hearing disturbance.

We have occasionally also seen a low tone deafness after spinal anesthesia in urological patients (Panning et al. 1983). These disturbances of hearing had developed almost symmetrically and were transitory (Fig. 50). The suprathreshold tests suggested a disturbance of function in the sense organ. Reflections on the possible cause of these hearing losses led back to the "pressure ear" (*Druckohr*), as Hommerich (1963) had called it. He also described hearing losses involving either the low tones only or all the frequencies, which in his cases were caused by increased intracranial pressure. It is possible that such or analogous events occur in spinal anesthesia, at least temporarily. Grant et al. (1985) attribute two cases of transient bilateral low frequency hearing loss following myelography not to spinal punction but to metrizamide.

3.9 Middle Ear Causes of Inner Ear Deafness

In this connection there is no need to deal with tympanogenic labyrinthitis, especially as no new clinical aspects of this disorder have been presented. Also the possibility that a sero- or mucotympanum can mimic a sensori-neural deafness – although in fact it only impedes the hydrodynamics of the inner ear by direct contact of the secretion with the round window membrane and possibly simultaneously with the footplate of the stapes (Münker 1977, Plath 1983) – shall only be pointed out once again. The attempt to explain the fall in bone conduction here by an impaired O_2-transfer from the middle ear mucous membrane to the inner ear (Morgenstern 1980) seems a little far-fetched. The idea of Paparella et al. (1979) that subclinical inflammations in the window niches might be the cause of a low tone sensori-neural deafness has been discussed at length (cf. Chap. 3.8). Inner ear damage caused by the application of ototoxic agents into the tympanic cavity was also discussed in the relevant chapter (cf. Chap. 3.2).

The effect of a round window rupture on inner ear function in the case of a sero- or mucotympanum, was investigated by Fukaja and Nomura (1983) (cf. Chap. 3.1.3.1). The possibility of an explosive rupture is said to exist particularly if a low pressure prevails in the middle ear. The escaping perilymph may mix with the secretion of the tympanic effusion and vice versa; the result is a high tone impairment of the inner ear.

Arnold (1974) pointed out the close relationships of the lymphatic drainage channels of the inner ear to those of the middle ear mucous membrane in the area of the windows. It seems likely that e.g. staphylococcal exotoxins from the middle ear by this pathway produce inflammatory cellular reactions initially in the scala tympani and then also in the aquaeductus cochleae (Schachern et al. 1981). If this route is assumed in extremely mild middle ear infections and a hydropic inner ear reaction (Paparella et al. 1979), it is all the more likely in a clinically obvious otitis media with impairment of the high tone region (Moore and Best 1980, and many others).

An involvement of the inner ear is said to exist even in bullous myringitis and indeed also in those cases in which the complement fixation reaction to virus antibodies remains negative (Stephen and Abramson 1979). With a positive reaction to varicella one would suspect a zoster infection of the inner ear to be an accompanying finding or the cause of the myringitis and the otalgia. Feinmesser et al. (1980) believe they have identified mycoplasma as the pathogen in one case with inner ear involvement (Fig. 51).

With increased blockage of the middle ear in otosclerosis the inner ear is also involved (Zechner 1977, Fikentscher et al. 1982). It remains unclear *how* this inner ear component develops. From the late results after stapedectomy it may be assumed that in relation to age, the bone conduction *does not deteriorate further* as compared with the stabilised postoperative value. (Smyth and Hassard 1978, Strauss and Strahl 1976, Virolainen et al. 1980, Dieroff 1981) – a result, however, which by itself does not allow any conclusions regarding the origin of the inner ear component in middle ear otosclerosis. Various factors have been made responsible for occasional inner ear high tone losses following stapedectomy: Acoustic or mechanical trauma, mild infection, activation of otosclerotic foci (Beickert 1979). Bockmüller (1983) considers the etiology to be not at all clarified. Cancura (1983) thinks he can explain the bone conduction high tone loss by the mechanics of the connective tissue prosthesis.

As regards the question of "otosclerotic" inner ear deafness *without any middle ear component* Freeman (1979) argued that in many cases of progressive inner ear deafness otosclerosis must be considered as a cause, and that corresponding foci in the capsule of the labyrinth could be detected by X-ray polyto-

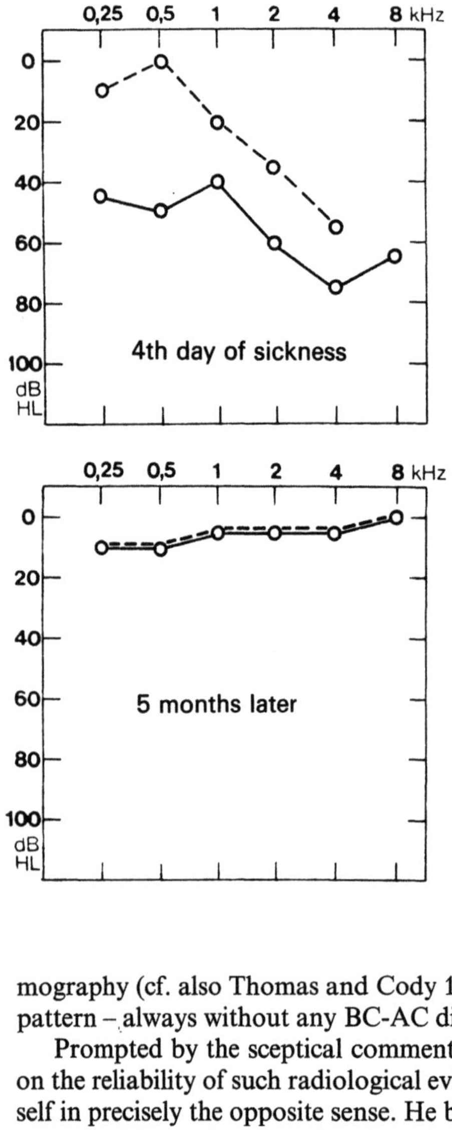

Fig. 51. *Above*: Audiogram of a bullous myringitis with combined middle and inner ear deafness. *Below*: After complete healing of the ear drum the *bone conduction also* returned to normal. (From Wetmore and Abramson 1979)

mography (cf. also Thomas and Cody 1981) – independent of the tone threshold pattern – always without any BC-AC difference.

Prompted by the sceptical comments of Applebaum and Shambaugh (1978) on the reliability of such radiological evidence Schuknecht (1979) expressed himself in precisely the opposite sense. He believes he has proved, on the basis of his extensive histological material, that a hearing loss *exclusively* due to inner ear disturbances cannot be caused by otosclerosis; if the otosclerotic alterations are severe enough to cause an inner ear deafness they would always have led to a fixation of the stapes, too.

Cochleo-tympanic bone scintigraphy (Bornemann et al. 1982) may perhaps contribute to this dispute; in the orientational studies so far published (n = 20) no otosclerotic foci have been discovered in progressive deafness due to inner ear disturbances. Or it will be possible, by peculiarities of the stapedius reflex, to identify a beginning ankylosis of the stapes in certain types of deafness apparently purely due to inner ear disturbances. Terkildsen et al. (1973) had described the negative on-off reactions in patients with a "minimal" BC–AC difference. Forquer and Sheehy (1981) claim to have seen the same reaction also in pure inner ear deafness, that is without any middle ear component. We have not been able to verify this (Lehnhardt et al. 1976).

The hope of finding a characteristic HLA-association for otosclerosis has not so far been fulfilled (Chobaut et al. 1982). Whatever criteria of an inner ear related otosclerosis might be put forward, we are still far from a *broad*, largely indiscriminate prophylactic administration of fluorides, as recommended by Causse and Causse (1980).

Middle ear disorders equally induce those types of inner ear deafness which appear quite regularly with osteogenesis imperfecta (Bergstrom 1981) and more distinctly with increasing age; their genesis, however, is completely unknown (Pedersen and Elbrond 1979, Riedner et al. 1980).

3.10 Immunological Diseases

We are grateful to Stephens et al. (1982) for a well arranged survey of those immunological diseases which are of interest to the ENT-specialist. If confined to those involving the inner ear, the only relevant auto-antibody-mediated illnesses are:

- the Vogt-Koyanagi-Harada syndrome
- "auto-immune deafness" and
- the generalised vasculitides, including
  Polyarteritis nodosa
  Behçet's syndrome
  Panchondritis
  Wegener's granulomatosis
  Giant cell temporal arteritis
  Cogan's syndrome

It appears necessary to place such a classification at the beginning in order to build up a differential diagnosis of these diseases which have, up to now, only slightly impinged on otology.

The *Vogt-Koyanagi-Harada syndrome* includes a granulomatous uveitis with generalised pigment disturbances, meningitic symptoms and inner ear deafness. Though the disease is seen almost exclusively in Japan it has pathophysiological importance insofar as antimelanin-antibodies could be demonstrated here (Hammer 1974). For this reason, the deafness, too, is considered to be a reaction to a loss of pigment in the cochlea. The hearing loss is reported to be mostly only trifling and "fluctuating", but possibly also extreme (Maxwell 1963).

Auto-immune inner ear deafness was described by McCabe (1979) as a separate clinical entity. He reported on 18 patients with inner ear deafness which for the most part had begun suddenly, was bilateral and progressive – sometimes with disturbances of equilibrium or also with facial paresis and destruction in the middle ear or in the mastoid (!). The course of the deafness is said to be pathognomonic, in so far as it progresses rapidly within weeks or months but develops more slowly than the "sudden hearing loss". The deafness may be distinguished from Menière's disease by the absence of fluctuation, and from syphilitic labyrinthitis by the negative serological tests. The facial palsy is reported to have always improved without any surgical measures. Only in one patient observed over ten years he was able to detect a vasculitis by histological examination and that was in the mucous membrane of the mastoid process. All the other laboratory results had been negative, with the exception of the lymphocyte aggregation inhibition assay (LAIA) against inner ear antigen which had been obtained from destructive operations of the labyrinth. This test had been carried out in six patients and had always shown a positive result. Nevertheless, the author stresses that the test is coarse and its specificity has not yet been proved. Furthermore, the CSF concentration of protein and IgM was said to be increased. An improvement in hearing had always been attainable, if the hearing loss had not been total. The treatment consisted in cyclophosphamide and dexamethasone. Since the hearing consistently got worse after discontinuing the medication, the author recommends its continuation for at least eight months, possibly for up to two years.

This report was taken up again, first of all by Kanzaki and O-Uchi (1981) who in four cases had also seen an improvement in hearing during the administration of corticoids. In some patients they were able to detect an abnormally high concentration of immune complex (IC), as is known from lupous nephritis. Meanwhile the same authors (1983) have reported on raised IC-levels in 53 patients with bilateral inner ear deafness. In 47 cases the cause of deafness was not known, in five patients the tests for syphilis had been positive and in one there was an aortitis. High IC values had been found only in four of the cases of deafness with uncertain etiology, as well as in the one with arteritis, and only these four patients responded to the steroid medication – however, two other patients *without* raised IC levels responded in the same way. All of them were women.

Elies et al. (1981) thought they could confirm the high levels of individual immune globulin fractions and/or the total protein in the CSF of patients with inner ear deafness and interpret them as an "inflammatory reaction with corresponding antigen-antibody involvement". In one case treated by them tissue antibodies against vascular endothelium had been identified by means of the indirect immuno-fluorescence test. These antibodies would have to be considered as an etiological marker for an infection or a virus-induced process. Antibodies against the basilar membrane of the guinea pig had also been detectable. Treatment with dexamethasone had produced a complete regression of bilateral deafness within 14 days (Elies 1983). In his statements Elies refers particularly to Arnold et al. (1976), Quick (1973) and Weidauer et al. (1976, 1977) who had been able to detect immune complex in the basilar membrane and in the vessels of the stria vascularis, as in Masugi-nephritis and in Alport's syndrome. Also in cases of progressive deafness of uncertain etiology Arnold (1984) has recently produced indirect immunofluorescent microscopic evidence of IgA antibodies in the patient's serum namely in formalin-fixated and EDTA-decalcified human temporal bones. The reactions were, among others, directed against the marginal cells of the stria vascularis and against the perilymphatic layer of Reissner's membrane. Arnold considers it a technical advantage that these reactions can be produced on the "fixed" inner ear; his pictures are actually very impressive.

Stephens et al. (1982) are more cautious and wish to await the results of further investigations in order to be able to decide whether auto-immune deafness actually represents an independent illness or merely a variant of the generalised vasculitides which happens to be located in the inner ear.

Periarteritis nodosa scarcely ever affects the inner ear directly, as it mainly involves the larger vessels, but either within the picture of *Wegener's granulomatosis* or as *Cogan's syndrome* (Zechner 1980). A *giant cell temporal arteritis* is only exceptionally seen in the inner ear, either (Pietersen and Carlsen 1966). In a description of the histological changes in periarteritis nodosa of the inner ear (Gussen 1977), it is interesting to read that among other things there was an endolymphatic hydrops, a finding which bears no relation to the sequels to a vascular occlusion (Kimura and Perlman 1958, Gussen 1976). Quite extraordinary, but apparently confirmed, is the coexistence of periarteritis nodosa and *otosclerosis* (Druss and Maybaum 1934, Stephens 1982). In Cogan's syndrome, too, otosclerosis is allegedly included in the histological differential diagnosis (Wolff et al. 1965).

A special form of periarteritis is Takajasu arteritis, a vasculitis of the aortic arch (Wada 1976). The deafness which is occasionally related to it is not a symptom of this disease (Currier et al. 1954, Wada 1976), at all events, the deafness described by Nomura and Kitamura (1979) in a Takajasu patient was not of vascular origin.

Behçet's syndrome, with lesions of the mucous membranes especially in the mouth, as well as with arthritic symptoms, also belongs to the vasculitides with perivascular infiltration of mononuclear leucocytes. According to an individual communication, 10 out of 16 Behçet patients had suffered from bilateral inner ear deafness – presumably as a late complication of this clinical condition (Brama and Faineru 1980). Corticosteroid immuno-suppressive treatment – if started in good time – may lead to an improvement of hearing in these cases (Krauer and Pfaltz 1981).

Finally, 25% of the panchondritides (relapsing polychondritis), which are included among the autoimmune diseases, are supposed to show an advanced hearing loss (n = 40) which is interpreted by some authors as a sequel to arteritis (Cody et al. 1971) and by others as a *viral* endolabyrinthitis which, on its part, followed from the susceptibility of autoimmune patients to viral infections (Hoshino et al. 1980).

The lesion which underlies *Wegener's granulomatosis* is a necrotising vasculitis, in the sense of an auto-immune disease. Just because of the fact that it is nowadays described as a pneumogenous granulomatosis (Wegener 1967), the involvement of the middle ear is easy to understand. The inner ear is affected shortly afterwards, clinically recognisable as a special, *subacutely* developing *combined* middle and inner ear deafness. The alterations of the ear drum are mild, at all events nowadays with corticosteroid and azathioprin medication. Indeed, this finding is numbered among the otorhinological cardinal symptoms of Wegener's granulomatosis (Survey by Lehnhardt 1977). The accompanying orbital, pulmonary or renal symptoms may vary a lot in appearance and will remain all the more discrete the earlier treatment is started. At least one of McCabe's cases, namely the one with the mastoiditis and facial palsy, would probably have to be classified as Wegener's disease – possibly also the other four patients with facial palsy.

With the possibilities of modern treatment, the clinical picture of Wegener's granulomatosis has changed so much that even *supposedly isolated* ear diseases are conceivable with such a mild otitis media that the inner ear deafness becomes the most prominent feature.

Well-documented and probably more uniform in its signs and symptoms is *Cogan's syndrome* with non-syphilitic interstitial keratitis and cochleovestibular symptoms (Cogan 1945). It appears mostly in the second and third decade (Haynes et al. 1980), but it was also observed in a 12-year-old boy (Kundell and Ochs 1980). Deafness develops relatively acutely and possibly on both sides; it is progressive. With unilateral symptoms and pains around the ear a herpes zoster oticus must be excluded by differential diagnosis, especially as even in Cogan's syndrome the ear drum may be injected and appear thickened (Pausch et al. 1982). The vestibular function, too, is often reduced or abolished (Haynes et al. 1981; Feldmann, personal communication). There is no doubt about this disease belonging to the generalised vasculitides, as is shown clearly by multiple vascular

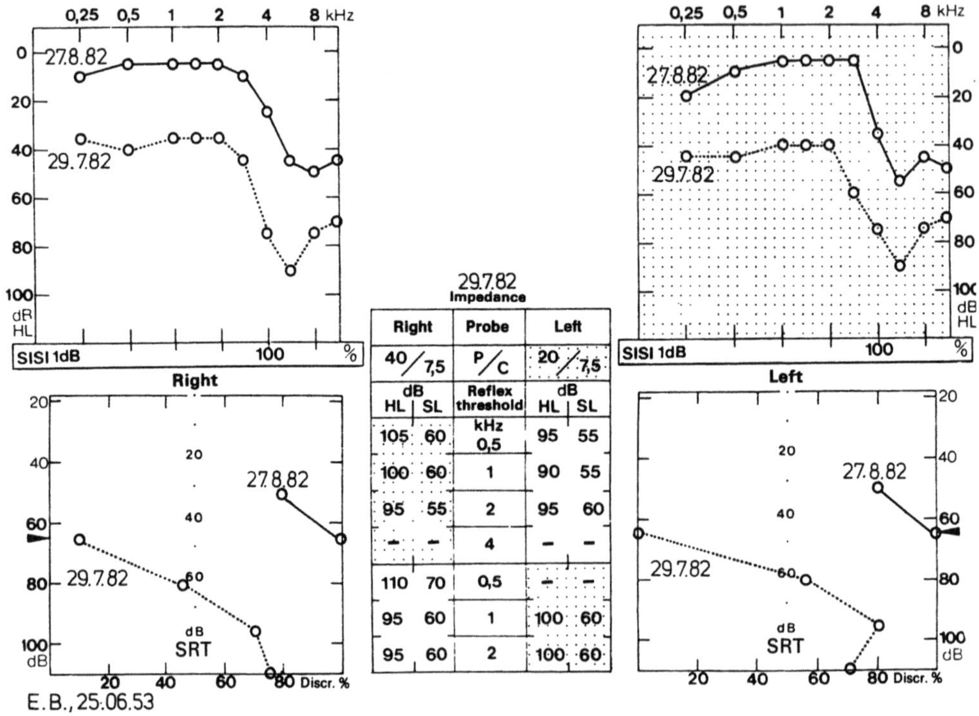

Right		Probe	Left	
40/7,5		P/C	20/7,5	
dB HL	SL	Reflex threshold kHz	dB HL	SL
105	60	0,5	95	55
100	60	1	90	55
95	55	2	95	60
–	–	4	–	–
110	70	0,5	–	–
95	60	1	100	60
95	60	2	100	60

Fig. 52. Cogan's syndrome. Improvement of hearing with prednison 50 mg/day and indometacin (Amuno®) 3 × 50 mg/day. At the same time the ophthalmological findings also regressed. The patient has now been symptom-free for one year. The hearing has remained unchanged. BC = AC

occlusions in the digital arteries (Pausch et al. 1982) or histological findings corresponding to periarteritis nodosa (Aupy et al. 1980). Only Nomoto et al. (1981) do not consider Cogan's syndrome to be an expression of *generalised* vasculitis.

In Cogan's syndrome deafness regularly affects all frequencies, but preferentially the high tone region (Wolff et al. 1965, Morgenstern and Arnold 1981, Bornholdt et al. 1982). The suprathreshold findings indicate an inner ear lesion, the potential reversibility and the histological findings an endolymphatic hydrops (Wolff et al. 1965, Zechner 1980). The prospects for successful treatment of the inner ear deafness depend predominantly on the time of onset of the medication: Corticosteroids and possibly azathioprin (Haynes et al. 1981, Krauer and Pfaltz 1981) (Fig. 52). However, therapy resistance has been observed in spite of an early start of treatment, even resulting in total deafness (Kantor 1981).

Thirty years after the first description of the syndrome named after him, Cogan tried to clarify the question as to which abnormal immunological reactions play a part in the pathophysiology of this disease. No clues have been found indicating any *unspecific* cell-linked or humoral immunological changes. However, he believed that in three of four patients he had identified the HLA W-17 which in a normal population is met with in only 3–10% (Char et al. 1975). At first, this finding seemed to have been confirmed (Del Carpio et al. 1976), finally, however, it did not prove to be correct, as indicated by a study of 11 patients (Cheson 1977, Kaiser-Kupfer et al. 1978, Heinemann et al. 1980).

The association of Cogan's syndrome with an HL-antigen would have been interesting in view of the fact that such an antigen is also suspected in some familial and etiologically unclear cases of infantile deafness. As regards these, Gross and Arndt-Hanser (1982) believe they have found above all the antigens B_{18} and BW_{16}. After the experiences with Cogan's syndrome, however, one should await the results of large-scale test series.

The inner ear disorder in Wegener's disease and in Cogan's syndrome is certainly due to an auto-immune reaction in the *vessel wall*. As regards the individual resulting reactions, there are nowadays detailed but also still speculative conceptions. The damaged vascular endothelium and the exposed subendothelial collagen, by interaction with the prostacyclin of the thrombocytes, might lead to a disequilibrium between prostacyclin and thromboxan and hence to microthrombi. In this process not only acetylsalicylic acid but also indomethazine intervenes (Bornholdt et al. 1982, Matthias 1983).

In contrast to this, McCabe interprets his bilateral, progressive inner ear deafness as an auto-immune reaction aimed *directly* at the *structures of the inner ear*. Such a clinical entity would meet the wishes of the otologists, because there would be a chance of therapeutic control, in the hope of an – at least partially – reversible hydropic disturbance of inner ear function.

It would be all the more inappropriate now, on the basis of such isolated observations, to declare the majority of inner ear hearing disturbances to be an immuno-pathological process and to "treat" them with corticoids – possibly even for years! Certainly we are caught in a dilemma between therapeutic helplessness and the inexorable fate of total deafness. However, the justification of the decision to accept the side-effects of the corticosteroids, which on their part also affect the vascular system, necessitates in every single case a thorough consultation with a competent internist. As long as there is no convincing evidence of an auto-immune process in "McCabe's deafness", one should more often decide on being cautious.

Incidentally, the *intellectual* concept of an auto-immune reaction in the inner ear is an older one, however, only referring to the *successive loss of hearing in the second ear* (Lehnhardt 1958). With this special symptom complex the antibody reaction might be directed against the antigen of the inner ear which was first deaf (cf. Fig. 39). However, in the patients concerned no antigen against cellular elements of the inner ear could be demonstrated (Beickert 1961). Up to the present time, such an auto-immune reaction has not been reproducible in animal experiments, either – possibly on account of the time factor, for the loss of hearing in the second ear usually develops in man only after an interval of 10–15 years.

Schuknecht et al. (1973) described the morphological findings of a deafness in the second ear thirteen years after that of the first one. According to these, the wide aquaeductus cochleae would have enabled virus circulating in the CSF to reach one inner ear first and later the second one – no indication therefore of an antigen-antibody reaction.

It might also be assumed that an auto-immune reaction even of *both ears* ensues from an earlier unilateral or bilateral *partial* lesion of the inner ear structures and thus leads to the clinical picture of auto-immune impairment of hearing. In the meantime such an auto-immune hearing loss could successfully be produced in rats and mice (Yoo et al. 1982). The hearing responses were recorded by means of brain stem AEP, and the perivascular reaction was observed by immunofluorescent microscopy. In addition, "spongiotic changes" in the sense of a capsular otosclerosis (!) had appeared.

The policy of "wait and see" as regards McCabe's postulates, should thus not be directed against the possible existence of an auto-immune deafness; reservations are, however, advisable on account of the hitherto lacking results of basic research work, as well as against the indiscriminate use of steroids.

References

Abramovich SJ, Gregory S, Slemick M, Stewart A (1979) Hearing loss in very low birth weight infants treated with neonatal intensive care. Arch Dis Child 54:421–426

Adams DA, Kerr AG, Smyth GDL et al. (1983) Congenital syphilitic deafness – a further review. J Laryngol Otol 97:399–404

Adler D, Fiehn W, Ritz E (1980) Inhibition of Na^+, K^+-stimulated ATPase in the cochlea of the guinea pig. A potential cause of disturbed inner ear function in terminal renal failure. Acta Otolaryngol (Stockh) 90:55–60

Afzelius LE, Aursnes J (1979) Structural changes in the organ of Corti of the guinea pig after obstruction of the arterial blood flow to the inner ear. Acta Otolaryngol (Stockh) 88:183–186

Alberti P, Symons F, Hyde ML (1979) Occupational hearing loss. The significance of asymmetrical hearing thresholds. Acta Otolaryngol (Stockh) 87:255–263

Albrecht W (1922) Über die Vererbung der konstitutionell sporadischen Taubstummheit, der hereditären Labyrinthschwerhörigkeit und der Otosclerose. Arch Ohr-Nas-Kehlk-Heilk 110:15–48

Albrecht W (1931) Über Konstitutionsprobleme in der Pathogenese der Hals-, Nasen- und Ohrenkrankheiten. Z Hals-Nas-Ohrenheilk 29:18

Alexander K (1977) Arterienerkrankungen. Fischer, Stuttgart New York

Allam F (1976) Ruptur der Membran des runden Fensters (Klinische Studie). Laryngol Rhinol Otol (Stuttg) 55:544–548

Allen GS, Ahn HS, Preziosi TJ et al. (1983) Cerebral arterial spasm – a controlled trial of nimodipine in patients with subarachnoid hemorrhage. N Engl J Med 308:619–624

Allen JB (1980) Cochlear micromechanics: a physical model of transduction. J Acoust Soc Am 68:1660–1670

Alström CH, Hallgren B, Nilsson LB, Åsander H (1959) Retinal degeneration combined with obesity, diabetes mellitus, and neurogenous deafness. Acta Psychiatr Scand [Suppl] 129:1–35

Althaus SR (1981) Perilymph fistulas. Laryngoscope 91:538–562

Altmann E, Klemm E, Brandt RH, Schmidt PKH (1980) Erste Ergebnisse der fibrinolytischen Behandlung des Hörsturzes und akuten Vestibularisausfalles. Dtsch Gesundh-Wesen 35:2038–2040

Anderson H, Wedenberg E (1970) Genetic aspects in hearing impairment in children. Acta Otolaryngol (Stockh) 69:77–88

Angelborg C, Hultcrantz E, Beausang-Linder M (1979) The cochlear blood flow in relation to noise and cervical sympathectomy. Adv Otorhinolaryngol 25:41–48

Angelborg C, Klockhoff J, Stahle J (1977) Urea and hearing in patients with Menière's disease. Scand Audiol 6:143–146

Anniko M (1976) Damage to Reissner's membrane in the guinea pig following acute atoxyl intoxication. Acta Otolaryngol (Stockh) 81:415–423

Anniko M, Wersäll J (1976) Damage to the stria vascularis in the guinea pig by acute atoxil intoxication. Acta Otolaryngol (Stockh) 80:415–423

Aporti F, Facci L, Pastorello A et al. (1981) Brain cortex gangliosides and (Na^+, K^+)ATPase system of the stria vascularis in guinea pig. Acta Otolaryngol (Stockh) 92:433–437

Appaix A, Demard F (1970) Oxygénothérapie hyperbare et surdités brutales de perception. Rev Laryngol Otol Rhinol (Bord) 91:951–972

Applebaum EL, Shambaugh GE Jr (1978) Otospongiosis (otosclerosis): polytomographic and histologic correlation. Laryngoscope 88:1761–1768

Aran JM (1971) The electrocochleogram. Recent results in children and some pathological cases. Arch Klin Exp Ohr-Nas-Kehlk-Heilk 198:128

Aran JM, Charlet de Sauvage R (1976) Clinical value of cochlear microphonic recording. In: Ruben O, Elberling C, Salomon G (eds) Electrocochleography. University Park Press, Baltimore, pp 55–56

Aran JM, Charlet de Sauvage R (1977) Evolution of CM, SP and AP during etacrynic acid intoxication in the guinea pig. Acta Otolaryngol (Stockh) 83:153–159

Aran JM, Erre JP, Guilhaume A, Aurousseau C (1982) The comparative ototoxicities of Gentamycin, Tobramycin and Dibekacin in the Guinea pig. A functional and morphological cochlear and vestibular study. Acta Otolaryngol [Suppl] (Stockh) 390

Arenberg IK, Dodson VN, Falls HF, Stern SD (1967) Alport's syndrome. Re-evaluation of the associated ocular abnormities and report of a family study. J Pediatr Ophthalmol 4:21–32

Arenberg IK, Goodfriend TL (1980) Indomethacin blocks acute audiologic effects of furosemide in Menière's disease. Arch Otolaryngol 106:383–386
Arenberg IK, Hermann LE, Swanson SN (1977) Prüfung der fluktuierenden Gehörverminderung mit der Glyzerinprobe und mit Kochsalzbelastung. Fül-Orr-Gége-Gyógyászat 23:249–253
Arenberg IK, May M, Stroud MH (1974) Perilymphatic fistula: an unusual cause of Menière's syndrome in a prepubertal child. Laryngoscope 84:243–246
Arentsschild O v (1972) Das alternde Ohr. Funktionelle Aspekte. HNO 20:108–112
Arnold W (1972) Ultrastrukturelle Untersuchungen zur Pathogenese des serösen Paukenergusses. Arch Klin Exp Ohr-Nas-Kehlk-Heilk 201:91
Arnold W (1974) Zur Frage der Produktion und Resorption der Perilymphe (Lymphabfluß des Innenohres). Laryngol Rhinol Otol (Stuttg) 53:774–790
Arnold W (1982) Ototoxizität durch Schleifen-Diuretika. Münch Med Wochenschr 124:271–274
Arnold W (1984) Möglichkeiten der immunfluoreszenzmikroskopischen Diagnostik am entkalkten menschlichen Felsenbein. Laryngol Rhinol Otol (Stuttg) 63:260–265
Arnold W (1984) Inner ear and renal diseases. Ann Otol Rhinol Laryngol 93, Suppl. 112:119–123
Arnold W, Ilberg C v (1972) Neue Aspekte zur Morphologie und Funktion des runden Fensters. Laryngol Rhinol Otol (Stuttg) 51:30–399
Arnold W, Morgenstern C, Thorn L, Schinko I (1978) Morphologische und funktionelle Veränderungen am Innenohr nach Vergiftung mit Ethacrynsäure und Atoxyl. Arch Otorhinolaryngol 218:179–190
Arnold W, Nadol JB Jr, Weidauer H (1981) Ultrastructural histopathology in a case of human ototoxicity due to loop diuretics. Acta Otolaryngol (Stockh) 91:399–414
Arnold W, Nadol JB, Weidauer H (1981) Temporal bone histopathology in human ototoxicity due to loop diuretics. Scand Audiol [Suppl] 14:201–213
Arnold W, Vosteen KH (1977) Akute Ertaubung als Folge der Ruptur eines Basilarisaneurysma. HNO 25:127–130
Arnold W, Vosteen KH (1979) Zur Physiologie von Perilymphe und Endolymphe. In: Berendes, Link, Zöllner (eds) Hals-Nasen-Ohrenheilkunde in Praxis und Klinik, 2. Aufl, Bd 5 Kap 4. Thieme, Stuttgart
Arnold W, Weidauer H, Seelig HP (1976) Experimenteller Beweis einer gemeinsamen Antigenität zwischen Innenohr und Niere. Arch Otorhinolaryngol 212:99–117
Arnvig J (1968) Transitory decreases of hearing after lumbar punction. A personal experience which throws some light on the function of the aquaeduct of the cochlea. Acta Otolaryngol (Stockh) 56:699–705
Asakuma S, Snow JB (1980) Effects of furosemide and ethacrynic acid on the endocochlear direct current potential in normal and kanamycin sulfate-treated guinea pigs. Otolaryngol Head Neck Surg 88:188–193
Asher DL, Sano I (1981) Perilymphatic communication routes in the auditory and vestibular system. Otolaryngol Head Neck Surg 89:822–830
Atzpodien W, Thuemler R, Kremer GJ (1979) Refsum-Syndrom (Heredopathia atactica polyneuritiformis). Therapiewoche 29:6389–6390
Aupy M, Orgogozo JM, Loisau P et al. (1980) Atteinte multiple des nerfs craniens relevant une periartrite noueuse. Relation avec le syndrome de Cogan. Rev Neurol (Paris) 136:59–65
Aursnes J (1982) Atotoxic effects of quaternary ammonium compounds. Acta Otolaryngol (Stockh) 93:421–433
Autio S, Norden NE, Öckermann PA, Riekkinen P, Rapola J, Louhimo T (1973) Mannosidosis: Clinical, fine-structural and biochemic findings in three cases. Acta Paediatr Scand 62:555–565
Axelsson A, Borg E, Hornstrand Ch (1983) Noise effects on the cochlear vasculature in normotensive and spontaneously hypertensive rats. Acta Otolaryngol (Stockh) 215:225
Axelsson A, Jerson T, Lindberg U et al. (1981) Das akustische Trauma bei halbwüchsigen Jugendlichen. Scand Audiol 10:91–96
Axelsson A, Jerson T, Lindgren F (1981) Noisy leisure time activities in teenage boys. Am Ind Hyg Assoc J 42:229–233
Axelsson A, Lindgren F (1977) Does pop music cause hearing damage? Audiology 16:432–437
Axelsson A, Sigroth K, Vertes D (1978) Hearing in diabetics. Acta Otolaryngol [Suppl] (Stockh) 356:1–23
Axelsson A, Vertes D (1982) Histological findings in cochlear vessels after noise. In: Hamernik RP, Henderson D, Salvi R (eds) New perspectives on noise-induced hearing loss. Raven Press, New York

Baba K et al. (1980) Sugar and lipoid metabolism in patients with bilateral sensorineural hearing defects. Variation of blood FFA level with 50 g-OGTT. ORL Tokyo 23, Nr. 2, engl. Abstr. 6; ref Zentralbl HNO 124 (1980/81) Nr. 5021
Bagger-Sjöbeck D, Filipek CS, Schacht J (1980) Characteristics and drug responses of cochlear and vestibular adenylate cyclase. Arch Otorhinolaryngol 228:217–222
Bahgat MS, Shenoi PM (1982) Sudden sensori-neural hearing loss treated by carbon dioxide and oxygen inhalation. A preliminary study. J Laryngol Otol 96:73–81
Bailey CM, Graham MD, Lawrence M (1982) Recovery from prolonged sensorineural hearing loss. Am J Otol 4:1–8
Ballantyne CJ (1966) Perceptive deafness in subjects with renal failure treatment with haemodialysis and polybrene. Proc 8. Internat Congr ORL, Tokyo, 402–403
Ballantyne J (1970) Iatrogenic deafness. J Laryngol Otol 84:967–1010
Ballantyne J (1973) Ototoxicity: A clinical review. Audiology 12:325–336
Bardadin T (1965) The influence of salicylate on the organ of hearing. Otolaryngol Pol 18:509, 517; ref Zentralbl Hals-Nas-Ohrenheilk 87:91
Barolin GS, Hodkewitsch EE, Höfinger E, Scholz H, Bernheimer H, Molzer B (1979) Klinisch-biochemische Verlaufsuntersuchungen bei Heredopathia atactica polyneuritiformis (Morbus Refsum) Fortschr Neurol Psychiatr 47:53–66
Barr B (1960) Nonorganic hearing problems in school children. Acta Otolaryngol (Stockh) 52:337–346
Barr B, Andersen H, Wedenberg E (1973) Epidemiology of hearing loss in childhood. Audiology 12:426
Barr B, Wedenberg E (1965) Prognosis of perceptive hearing loss in children with respect to genesis and the use of hearing aid. Acta Otolaryngol (Stockh) 59:462–474
Barr DP, Reader GG, Wheeler CH (1950) Cryoglobulinemia. I. Report of two cases with discussion of clinical manifestations, incidence and significance. Ann Intern Med 32:6–29
Barsano CP, Groot LJ de (1979) Pendred's syndrome. In: Evered D, Hall WB (eds) Clinics in Endocrinology and Metabolism, Vol 8, No 1, Kap 10. Saunders, London
Batsakis JG, Nishiyama RH (1962) Deafness with sporadic goiter. Pendred's syndrome. Arch Otolaryngol 76:401–406
Battmer RD, Lehnhardt E (1984) Beziehungen zwischen der Dauertonschwelle und dem Einsilberverstehen bei Innenohrhochtonschwerhörigkeit. HNO 32:69–73
Bausch J (1983) Wirkung und Nebenwirkung hormonaler Antikonzeptiva im Bereich von Nase, Hals und Ohr. HNO 31:409–414
Beagley HA (1974) Can we use the cochlear microphonic in electrocochleography? Rev Laryngol Rhinol Otol (Bord) 95:531–536
Beagley HA, Gibson WPR (1978) Electrocochleography in adults. In: Naunton, Fernandes (eds) Evoked electrical activity in the auditory nervous system. Academic Press, New York, pp 259, 274
Beal DD (1968) Effect of endolymphatic sac ablation in the rabbit and cat. Acta Otolaryngol 66:333
Beal DB, Hemenway WG, Lindsay JR (1967) Inner ear pathology of sudden deafness. Arch Otolaryngol 85:591–598
Beaugard ME, Asakuma S, Snow JB (1981) Comparative ototoxicity of chloramphenicol and kanamycin with ethacrynic acid. Arch Otolaryngol 107:104–109
Beck Chl (1961) Das Pigment der Stria vascularis. Arch Ohr-Nas-Kehlk-Heilk 179:51–58
Becker W, Matzker J (1961) Akustischer Unfall. Laryngol Rhinol Otol (Stuttg) 40:49
Beckmann G (1962) Das hörgestörte Kind. Der gegenwärtige Stand der Pädoaudiologie aus oto-audiologischer Sicht. Arch Ohr-Nas-Kehlk-Heilk 180:1
Beentjes BI Jr (1972) The cochlear aquaeduct and the pressure of cerebrospinal and endolabyrinthine fluids. Acta Otolaryngol (Stockh) 73:112–120
Behbehani A, Kastenbauer E (1978) Zur Ruptur und Läsion der Labyrinthfenster. Laryngol Rhinol Otol (Stuttg) 57:983–986
Beickert P (1956) Plötzlich auftretende einseitige Ertaubung und ihre Behandlung (psychoemotionelle und zervikale Genese). Laryngol Rhinol Otol 35:384–395
Beickert P (1961) Zur Frage der Empfindungsschwerhörigkeit durch Autoallergie. Laryngol Rhinol Otol (Stuttg) 40:837
Beickert P (1979) Otosklerose (Otospongiose). In: Berendes, Link, Zöllner (Hrsg) Hals-Nasen-Ohrenheilkunde in Praxis und Klinik, 2. Aufl, Bd 5, Ohr 1, Kap 19. G. Thieme, Stuttgart
Beickert P, Terayama Y (1965) Reaktionen am Corti-Organ auf Sympathicusinnervation. (Zur Wirkung des Ephedrins.) Arch Klin Exp Ohr-Nas-Kehlk-Heilk 185:725–731

Beighton P, Hamersma H (1980) Frontometaphyseal dysplasia: Autosomal dominant or X-linked? J Med Genet 17:53–56

Békésy G v (1951) The coarse pattern of the electrical resistance of the cochlea of the guinea pig (electroanatomy of the cochlea). J Acoust Soc Am 23:18–28

Békésy G v (1951) DC potentials and energy balance of the cochlear partition. J Acoust Soc Am 23:576

Belal A (1979) The effects of vascular occlusion on the human inner ear. J Laryngol Otol 93:955–968

Bentzen O (1961) Skin anomalies in otosclerosis. 7. Congr Oto-Rhino-Laryngol Paris. Excerpta Med Int Congr Series 35:40–41

Bentzen O (1967) The otosclerotic syndrome. Acta Otolaryngol [Suppl] (Stockh) 224:124–132

Berg M, Pallasch H (1981) Sudden deafness and vertigo in children and juvenils. Adv Otorhinolaryngol 27:70–82

Berger K (1965) Nonorganic hearing loss in children. Laryngoscope 75:447–457

Bergholtz LM, Hooper RE, Mehta DC (1977) Electrocochleographic response patterns in a group of patients mainly with presbyacusis. Scand Audiol 6:3–11

Bergmann K, Haupt H, Scheibe F, Rogge I (1979) Der Verschluß des Aquaeductus cochleae für Perilymphuntersuchungen am Meerschweinchen. Arch Otorhinolaryngol 224:257–265

Bergsmark J, Djupesland G (1968) Heredopathia atactica polyneuritiformis (Refsum's disease). An audiological examination of two patients. Eur Neurol 1:122–130

Bergstrom L (1980) Pendred's syndrome with atypical features. Ann Otol Rhinol Laryngol 89:135-139

Bergstrom L (1981) Fragile bones and fragile ears. Clin Orthop 159:58–63

Bergstrom L, Thompson P, Sondo J et al. (1981) Renal disease. Its pathology, treatment, and effects on the ear. Arch Otolaryngol 106:567–572

Bergstrom L, Thompson P, Wood RP (1979) New patterns in genetic and congenital otonephropathies. Laryngoscope 89:177–194

Bernasconi A, Civardi F, Magri M (1983) Osservazioni sul comportamento della funzionalità uditiva in pazienti dializzati. Vortrag 2. Internat. Sympos. on Audiological Medicine, Sirmione 10–13 April

Bernath, Kellerhals, Jannett (1981) Untersuchung über die sogenannte altersbedingte Innenohrschwerhörigkeit. HNO 29:39

Berndt H, Wagner H (1979) Influence of thyroid state and improved hypoxia tolerance on noise-induced cochlea damage. Arch Otorhinolaryngol 224:125–128

Bernhard PA (1981) Freedom from ototoxicity in aminoglycoside treated neonates: a mistaken notion. Laryngoscope 91:1985–1994

Bernstein JM, Silverstein H (1966) Anterior cerebellar and labyrinthine arteries. A study in the cat. Arch Otorhinolaryngol 83:422–435

Berry RA (1975) Sickle cell anemia: audiological findings. J Am Audiol Soc 1:61–63

Bertram G, Luckhaupt H (1983) Ergebnisse unspezifisch durchblutungsfördernder Therapiemaßnahmen beim Hörsturz. Vortrag Westdtsch HNO-Ärzte Recklinghausen

Bess FH, Josey AF, Humes LF (1979) Performance intensity functions in cochlear and eighth nerve disorders. Am J Otol 1:27–31

Bichler E, Wieser M (1983) Experimental lipidosis of the inner ear. Morphological and functional results. Acta Otolaryngol (Stockh) 95:307–313

Biesalski HK, Gross M, Ehrenthal W, Harth H (1981) Bestimmung von Vitamin A (Retinol) und retinolbindendem Protein (RP) im Serum hörgestörter Kinder. Laryngol Rhinol Otol (Stuttg) 60:631–635

Bilger RC (1958) Intensive determinations of remote masking. J Acoust Soc Am 30:817–824

Bilger RC, Hirsh IJ (1956) Masking of tone by bands of noise. J Acoust Soc Am 28:623–630

Blumina MG, Moskovkina AG (1981) Frequency and types of genetic neurosensory hypoacusis inheritance in children. Vestn ORL (Mosk) Nr 3, 21–25; ref Zentralbl Hals-Has-Ohrenheilk 128 (1982) Nr 2251

Blumina MG, Moskovkina AG (1981) A new form of dominant-hereditary neurosenory amplyacousis. Vestn. ORL (Mosk) Nr 5, 12–14d; ref. Zentralbl Hals-Nas-Ohrenheilk 128 Nr 1733

Bocca E (1959) Le problème de la surdité sénile. J Fr Otorhinolaryngol 8:801

Bockmühl F (1983) Mögliche Ursachen des Hochtonverlustes nach Stapesplastik. Vortrag Österreich HNO-Kongr St. Pölten 28. 9.–1. 10. 83

Bodo G, Rozsa L, Shea JJ (1983) Temporary loss of hearing after salt loading in glycerol test. Am J Otol 5:16–19

Boenninghaus HG (1959) Ungewöhnliche Form einer Hörstörung nach Lärmeinwirkung und Fehlbelastung der Halswirbelsäule. Laryngol Rhinol Otol (Stuttg) 38:585

Boenninghaus HG, Feldmann H, Steimann G (1967) Ein Beitrag zur Entstehung von Schwindel und Hörstörung bei Menièrescher Krankheit und Lermoyezschem Syndrom. Laryngol Rhinol Otol (Stuttg) 46:709–727

Boenninghaus HG, Guelzow J (1981) Operationsindikation bei Fensterruptur und Hörsturz. Laryngol Rhinol Otol (Stuttg) 60:49–52

Bohne BA, Clark WW (1982) Growth of hearing loss and cochlear lesion with increasing duration of noise exposure. In: Hamernik RP, Henderson D, Salvi R (eds) New perspectives on noise induced hearing loss. Raven Press, New York, pp 283–302

Bomholt A, Knudsen JB, Permin H, Tommerup B, Cormsen J (1982) Profound sensorineural hearing loss in polyarteritis nodosa. An atypical case of Cogans's syndrome. Arch Otorhinolaryngol 236 (1982) 53–58

Bonding P (1979) Critical bandwith in loudness summation in sensorineural hearing loss. Br J Audiol 13:23–30

Bonding P (1979) Critical bandwith in patients with a hearing loss induced by salicilates. Audiology 18:133–144

Booth CW, Chen K, Nadler HL (1975) Radiological and biochemical abnormalities in mannosidosis. Pediatr Res 9:312

Booth JB (1982) Medical management of sensorineural hearing loss. I. Late syphilis; cardiovascular system; endocrine system; renal system. J Laryngol Otol 96:673–684

Booth JB (1982) Medical management of sensorineural hearing loss. II. Musculo-skeletal system. J Laryngol Otol 96:773–795

Borg E (1979) Physiological aspects of the effects of sound on man and animals. Acta Otolaryngol [Suppl] (Stockh) 300:80–83

Borg E, Nilsson R, Engström B (1983) Effect of the acoustic reflex on inner ear damage induced by industrial noise. Acta Otolaryngol (Stockh) 96:361–369

Bornemann H, Bornemann C, Franke KD, Hundeshagen H (1982) Cochleomeatale Szintigraphie zur Darstellung von Tumoren des inneren Gehörgangs. Arch Otorhinolaryngol 235:501–502

Bosatra A, Poli P, Bianchi M, Calabrese S, Giansante C (1983) Platelet aggregation and coagulation-factors in cases of acute cochleo-vestibular syndromes. Vortrag 2. internat. Sympos. on Audiological Medicine, Sirmione 10–13 April

Bosher SK (1981) The nature of the ototoxic actions of ethacrynic acid upon the mammilian endolymph system. I. Functional aspects. Acta Otolaryngol (Stockh) 89:407–418

Bosher SK, Smith C, Warren RL (1973) The effects of ethacrynic acid upon the cochlear endolymph and stria vascularis. Acta Otolaryngol 75:184–191

Brama I, Fainaru M (1980) Inner ear involvement in Behcet's disease. Arch Otolaryngol 106:215–217

Brenner JR, Spring BD, Sebastian A, McSherry EM, Genant H, Palubinskas AJ, Morris RC (1982) Incidence of radiographically evident bone disease, nephrocalcinosis, and nephrolithiasis in various types of renal tubular acidosis. N Engl J Med 307:217–221

Brinkman WFB (1979) Does presbyacusis exist? Ned Tjidschr Gerontol 10:139–143

Brodehl J (1982) Hereditäre Nephropathie Alport. In: Losse, Renner (Hrsg) Klinische Nephrologie in zwei Bänden, Bd III, Kapitel 52. Thieme, Stuttgart

Brookes GB (1983) Vit. D deficiency – a new cause of cochlear deafness. J Laryngol Otol 07:405–420

Brown JJ, Brummett RE, Fox KE et al. (1980) Combined effects of noise and kanamycin. Cochlear pathology and pharmacology. Arch Otolaryngol 106:744–750

Brown JJ, Vernon JA, Fenwick JA (1982) Reduction of acoustically-induced auditory impairment by inhalation of carbogen gas. I. Permanent noise-induced cochlear damage. Acta Otolaryngol (Stockh) 93:319–328

Brummett RE (1980) Drug-induced ototoxicity. Drugs 19:412–428

Brummett RE (1983) Ototoxicity resulting from the combined administration of potent diuretics and other agents. Scand Audiol [Suppl] 14:215–224

Brummett R, Smith CA, Ueno Y, Cameron S, Richter R (1977) The delayed effects of ethacrynic acid on the stria vascularis of guinea pigs. Acta Otolaryngol (Stockh) 83:98–112

Brunell PA, Brickmann A, O'Hare D (1968) Ineffectiveness of isolation of patients as a method of preventing the spread to mumps: Failure to the mumps-skin-test to predict immune status. N Engl J Med 279:1357–1361

Brusis T, Kesternich P, Lang R (1982) Das Gehör von Hypertonikern. Arch Otorhinolaryngol 235:637–639
Brusis T, Busmann R, Carstens V (1981) Das Gehör bei Koronarkranken. Arch Otorhinolaryngol 231:672–674
Buch NH, Tygstrup J, Jörgensen MB (1966) Erythroblastosis fetalis and the hearing organ. Acta Otolaryngol (Stockh) 61:387–397
Bujara K, Bruck U, Dreyer M et al. (1982) Optikusatrophie, Typ I-Diabetes mellitus und Schallempfindungsstörung. Ein familiäres Syndrom. Klin Monatsbl Augenheilkd 180:559–562
Bumm P, Krüger B, Lang E (1980) Überschwellige Befunde des Ton- und Sprachgehörs bei Presbyakusis. Arch Otorhinolaryngol 223:397–399
Burdick ChK (1981) Hearing loss from low-frequency noise. In: Hamernik RP, Henderson D, Salvi R (eds) New perspectives on noise-induced hearing loss. Raven Press, New York, pp 321–329
Burdick ChK, Patterson JH, Mozo BT, Camp RT Jr (1977) Threshold shifts in chinchillas exposed to low-frequency noise. J Acoust Soc Am 61:78A
Burgeat M, Hirsh IJ (1961) Shifts in masking with time. J Acoust Soc Am 33:963–965
Butt H, Berghorn K (1980) Familiäres Auftreten eines QT-Syndroms mit und ohne Schwerhörigkeit. Herz Kreisl 12:89–92
Buttler RA, Albrite JP (1956) The pitch-discriminate function of the pathological ear. Arch Otolaryngol 63:411
Byl F (1974) Thirty-two cases of sudden profound hearing loss (SPHL) occurring in 1973; incidence and prognostic findings. Talk presented at 79th Annual Meeting American of Ophthalmology and Otolaryngology, Dallas, Oct 6–10
Byl FM (1977) Seventy-six cases of presumed sudden hearing loss occuring in 1973; prognosis and incidence. Laryngoscope 87:817
Bystrzanowska T, Fitowski Z, Swiesiulska H (1971) The effect of age on the auditory fatigue. Otolaryngol Pol 25:17–24; ref Zentralbl Hals-Nas-Ohrenheilk 104 (1971/72) 499
Cancura W (1983) Diskussion z. Vortrag Bockmühl. Österreich HNO-Kongr St. Pölten 28.9.–1.10.1983
Carfi F, Siclari S, Liuzzo A et al. (1980) L'incidenza della ipertensione arteriora essenziale nella determinazione di turbe funzionali dell' orecchio interno. Nuova Clin ORL 32:135–137; ref Zentralbl Hals-Nas-Ohrenheilk 126 (1981) Nr 3402
Carlborg B (1981) On physiological and experimental variation on the perilymphatic pressure in the cat. Acta Otolaryngol (Stockh) 91:19–28
Carlborg B, Densert B, Densert O (1982) Functional patency of the cochlear aqueduct. Ann Otol Rhinol Laryngol 91:209–215
Carlier E, Pujol R (1980) Supra-normal sensitivity to ototoxic antibiotic of the developing rat cochlea. Arch Otorhinolaryngol 226:129–133
Carotti A, Mitri T de, Novello G, Anibaldi G (1983) The dislipidemic disease as risk factor in auditory function damage. Vortrag 2. Internat. Sympos. on Audiological Medicine, Sirmione, 10–13 April
Carter NL (1980) Eye colour and susceptibility to noise-induced permanent threshold shift. Audiology 19:86–93
Caruso VG, Winkelmann P, Correia MJ, Miltenberger GE, Love JT (1977) Otologic and neurologic injuries in divers: Clinical study on nine commercial and two sport divers. Laryngoscope 87:508
Cassidy B, Brown K, Cohen M, De Maria W (1965) Hereditary renal dysfunction and deafness. Pediatrics 35:967–979
Causse JB (1980) Etiology and therapy of cochlear drops following stapedectomy. Am J Otol 1:221–224
Causse J, Causse JB (1980) Note thérapeutique concernant l'utilisation du fluorure de sodium dans l'otospongiose. Cah ORL Chir Cervicofac 15:427–428, 430–432, ref Zentralbl Hals-Nas-Ohrenheilk 125 (1981) Nr 1915
Causse JR, Cause JB (1980) L'otospongiose, maladie familiale. Sa detection precoce. Son traitement medical. Ann Otolaryngol Chir Cervicofac 97:325–351
Caussé R (1949) Action toxique vestibulaire et cochléaire de la streptomycine au point de vue expérimental. Ann Otolaryngol Chir Cervicofac 10/11:518
Cervellera G, Quaranta A, Amoroso C (1980) Clinical experience with remote masking. Audiology 19:404–410
Cervellera G, Quaranta A, Cassano P (1978) Le „remote masking": un test de surdité de transmission cochléaire. Audiology 17:317–323
Chan V, Wang C, Yeung RTT (1979) Dissociated thyroxine, triiodothyronine and reverse triiodothyronine levels in patients with familial goiter due to iodide organification defects. Clin Endocrinol (Oxf) 11:257–265

Char DH, Cogan DG, Sullivan WR (1975) Immunological study of non-syphilitic interstitial keratitis with vestibuloauditoy symptoms. Am J Ophthalmol 80:491

Cheson BD, Jarevoy MR (1977) Cogan's syndrome and BW17 revisited. N Engl J Med 297:62

Chiricosta A, Jindal SL, Metuzals J, Koch B (1970) Nephropathia with hematuria (Alport's syndrome). Can Med Assoc J 102:396–401

Chobaut JC, Bertrand D, Raffoux C et al. (1982) HLA antigens in otosclerosis. Am J Otol 3:241–242

Chole R (1978) Experimental studies on the role of vitamin A in the guinea pig cochlea. Otolaryngol Head Neck Surg 86:595

Chole RA (1980) Autoradiographic localization of vitamin A in the stria vascularis of the rat cochlea. Acta Otolaryngol (Stockh) 106:745

Chou JTY, Hellenbrecht D (1979) Further studies of the membrane potential of the stria cells of the guinea pig in vitro. Acta Otolaryngol (Stockh) 88:187–197

Chüden HG (1979) Ruptur der runden Fenstermembran. HNO 27:227–231

Chüden HG (1983) Hearing disorders in renal diseases. Vortrag 2. Intern Symp Audiological Medicine, Sirmione, 10–13 April

Chüden HG, Mickte W, Stehr K (1978) Hörstörungen bei endemischer Mumpserkrankung. Laryng Rhinol Otol (Stuttg) 57:745–750

Chung DY (1980) Meanings of a double-notch audiogram. Scand Audiol 9:29–32

Chung DY, Gannon PR, Wilson GN, Mason K (1981) Shooting, sensorineural hearing loss, and worker's compensation. J Occupat Med 23:480–484

Chung DY, Wilson GN, Gannon RP (1983) Lateral differences in susceptibily to noise damage. Audiology 22:199–205

Churg J, Sherman RL (1973) Pathologic characteristics of hereditary nephritis. Arch Pathol Lab Med 95:374–379

Clare NM, Montiel MM, Lifschitz MD, Bannayan GA (1979) Alport's syndrome associated with macrothromboipathic thrombocytopenia. Am J Clin Pathol 72:111–117

Clark SK, Rees TS (1977) Posttraumatic endolymphatic hydrops. Arch Otolaryngol 103:725–726

Clark WW, Bohne BA (1978) Animal model for the 4-kHz tonal dip. Ann Otol Rhinol Laryngol [Suppl] 51:1–16

Claux J, Coll J (1979) La place des abiotrophies dans l'etiologie des surdités de l'enfant. J Fr Otorhinolaryngol 28:55

Coats AC, Alford BR (1981) Meniére's disease and the summating potential. Arch Otolaryngol 107:469–473

Cody DT, Sones DA (1971) Relapsing polychondritis: audiovestibular manifestations. Laryngoscope 81:1208–1222

Cogan DG (1945) Syndrome of nonsyphilitic interstitial keratitis and vestibuloauditory symptoms. Arch Ophthalmol Otolaryngol 33:145

Cohen T, Brand-Auraban A, Karshai C, Jacobi A, Gay J, Tsitsianov J, Shapiro T, Jatziv S, Ashkenazi A (1973) Familial infantile renale tubular acidosis and congenital nerve deafness: an autosomal recessive syndrome. Clin Genet 4:275–278

Colclasure JB, Graham SS (1981) Intracranial aneurysm occurring as sensorineural hearing loss. Otolaryngol Head Neck Surg 89:283–287

Coles RRA (1976) Cochleo-vestibular disturbances in diving. Audiology 15:273–278

Comis SD, Leng G, Pratt SR (1981) The effects of furosemid, bumetanide and piretanide on the guinea pig cochlea and auditory nerve. Scand Audiol Suppl 14:85–94

Conrad ME Jr, Crosby WH (1960) Massive nitrogen Mustard therapy in Hodgkin's disease with protection of bone marrow by tourniquets. Blood 16:1089–1103

Corso JF (1977) Presbyacusis, hearing aids and aging. Audiology 16:146–163

Corso JF (1980) Age correction factor in noise-induced hearing loss: a quantitative model. Audiology 19:221–232

Costa OA (1967) Inner ear pathology in experimental diabetes. Laryngoscope 77:68–75

Cram DL, Resneck JS, Jackson WB (1979) A congenital ichthyosiform syndrome with deafness and keratitis. Arch Dermatol 115:467–471

Crammond GW, Gabb P (1980) Impaired hearing in the elderly. Br Med J 280:612

Cremers CWRJ (1979) Autosomal recessive non-syndromal progressive sensorineural deafness in childhood. A separate clinical and genetic entity. Int J Pediatr Otorhinolaryngol 1:193–199

Cremers CWRJ, Monnens LAH, Marres EHMA (1980) Renal tubular acidosis and sensorineural deafness. Arch Otolaryngol 106:287–289

Crifo S, Antonelli M, Gagliardi M et al. (1980) Ototoxicity of aminoglycoside antibiotics in long-term treatment for cystic fibrosis. Int J Pediatr Otorhinolaryngol 2:251–253
Crowe SJ, Guild SR, Polvogt LM (1934) Observations on the pathology of high-tone deafness. Bull John Hopkins Hosp 54:315
Cummings ChW (1968) Experimental observations on the ototoxicity of nitrogen mustard. Laryngoscope 78:530–538
Cunningham DR, Goetzinger CP (1974) Extra-high frequency hearing loss and hyperlipidemia. Audiology 13:470–484
Dahle AJ, McCollister FP, Stagno S et al. (1979) Progressive hearing impairment in children with congenital cytomegalovirus. J Speech Hear Disord 44:220–229
Dallos P, Santos-Sacchi JS, Flock Å (1982) Intracellular recordings from cochlear outer hair cells. Science 218:582–584
Dallos P, Wang ChY (1974) Bioelectric correlates of kanamycin intoxication. Audiology 13:277–289
Dauman R, Cros AM, Mehsen M, Cazals Y (1983) Hemodilution in sudden deafness: first results. Arch Otorhinolaryngol 238:97–102
Davey PG, Jabeen FJ, Harpur ES, Shenoi PM, Geddes AM (1983) A controlled study of the reliability of pure tone audiometry for the detection of gentamicin auditory toxicity. J Laryngol Otol 97:27–36
Davies MG, Marks R, Dykes PJ, Reynolds D (1977) Epidermal abnormalities in Refsum's disease. Br J Dermatol 97:401–406
Davis EC, Nilo ER (1964) Hearing improvement induced by phlebotomy in polycythemia. Laryngoscope 75:1847–1852
Davis GL (1979) Congenital cytomegalovirus and hearing loss: Clinical and experimental observations. Laryngoscope 89:1681–1688
Davis GL (1981) In vitro models of viral-induced congenital deafness. Am J Otol 3:156–160
Davis H (1957) Biophysics and physiology of the inner ear. Physiol Rev 37:1
Davis RR, Brummett RE, Bendrick TW et al. (1982) The ototoxic interaction of viomycin, capreomycin and polymycin B with ethacrynic acid. Acta Otolaryngol (Stockh) 93:211–217
Dawes JDK, Watson RT (1979) Perilymph fistula. Clin Otolaryngol 4:291–302
Deatherage BH, Bilger RC, Eldredge DH (1957a) Remote masking in selected frequency regions. J Acoust Soc Am 29:512–514
Deatherage BH, Davis H, Eldredge DH (1957b) Physiological evidence of the masking of low frequencies. J Acoust Soc Am 29:132–137
Debruyne F, Vaderschueren-Lodeweyckx M, Bastijns P (1983) Hearing in congenital hypothyreoidism. Audiology 22:404–409
Deer BC, Hunter-Duvar J (1982) Salicylate ototoxicity in the chinchilla: a behavioral and electron microscopic study. J Otolaryngol 11:260–264
Del Carpio J, Espinoza LR, Osterland CK (1976) Cogan's syndrome and HLA BW 17. N Engl J Med 295:1262
Demaertelaere L, van Opstal M (1981) Behandlung von akustischen Traumen mit hyperbarem Sauerstoff. Acta Otorhinolaryngol Belg 3:303–314; ref Zentralbl Hals-Nas-Ohrenheilk 128 (1982) Nr 3841
Dencker L, Lindqvist NG, Ullberg S (1973) Mechanism of drug-induced chronic lesions role of drug accumulation on the melanin of the inner ear. Experientia 29:1362–1367
Densert O, Carlborg B, Stagg J (1978) Pressure-regulating mechanisms in the inner ear. ORL 40:319–324
Densert O, Carlborg B, Stagg J (1981) Transmission of low frequency steps to the perilymphatic fluid. Acta Otolaryngol (Stockh) 91:55–64
Deol MS (1970) The relationship between abnormalities of pigmentation and of the inner ear. Proc Roy Soc Lond A 175:201–217
Desjardins R, Guerguergian AJ, Dube J et al. (1982) Meningitis and congenital fistula of the internal ear. J Otolaryngol 11:97–100
Desrochers CS, Schacht J (1982) Neomycin concentrations in inner ear tissues and other organs of the guinea pig after chronic drug administration. Acta Otolaryngol (Stockh) 93:233–236
Dey FL (1970) Auditory fatigue and predicted permanent hearing defects from rock-and-roll music. N Engl J Med 282:467–470

Diamant H (1958) The toxic action of some compounds on the inner ear and its vestibular connections. An experimental investigation with reference to nitrogen mustards and sodium arsanilate (atoxyl). Arch Otolaryngol 67:546
Dieroff HG (1973) Zum Wert der Richtungsaudiometrie für die Abgrenzung zentraler Hörschadensanteile bei der Lärmschwerhörigkeit. Laryngol Rhinol Otol (Stuttg) 52:681–686
Dieroff HG (1975) Lärmschwerhörigkeit. Leitfaden der Lärmhörschadenverhütung in der Industrie. Urban & Schwarzenberg, München Berlin Wien
Dieroff HG (1976) Erfahrungen mit der Hochfrequenzaudiometrie und ihre Einsatzmöglichkeit. Laryngol Rhinol Otol (Stuttg) 55:739–743
Dieroff HG (1976) Possibilities of improving the diagnosis of noise-induced hearing damage by means of directional audiometry, the dichotic speech discrimination test, and the EEG. Audiology 15:152–162
Dieroff HG (1976) Der Nachweis der aufsteigenden Degeneration des Hörnerven bei der Lärmschädigung durch audiometrische Methoden. Z Gesamte Hyg 22:360–363
Dieroff HG (1979) Der unterschiedliche Schadmechanismus bei Dauer- und Impulslärmbelastung in der Industrie und seine Bedeutung für die Praxis. Z Gesamte Hyg 25:143–147
Dieroff HG (1979) Unterschied im Hörschadenmechanismus bei Dauer- und Impulslärm. OAL-Fachtagung 1979 „Lärmbekämpfung Medizin, Technik, Recht", pp 4–11
Dieroff HG (1982) Zum derzeitigen Entwicklungsstand der Hochfrequenzaudiometrie und deren Anwendungsmöglichkeit. HNO-Praxis 7:1–8
Dieroff HG (1982) Behavior of high-frequency hearing in noise. Audiology 21:83–92
Dieroff HG (1982) Zum Problem der Frühveränderung im Innenohr durch Lärmexposition und das Verhalten der Schwelle im Normalhörbereich. XII. AICB-Kongreß „Erfolge und Prognosen der Lärmbekämpfung", pp 61–64
Dietzel K, Kleinfeldt D, Dahl D (1971) Klinische und tierexperimentelle Untersuchungen über die Leistungssteigerung des Innenohrs nach Stellatum-Blockade. Wiss Z Univ Halle 20:34–37
Dilling JM, Makishim T, Snow JB (1973) Effect of ethacrynic acid on endolymphatic DC potential. Arch Otolaryngol 98:183
Dishoeck HAE van, Biermann TA (1957) Sudden perceptive deafness ad viral infection (report of the first hundred patients). Ann Otol Rhinol Laryngol 66:963–980
Djupesland G, Flottorp G, Degré M, Stien R, Skrede S (1979) Cochlear hearing loss and viral infection. Acta Otolaryngol (Stockh) 87:247–254
Dodson HC, Banister LH (1982) The effects of combined gentamycin and white noise on the spiral organ of young guinea pigs. A structural study. Acta Otolaryngol 94:193, 202
Dokianakis G, Ferekidis E, Pantazopoulos P (1978) Hypothyreose und Schwerhörigkeit. Arch Otorhinolaryngol 219:351–353
Donaldson JA (1979) Heparin therapy for sudden sensorineural hearing loss. Arch Otolaryngol 105:351–352
Donckerwolcke RA, Bierrliet JP van, Koorevaar G, Kuijten RH, Stekelenburg GJ van (1976) The syndrome of renal tubular acidosis and nerve deafness. Acta Paediatr Scand 65:100–104
Druss JG, Maybaum JL (1934) Periarteritis nodosa of the temporal bone. Arch Otolaryngol 19:502, 507
D'Souza SW, McCartney E, Nolan M, Taylor IG (1981) Hearing, speech, and language in survivors of severe perinatal asphyxia. Arch Dis Child 56:245–252
Duclos JC, Dubreuil C (1979) Les aspects actuels de la surdité professionnelle. Bull Audiophonol Besancon 9:129–155
Dunger DP, Brenton DP, Cain AR (1980) Renal tubular acidosis and nerve deafness. Arch Dis Child 55:221–225
Durska-Zarzewska A, Zarzewski A (1971) Hörprüfungs-Spätergebnisse bei Patienten nach Therapie mit hohen Streptomycindosen. Wiss Z Univ Halle 20:164–167
Duvall AJ, Sanit PA, Hukee MJ (1980) Cochlear fluid balance. A clinical research overview. Ann Otol Rhinol Laryngol 89:335–341
Eeckhaut J van den, Mangen R, Depover R, Freund M, Meyer R de (1983) Genetic inheritance of perceptive deafness associated with hypertension and hyperlipidemia in a family of ten adults and seventeen adults. Vortrag 2. Intern Symp Audiological Medicine. Sirmione 10–13 April
Eggemann G, Bruchmüller W (1968) Die Kohlensäureanhydrase im Innenohr des Meerschweinchens und ihre Hemmung. Arch Klin Exp Ohr-Nas-Kehlk-Heilk 190:450–456

Eggermont JJ (1974) The temperature dependency of cochlear adaptation and masking in guinea pig. Audiology 13:147–161
Eggermont JJ (1976) Electrocochleography. In: Keidel, Neff (eds) Handbook of sensory physiology, vol V, part 3. Springer, Berlin Heidelberg New York, pp 625–705
Eggermont JJ (1976a) Electrophysiological study of the normal and pathological human cochlea. I. Presynaptic potential. Rev Laryngol Rhinol Otol [Suppl] (Bord) 99:487–495
Eggermont JJ (1976b) Electrophysiological study of the normal and pathological human cochlea. III. Neural responses. Rev Laryngol Rhinol Otol [Suppl] (Bord) 99:497–506
Eggermont JJ (1976c) Summating potentials in electrocochleography: Relation to hearing disorders. In: Ruben O, Elberling C, Salomon G (eds) Electrocochleography. University Park Press, Baltimore, pp 67–87
Eggermont JJ (1977a) Electrocochleography and recruitment. Ann Otol Rhinol Laryngol 86:138–149
Eggermont JJ (1977b) Summating potential in Menière's disease. Arch Otorhinolaryngol 222:63–75
Eggermont JJ, Odenthal DM (1974) Action potentials and summating potentials in the normal human cochlea. Acta Otolaryngol [Suppl] (Stockh) 316:39
Eggermont JJ, Odenthal DW, Spoor A (1973) Frequency selective masking in electrocochleography. Presented at X. World Congr. of ORL, Venice, Italy. Excerpta Medica Congr. Series 276:132
Ehrly AM (1981) Gesamtblutviskosität, Erythrocytenverformbarkeit und Erythrocytenaggregation. Dtsch Med Wochenschr 106:35
Eibach H, Börger U (1980) Therapeutic results in acute acoustic trauma. Arch Otorhinolaryngol 226:177–186
Eichhorn M, Martin G (1984) Verlauf und Prognose beim Hörsturz. HNO 32:341–345
Eisdorfer C, Wilkie F (1972) Auditory changes in the aged: A followup study. J Am Geriatr Soc 20:377–382
Eiseman ML, Sharma GK (1979) The Wildervanck syndrome: Cervico-oculoacoustic dysplasia. Otolaryngol Head Neck Surg 87:892–897
Elberling C, Salomon G (1973) Cochlear microphonics recorded from the ear canal in man. Acta Otolaryngol (Stockh) 75:489–495
Elies W (1978) Differentialdiagnostische Erwägungen zum Morbus Menière: Die basiläre Impression. Arch Otorhinolaryngol 219:358–359
Elies W (1983) Beiträge zu Ätiologie und Pathogenese ein- und doppelseitiger cochleo-vestibulärer Störungen. Habilitationsschrift Aachen
Elies W (1983) Ein Fall von erfolgreicher Dexa-Methasonbehandlung bei beidseitiger, chronisch-progredienter Innenohrschwerhörigkeit. HNO 31:443–444
Elies W, Mitzkat K, Bosch T (1980) Cochleo-vestibuläre Befunde bei „HWS-Syndrom" und idiopathischer Skoliose. Arch Otorhinolaryngol 227:496–499
Elies W, Plester D (1980) Basilar impression. A differential diagnosis of Menière's disease. Arch Otolaryngol 106:232–233
Elies W, Wolff G, Seuffer R (1981) Liquoreiweißbefunde bei Hörsturz und chronisch progredienter Innenohrschwerhörigkeit. Arch Otorhinolaryngol 231:679
Elverland H, Mair IWS (1983) Recurrent meningitis, congenital anacusis and Mondini anomaly. Acta Otolaryngol (Stockh) 95:147–151
Emmett JR, Shea JJ (1979) Diatrizoate meglumine (hypaque) treatment for sudden hearing loss. Laryngoscope 89:1229–1238
Emmett JR, Shea JJ (1980) Traumatic perilymph fistula. Laryngoscope 90:1513–1520
Epstein CJ, Sahud MA, Piel CF, Goodman JR, Bernfield MR, Kushnev JH, Albin AR (1972) Hereditary macrothrombozythopathia and deafness. Am J Med 52:299–310
Escher F (1948) Die otologische Beurteilung des Schädeltraumatikers. Pract oto-rhino-laryng (Basel) 10, Suppl. 1
Evans EF (1972) Does frequency sharpening occur in the cochlea? Symp Hearing Theory, IPO Eindhoven, pp 27–34
Evans EF (1974) The effects of hypoxia on the tuning of single fibres in the cochlear nerve. J Physiol (Lond) 238:65–67
Evans EF (1975) The sharpening of cochlear frequency selectivity in the normal and abnormal cochlea. Audiology 14:419–442
Evans EF (1978) Peripheral auditory processing in normal and abnormal ears: Physiological considerations for attempts to compensate for auditory deficits by acoustic and electrical prosthesis. Scand Audiol [Suppl] 1978:9–47

Eviatar L, Eviatar A (1981) Aminoglycoside ototoxicity in the neonatal period: Possible etiologic factor in delayed postural control. Otolaryngol Head Neck Surg 89:818–821
Falbe-Hansen J (1941) Clinical studies on the effect of salicylate acid and quinine on the human ear. Acta Otolaryngol [Suppl] (Stockh) 44:50–74
Falser N (1981) Experimental infection of the guinea pig inner ear with Toxoplasma gondii. Arch Otorhinolaryngol 233:219–225
Farmer JC, Thomas WG, Youngblood DG, Bennett PB (1976) Inner ear decompression sickness. Laryngoscope 86:1315–1327
Farrior B (1966, 1967, 1968) zit nach Farrior und Endicott (1971)
Farrior B, Endicott JN (1971) Congenital mixed deafness: Cerebrospinal fluid otorrhea. Ablation of the aquaeduct of the cochlea. Laryngoscope 81:684–699
Fastl H, Schorn K (1981) Discrimination of level differences by hearing-impaired patients. Audiology 20:488–502
Federspil P (1972) Über das Haarzellschädigungsmuster nach parenteraler Gentamycin-Applikation beim Meerschweinchen. Laryngol Rhinol Otol (Stuttg) 51:845–866
Federspil P (1979) Antibiotikaschäden des Ohres, dargestellt am Beispiel des Gentamyzins. JA Barth, Leipzig
Federspil P (1981) Experimentelle Untersuchungen zur Ototoxizität der Aminoglykosid-Antibiotika und ihre klinische Bedeutung. Laryngol Rhinol Otol (Stuttg) 60:553–557
Federspil P (1982) Ototoxizität von Antibiotika unter besonderer Berücksichtigung der Lokalbehandlung. In: Ganz H, Schätzle W (Hrsg) HNO Praxis Heute, Nr 2. Springer, Berlin Heidelberg New York, S 1–33
Federspil P, Schätzle W, Kayser M, Sack K (1980) Zur Minderung der Ototoxizität und Nephrotoxizität des Tobramycins. Arch Otorhinolaryngol 223:238–240
Fee GA (1968) Traumatic perilymphatic fistulas. Arch Otolaryngol 88:477–480
Feinmesser M, Sohmer H (1965) Influence of streptomycin and dihydrostreptomycin on the cochlear potentials of the guinea pig. Ann Otol Rhinol Laryngol 74:48–58
Feinmesser M, Weisser MJ, Levi H, Weiss S (1980) Bullous myringitis: Its relation to sensorineural hearing loss. J Laryngol Otol 94:643–647
Feldmann H (1960) Untersuchungen zur Diskrimination differenter Schallbilder bei simultaner, monauraler und binauraler Darbietung. Arch Ohr-Nas-Kehlk-Heilk 176:601–605
Feldmann H (1980) Das Refsum-Syndrom, klinische und audiologische Befunde einer eigenen Beobachtung. Arch Otorhinolaryngol 227:379–382
Feldmann H (1981) Refsum-Syndrom. Heredopathia atactica polyneuritiformis in der Sicht des HNO-Arztes. Laryngol Rhinol Otol (Stuttg) 60:235–240
Feldmann H (1981) Sudden hearing loss: A clinical survey. Adv Otorhinolaryngol 27:40–69
Feldmann H (1981) Der symptomatische Hörsturz. Vortrag/Tagung 60. Geburtstag von Prof. Boenninghaus 30. 4. 81 (unveröff)
Ferekidis E, Papafrangos K, Symvoulidis A, Candiloros D, Pantazopoulos P (1980) Über die urämische Hörstörung. Arch Otorhinolaryngol 223:235–237
Ferguson AC, Rance CP (1972) Hereditary nephropathy with nerve deafness (Alport's syndrome). Am J Dis Child 124:84–88
Fiebach A, Plath P (1983) Differentialdiagnostische Überlegungen zum Hörsturz: Ruptur der runden Fenstermembran. HNO 32:132–135
Fiedler H (1984) Klinische Studie über die Verwendung von Urografin in der Behandlung des Hörsturzes: Notwendige Voruntersuchungen, Resultate und Kritik. HNO 32:338–340
Fikentscher R, Albrecht R, Jakobi H (1982) Beziehungen zwischen Innenohrfunktion und verschiedenen klinischen Merkmalen bei Otosklerose. HNO-Praxis 7:109–113
Finitzo-Hieber T, McCracken GH, Roeser RJ, Allen DA, Chrane DF, Morrow J (1979) Ototoxicity in neonates treated with gentamicin and kanamycin: Results of a four-year controlled follow-up study. Pediatrics 63:443–450
Fiorino FG, Bonani G, Coletti V, Facchinetti R, Sittoni V (1983) Hearing abnormalities in diabetes mellitus. Vortrag 2. Intern Symp Audiological Medicine, Sirmione 10–13 April
Fisch L (1959) Deafness as part of an hereditary syndrome. J Laryngol Otol 73:355
Flach M, Uhlemann B, Knothe J, Steinert R (1969) Elektrophysiologische Untersuchungen zur Frage einer Innenohrschädigung durch örtliche Anwendung proteolytischer Fermente (a-Chymotrypsin). Arch Klin Exp Ohr-Nas-Kehlk-Heilk 195:17–24

Fleischer K (1956) Histologische und audiometrische Studie über alternsbedingten Struktur- und Funktionswandel des Innenohres. Arch Ohr-Nas-Kehlk-Heilk 170:142–167

Fleischer K (1972) Das alternde Ohr: Morphologische Aspekte. HNO 20:103–107

Flint EF (1983) Severe childhood deafness in Glasgow, 1965–1979. J Laryngol Otol 97:421–425

Flottorp G, Foss I (1979) Development of hearing in hereditarily deaf white mink (Hedlund) and normal mink (standard) and the subsequent deterioration of the auditory response in Hedlund mink. Acta Otolaryngol (Stockh) 87:16–27

Forman-Franco B, Karayalcin G, Mandel DD, Abramsom AL (1982) The evaluation of auditory function in homozygous sickle cell disease. Otolaryngol Head Neck Surg 90:850–856

Forquer BD (1979) The stability of and the relation between the acoustic reflex and uncomfortable loudness levels. J Am Audiol Soc 5:55–59

Fotin AG, Ageeva SA (1981) Audition damage aspects in hypothyrosis. Vestn ORL (Mosk) Nr 3:18–21; ref Zentralbl Hals-Nas-Ohrenheilk 128 (1982) Nr 2250

Fowler EP (1950) Sudden deafness. Ann Otol Rhinol Otol 66:980–987

Fox KE, Brummett RE, Brown R, Himes D (1980) A comparative study of the ototoxicity of gentamicin and gentamicin C_1. Arch Otolaryngol 106:44–49

Francois J (1979) Albinism. Ophthalmologica 178:19–31

Franke K (1978) The structure of the round window membrane studied by thin-section-freeze-fracture and scanning electron microscopic techniques. Arch Otorhinolaryngol 219:362–363

Franke K (1979) Fine structure of tissue lining the cochlear perilymphatic space against the bony labyrinthine capsule. Arch Otorhinolaryngol 222:161

Fraser GR (1964) Profound childhood deafness. J Med Genet 1:118

Fraser GR (1965) Association of congenital deafness with goiter (Pendred's syndrome). A study of 207 families. Ann Hum Genet 28:201–249

Fraser GR (1971) The role of genetic factors in the causation of human deafness. Audiology 10:212–221

Fraser GR (1974) Epidemiology of profound childhood deafness. Audiology 13:335–341

Fraser JG, Harborow PC (1975) Labyrinthine window rupture. J Laryngol Otol 89:1–7

Freeman J (1979) Progressive sensorineural hearing loss and cochlear otosclerosis: A prospective study. Laryngoscope 89:1487–1521

Freeman P (1975) Rupture of the round window membrane. Acta Otorhinolaryngol Belg 29:783–794

Freeman P (1978) Rupture of the round window membrane. Otolaryngol Clin North Am 11:81–93

Frei J (1980) Gehörschäden durch elektroverstärkte Musik. 7. Audio-Symposium 1980. Bommer-INTL AG Rexton, Zürich, pp 143–151

Friedman EM, Luban NLC, Herer GL, Williams I (1980) Sickle cell anemia and hearing. Ann Otol Rhinol Laryngol 89:342–347

Friedrich G, Pilger E (1981) Lipoproteinmuster bei cochleovestibulären Störungen. Arch Otorhinolaryngol 232:101–105

Friedrich G, Wolf G (1984) Prognostisch relevante Faktoren beim Hörsturz. HNO 32:74–80

Fritz W, Hörmann K, Brassow W, Koehn W (1980) Zur Ätiologie des Hörsturzes. Arch Otorhinolaryngol 227:370–372

Fritze W (1981) Eine Methode zur Prognose des chronischen Lärmschadens. Laryngol Rhinol Otol (Stuttg) 60:512–516

Fritze W, Gedlicka W (1982) Ein Verfahren zur Prognose des chronischen Lärmschadens. Österreich HNO-Kongr 1981:226–228

Frühwald H, Köllner W, Prohaska O (1979) Lokale pO_2-Messungen in der Perilymphe der Meerschweinchenkochlea bei Sauerstoff- und Sauerstoff-/Kohlendioxyd-Inhalationen. Laryngol Rhinol Otol (Stuttg) 58:731–736

Fues CP, Heumann H, Steinbach E (1983) Schädigung des Innenohres beim Kaninchen durch Anwendung von 2-Cyanoacryl im Mittelohr. Arch Otorhinolaryngol Suppl II/1983:183–186

Fujita S, Fujiwara N, Ohba N (1980) Norrie's disease: Report of cases in two Japanese families. Jap J Ophthalmol 24:22–28

Fujita S, Hayden RC Jr (1969) Alport's syndrome. Arch Otolaryngol 90:75–88

Fukaya T, Nomura Y (1983) Experimental round window rupture with middle ear effusion. Acta Otolaryngol [Suppl] (Stockh) 393:20–24

Galetti G, Mattiolo R, Bergamini G et al. (1931) Revisione critica della istomorfologia della malattia di Menière e ipotesi sulla sede e sui meccanismi del fenomeno del recruitment. Otorinolaringologia (Torino) 31:89, 94; ref Zentralbl Hals-Nas-Ohrenheilk 128 (1982) Nr 929

Galle E, Siegel G (1979) The permeability of ^{51}Cr between cerebrospinal fluid and internal ear. Arch Otorhinolaryngol 224:85–88

Ganguin G, Rempt E (1970) Streptomycinbehandlung in der Schwangerschaft und ihre Auswirkung auf das Gehör des Kindes. Laryngol Rhinol Otol (Stuttg) 49:496–503
Gedda L, Gruno G (1974) Aspetti genetici della presbyacusia. Acta Genet Med Gemellol 23:303–305
Genka T, Kusumi A, Kiyuna C, Shikina Y, Noda Y (1981) Ryukyu Univ J Health Sci Med 3:358–364
Gersdorf MCH (1978) Modifications du réflexe acoustico-facial chez l'homme en fonction de l'age, par étude impédancemetrique. Audiology 17:260–270
Gerwin JM, LaCoste P (1981) The acoustic stapedial reflexe as a prognostic indicator in sudden onset sensorineural hearing loss. Otolaryngol Head Neck Surg 90:857–861
Gibberd FB (1980) Heredopathia atactica polyneuritiformis (Refsum's disease) and its management with plasma exchange. Plasma Ther 1:17–26
Gibberd FB, Billimoria NGR, Page NGR, Retsas S (1979) Heredopathia atactica polyneuritiformis (Refsum's disease) treated by diet and plasma-exchange. Lancet 1:575–578
Gibbin KP, Davis CG (1981) A hearing survey in diabetes mellitus. Clin Otolaryngol 6:345–350
Gibson WPR, Moffat DA, Ramsden RT (1977) Clinical electrocochleography in the diagnosis and management of Menière's disorder. Audiology 16:389–401
Giebel W (1982) Das dynamische Verhalten der Innenohrflüssigkeiten. Laryngol Rhinol Otol (Stuttg) 61:481–488
Gignoux M, Martin H, Cajfinger H (1966) Troubles cochleo-vestibulaires après tentative de suicide a l'aspirine. J Fr Otorhinolaryngol 15:631–635
Gilad O, Glorig A (1979) Presbyacusis: The aging ear. J Am Audiol Soc 4:195–206
Gladney JH, Shepherd DJC (1970) Labyrinthine dysfunction in latent and early manifest diabetes. Ann Otol Rhinol Laryngol 79:984–991
Glorig A (1973) Clinical manifestations of ototoxicity and noise. Adv Otorhinolaryngol 20:213
Glorig A, Davis H (1961) Age, noise and hearing loss. Ann Otol Rhinol Laryngol 70:556–571
Glorig A, Roberts J (1965) Hearing levels of adults by age and sex. United States 1960, 1962 National Center for Health Statistics HEW Series 11, No 11, US Government Printing Office, Washington
Gofman L, Bátsi I (1980) Hereditary nephritis and impaired hearing. Fül-Orr-Gége-Gyógyászat 26:142–147; ref Zentralbl Hals-Nas-Ohrenheilk 125 (1981) Nr 1893
Goldstein JL, Fialkow PJ (1973) The Alström syndrome. Medicine 52:53–71
Goodhill V (1971) Sudden deafness and round window rupture. Laryngoscope 81:1462
Goodhill V (1980) Traumatic fistulae. J Laryngol Otol 94:123–128
Goodhill V (1981) Intranasal forces and labyrinthine deformations and fistulae. Rhinology 19:187–193
Goodhill V, Harris I, Brockmann SJ, Hants O (1973) Sudden deafness and labyrinthine window ruptures. Ann Otol Rhinol Laryngol 82:2–12
Gorlin RJ, Tisner TJ, Feinstein S, Duvall AJ (1979) Usher's syndrome type III. Arch Otolaryngol 105:353–354
Gorlina AA, Kuminov OD, Chupyi LV (1980) Hyperbaric oxygenation in multiple modality treatment of neurosensory amblyacusis of vascular genesis. Vestn ORL (Mos) Nr 5:12–14; ref Zentralbl Hals-Nas-Ohrenheilk 126 (1981) Nr 2594
Gosselin EJ, Yanick P Jr (1976) Audiologic and metabolic findings in 90 patients with fluctuant hearing loss. J Am Audiol Soc 2:15–18
Goulon M, Gajdos PU, Chesneau AM, Raphael JC (1977) Maladie de Refsum, Thiebaut, Klenk et Kahlke. Etude anatomo-clinique d'un cas. Ann Med Interne (Paris) 128:869–876
Goyer RA, Reynold J Jr, Burke J, Burkholder P (1968) Hereditary renal disease with neurosensory hearing loss, prolinuria, and ichthyosis. Am J Med Sci 256:166–179
Granitz DW, Byers VW (1976) Typing of Békésy audiograms. Audiology 15:215–221
Grant MG, Weiss KS, Novak MA, Tobin WD (1985) Transient hearing loss with metrizamide. Laryngoscope 95:67–69
Gray HW, Hooper LA, Greig WR (1973) An evaluation of the twenty-minute perchlorate discharge test. J Clin Endocrinol 37:351–355
Gray RF, Barton RPE (1981) Round window rupture. J Laryngol Otol 95:165–177
Gregg JB, Shaeffer JH (1964) Unilateral inner ear deafness complicating infectious mononucleosis. South Dakota J Med Pharm 17:22–23
Grewal DS, Hiranandani NL, Pusalkar AG (1983) Traumatic perilymph fistulae of the round and oval window. J Laryng Otol 97:1149–1155
Grisanti G (1967) Presbiacusia, memoria tonale e capacità discriminative di frequenza. Atti Clin ORL Univ Palermo 12; ref Zentralbl Hals-Nas-Ohrenheilk 98 (1969) 507
Groot LJ de, Stamburry JB (1959) The syndrom of genital goiter with Butanol insoluble serum. Am J Med 27:586

Gross I, Hahn K, Biesalski HK (1981) Die Diagnose des Pendred-Syndroms bei Kindern mit Hilfe des Depletions-Testes mit ^{123}-Jod. HNO 29:95–97
Gross M (1981) Differentialdiagnose der Syndrome mit Schwerhörigkeit und Retinopathia pigmentosa. Laryngol Rhinol Otol (Stuttg) 60:446–449
Gross M, Arndt-Hauser Ä (1982) HLA-Antigene und Schallempfindungsschwerhörigkeit. Laryngol Rhinol Otol (Stuttg) 61:316–318
Großenbacher R (1976) Pathologie des runden Fensters bei akuter Ertaubung. HNO 24:227–232
Grundfast KM, Bluestone CD (1978) Sudden or fluctuating hearing loss and vertigo in children due to perilymph fistula. Ann Otol Rhinol Laryngol 87:761–771
Gryczynski M (1981) Age effect on differentiation of small changes in tone frequency. Otolaryngol Pol 35:35–41; ref Zentralbl Hals-Nas-Ohrenheilk 128 (1982) Nr 1785
Gstaltner H (1961) Forme fruste einer Parotitis epidemica mit plötzlicher Ertaubung. Mschr Ohrenheilk 95:425–428
Gülzow J (1980) Die Ruptur der runden Fenstermembran. Arch Otorhinolaryngol 227:365–367
Guibaud P, Parchioux B, Langue J et al. (1979) Acidose renale tubulaire distale avec surdité. A propos de 3 observations. Bordeaux Med 12:865–869
Guindi GM (1981) Congenital labyrintho-tympanic fistula: A recently recognized entity in children. J Otolaryngol 10:67–71; ref Zentralbl Hals-Nas-Ohrenheilk 12 (1982) Nr 1735
Gussen R (1976) Sudden deafness of vascular origin: A human temporal bone study. Ann Otol Rhinol Laryngol 85:94–100
Gussen R (1977) Polyarteritis nodosa and deafness: A human temporal bone study. Arch Otorhinolaryngol 217:263–271
Gussen R (1981) Sudden hearing loss associated with cochlear membrane rupture. Two human temporal bone reports. Arch Otolaryngol 107:598–600
Habu K, Kuroda T, Hirayama H (1979) Correlation between the changes of neuro-otological and neurological findings of the patients with organic mercury compounds poisoning during long term process. Otol Fukuoka 25:1363–1370; ref Zentralbl Hals-Nas-Ohrenheilk 123 (1980) Nr 3293
Hallermann W, Plath P (1971) Der Einfluß des Alters auf die Diskriminationsfähigkeit des Hörorgans. HNO 19:26–32
Hallpike CS (1967) Observations on the structural basis of two rare varieties of hereditary deafness in myotactic, kinesthetic and vestibular mechanisms. Ciba Foundation Symposium p 285, hrsg AVS de Reuch, J. Knight Churchill, London
Hamann KF (1981) Mögliche virale Genese von Innenohrerkrankungen. Laryngol Rhinol Otol 60:591–592
Hamernik RP, Henderson D, Coling D, Salvi R (1981) Influence of vibration on asymptotic threshold shift produced by impulse noise. Audiology 20:250–269
Hamet P, Kuchel O, Nowaczynski W, Rojo-Ortega JM, Saski C, Genest J (1973) Hypertension with adrenal, genital, and renal defects. Arch Int Med 131:563–569
Hammer H (1974) Cellular hypersensitivity to ureal pigment confirmed by leucocyte migration tests in sympathetic ophthalmia and the Vogt-Koyanagy-Harada-syndrome. Br J Ophthalmol 58:773–776
Handrock M (1978) Die Reaktionsform der Kochlea beim experimentell induzierten Hörsturz. Laryngol Rhinol Otol (Stuttg) 57:881–891
Handrock M (1982) Ototoxische Medikamente. Vortrag 16. Fortbildungsveranstaltung für HNO-Ärzte, Essen 30. 10. 1982
Handrock M, Fischer RL (1979) Die Bedeutung des Sympathikotonus auf den temporären und bleibenden Hörverlust nach Beschallung. Z Hörgeräte-Akustik; Sonderheft 1979, 18:45–52
Handrock M, Fisher R, Ising H, Dombrowski M (1981) Die Bedeutung des Magnesiumstoffwechsels für die Entstehung der Lärmschwerhörigkeit. Arch Otorhinolaryngol 231:707–710
Handrock M, Matthias R (1982) Nikotin, eine ototoxische Substanz? Arch Otorhinolaryngol 235:659–662
Hannley M, Jerger J (1981) PB rollover and the acoustic reflex. Audiology 20:251–258
Hansen E, Bachen NI, Flage T (1979) Refsum's disease. Eye manifestations in a patient treated with low phytol acid diet. Acta Ophthalmol 57:899–913
Hanzelik E, Pepperkorn M (1969) Deafness after ethacrynic acid. Lancet 1:416
Harada T, Sando I, Myers EN (1979) Temporal bone histopathology in deafness due to cryptococcal meningitis. Ann Otol Rhinol Laryngol 88:630–636
Harada T, Sando I, Stool SE, Myers EN (1980) Temporal bone histopathologic features in Fanconi's anemia syndrome. Arch Otolaryngol 106:275–279

Harnack GA v, Horst W, Lenz W (1961) Das erbliche Syndrom: Innenohrschwerhörigkeit und Jodfehlverwertung mit Kropf. Dtsch Med Wochenschr 88:2421, 2428

Harrison RV, Evans EF (1979) Some aspects of temporal coding by single cochlear fibres from regions of cochlear hair cell degeneration in the guinea pig. Arch Otorhinolaryngol 224:71–78

Haubrich J (1975) Tierexperimentelle histologisch-histochemische Untersuchungen zur Formalgenese der hypothyreotisch bedingten Schwerhörigkeit. Acta Otolaryngol [Suppl] (Stockh) 332:1–56

Haug HP, Giebel W, Breuninger H (1978) Die Ausbreitung von Tetrazyklin im Innenohr nach unterschiedlicher Applikation im Mittelohr. Arch Otorhinolaryngol 218:229–238

Hauser J (1974) Néphropathie chronique héreditaire avec surdité et atteinte oculaire. Schweiz Med Wochenschr 104:762–772

Hawkins JE Jr (1973) Comparative otopathology: Aging, noise, and ototoxic drugs. Adv. Otorhinolaryngol 20:125–141

Hawkins JE, Johnson LG, Aran JM (1969) Comparative test of gentamycin ototoxicity. J Infect Dis 119:417–426

Hawkins JE, Marques DM, Clark CS, Preston RE (1975) Ototoxic potentation between ethacrynic and aminoglycoside antibiotics in guinea pigs. J Acoust Soc Am [Suppl] 1:60

Hayes D, Jerger J (1979) Aging and the use of hearing aids. Scand Audiol 8:33–40

Hayes E, Babin R, Platz C (1980) The otologic manifestation of mucopolysaccharidoses. Am J Otol 2:65–69

Haynes BF, Kaiser-Kupfer MI, Mason P, Fauci AS (1980) Cogan's syndrome: Studies in thirteen patients, long-term follow up, and a review of the literature. Medicine (Baltimore) 59:426–441

Haynes BF, Pikus A, Kaiser-Kupfer M, Fauci AS (1981) Successful treatment of sudden hearing loss in Cogan's syndrome with corticosteroids. Arthrit Rheumat 24:501–503

Heermann J, Dammad H, Sperna H (1976) Perilymphschwall aus Perforation des runden Fensters nach leichtem Schädeltrauma bei vermutlich weitem Aquaeductus cochleae. Laryngol Rhinol Otol (Stuttg) 55:549–550

Heidland A, Wigand ME (1970) Deafness from furosemid. Ann Intern Med 73:858

Heidland A, Wigand ME (1976) Einfluß hoher Furosemiddosen auf die Gehörfunktion bei Urämie. Klin Wochenschr 48:1052–1056

Heinemann MH, Soloway SM, Lesser RL (1980) Cogan's syndrome. Ann Ophthalmol 12:667–674

Helle R (1983) Bestimmung der psychoakustischen Tuningkurven – ein Verfahren zur Messung des Frequenz-Selektions-Vermögens des Gehörs. Audiol Akust 22:30–50

Helson L, Okoukws E, Aubon L, Cvitkovic E (1978) Cis-platinum ototoxicity. Clin Toxicol 13:469–478

Henderson D, Hamernik RP (1982) Asymptotic threshold shift from impulse noise. In: Hamernik RP, Henderson D, Salvi R (eds) New perspectives on noise-induced hearing loss. Raven Press, New York, pp 265–281

Hennebert D (1955) L'integration de la preception auditive et l'audition alternante. Acta Otorhinolaryngol Belg 9:344

Henry KR, Guess MB, Chole RA (1983) Hyperthermia increases aminoglycoside ototoxicity. Acta Otolaryngol (Stockh) 95:323–327

Hesch RD (1982) Therapeutische Überlegungen zu vaskulären Innenohrerkrankungen. HNO 30:365–374

Heyden HW v, Schröder M, Scherpe A et al. (1984) Ergebnisse der primären Chemotherapie bei 44 Patienten mit fortgeschrittenen Plattenepithelkarzinomen des Kopf-Hals-Bereiches. HNO 32:

Hildesheimer M, Rubinstein M, Nuttal AM et al. (1982) Influence of blood viscosity on cochlear action potentials and oxygenation. Hearing Res 8:187–198

Himelfarb M, Kroin J, Strelioff D (1979) Evidence for intracochlear impedance changes following ethacrynic acid administration. Otolaryngol Head Neck Surg 87:880, 887

Hirashima N (1978) Treatment of sudden deafness with sodium salts of triiodobenzoic acid derivates. Ann Otol Rhinol Laryngol 87:29–31

Hirasugi Y, Yatomi T, Yagi M et al. (1979) A case of fluctuating hearing loss. Audiol Jap 22:239–242

Höft J (1969) Die Permeabilität und die Beeinflussung der Permeabilität der Membran des runden Fensters durch Pantocain (Tetracain). Arch Ohr-Nas-Kehlk-Heilk 193:128–137

Hörmann K, Held KR (1980) Zur Abklärung genetisch bedingter Schwerhörigkeit. 5 Fälle von Pendred-Syndrom. HNO 28:206–208

Hörmann K, Fritz W, Lemke Th (1980) Viskosität des Blutes unter Hörsturztherapie. Arch Otorhinolaryngol 277:383, 385

Hoke M (1973) Über den Nachweis der Mikrofonpotentiale beim Menschen. Habilitationsschrift Münster
Hoke M (1976) Cochlear microphonics in man and its probable importance in objective audiometry. In: Ruben O, Elberling C, Salomon G (eds) Electrocochleography. University Park Press, Baltimore, pp 41–54
Hoke M, Lütkenhöner B (1981) Electrophysiological finding in patient with sudden deafness: A survey. Adv Otorhinolaryngol 27:83–99
Hommerich K, Intracranieller Druck und Cochlearfunktion. In: Schaefer H (Hrsg) Einzeldarstellungen aus der theoretischen und klinischen Medizin. A. Hüthig Verlag, Heidelberg, Bd 17
Hood JD, Poole JP, Freedman L (1976) The influence of eye colour upon temporary threshold shift. Audiology 15:449–464
Hoshino T, Ishii T, Kodama A, Kato I (1980) Temporal bone findings in a case of sudden deafness and relapsing polychondritis. Acta Otolaryngol 90:257–261
House HP (1967) The fistula problem in otosclerotic surgery. Laryngoscope 77:1410–1426
Howarth AE, Lloyd HED (1966) Perceptive deafness in hypothyreodism. Brit Med J II, 431–433
Hudspeth AJ (1983) Die Haarzellen des Innenohres. Spektrum der Wissenschaft, pp 108–119
Hülse M, Boll B (1979) Literatur-Dokumentation zur Presbyacusis. Forschungsbericht Nr. 222 der Bundesanstalt für Arbeitsschutz und Unfallforschung Dortmund
Hülse M, Irion H (1982) La presbyacousie, une maladie bien définie? Audiophonol (Besancon) 15:225–237
Hülse M, Meyer JH (1981) Psychogene Taubheit, ein differentialdiagnostisches Problem des Hörsturzes. Laryngol Rhinol Otol (Stuttg) 60:53–58
Huizing EH, Wijngaart WSIM van den, Verschuure J (1983) A follow-up study in a family with dominant progressive inner ear deafness. Acta Otolaryngol (Stockh) 95:620–626
Hultcrantz E (1979) The effect of noise on cochlear blood flow in the conscious rabbit. Acta Physiol Scand 106:29–37
Hultcrantz E, Angelborg C, Beausang-Linder M (1979) Noise and cochlear blood flow. Arch Otorhinolaryngol 224:103–106
Hultcrantz E, Larsen HC, Angelborg C (1980) The effects of CO_2-breathing on cochlear blood flow. Arch Otorhinolaryngol 228:211–215
Hultcrantz E, Larsen HC, Angelborg C (1980) Effects of CO_2 inhalation on cochlear blood circulation. ORL 42:304–312
Hultcrantz E, Nuttall AL, Brown MCh, Lawrence M (1982) The effect of cervical sympathectomy on cochlear electrophysiology. Acta Otolaryngol (Stockh) 94:439–444
Humphries KN, Ashcroft PB, Douek EE (1977) Extra-tympanic electrocochleography. Acta otorhinolaryngol 83:303–309
Hutchinson JH, Howell RA (1953) Cryoglobulinemia: Report of a Case associated with gangrene of the digits. Ann Intern Med 39:350–357
Hvidberg-Hansen J, Balslev-Jørgensen M (1968) The inner ear in Pendred's syndrome. Acta Otolaryngol (Stockh) 66:129–135
Hyde ML, Alberti PW, Morgan PP, Symons F, Cummings F (1980) Puretone thresholds estimation from acoustic reflex thresholds – a myth? Acta Otolaryngol (Stockh) 89:345–357
Igarashi H (1982) An aspect of treatment of sensorineural hearing defect. Otorhinolaryngol (Tokyo) 25:42–47; ref Zentralbl Hals-Nas-Ohrenheilk 129 (1983) Nr 2077
Igarashi M, Macrae D, O-Uchi T et al. (1981) Cochleo-saccular degeneration in one of three sisters with hereditary deafness, absent gastric motility, small bowel diverticulitis and progressive sensory neuropathy. ORL 43:4–16
Igarashi M, Weber SC, Alford BR, Coats AC, Jerger J (1975) Temporal bone findings in cryotococcal meningitis. Arch Otolaryngol 101:577–583
Ijaiya K, Roth B, Gladtke E, Puyn U (1979) Diabetes insipidus, Diabetes mellitus, Optikusatrophie und Schwerhörigkeit: DIDMOAD-Syndrom. Klin Pädiatr 191:572–577
Ilberg C v (1968) Elektronenmikroskopische Untersuchungen über Diffusion und Resorption von Thoriumdioxyd an der Meerschweinchenschnecke. Arch Klin Exp Ohr-Nas-Kehlk-Heilk 190:425, 426; 192:16, 384
Ilberg C v (1968) Elektronenmikroskopische Überprüfung der Zugangswege zum Cortischen Organ. Arch Klin Exp Ohr-Nas-Kehlk-Heilk 191:540
Illum P (1972) The Mondini type of cochlear malformation. A survey of the literature. Arch Otolaryngol 96:305–311

Illum P, Kiaer HW, Hvidberg-Hansen J, Sondergaard G (1972) Fifteen cases of Pendred's syndrome: Congenital deafness and sporadic goiter. Arch Otolaryngol 96:297–304
Insley J, Astley R (1974) A bone dysplasie with deafness. Br J Radiol 47:241–251
Ising H, Günther T, Handrock M et al. (1981) Magnesium und Lärmwirkungen. Magnesium-Bulletin Vol. 3/1 a:155–164
Ising H, Handrock M, Günther T, Fischer R, Dombrowski M (1982) Increased noise trauma in guinea pig through Magnesium deficiency. Arch Otorhinolaryngol 236:139–146
Jacklin HN (1980) Falciform fold, retinal detachment, and Norrie's disease. Am J Ophthalmol 90:76–80
Jackson GG (1977) Present status of aminoglycoside antibiotics and their safe, effective use. Clin Ther 1:371
Jacobson JT, Mencher GT (1981) Intensive care nursery noise and its influence on newborn hearing screening. Int J Pediat ORL 3:45–54
Jaffe BF (1967) Sudden deafness – an otologic emergency. Arch Otolaryngol 86:55–60
Jaffe BF (1970) Sudden deafness, a local manifestation of systemic disorders: Fat emboli, hypercoagulation and infections. Laryngoscope 80:788–801
Jaffe BF (1978) Viral causes of inner ear deafness. Otolaryngol Clin North Am 11:63–69
Jahn AF, Noyek AM (1981) Hereditary hearing losses with delayed onset: Mechanism of expression. Otolaryngol Clin North Am 14:69–64
Jahnke K, Gorgas K (1974) The permeability of blood vessels in the guinea pig: I. Vessels of the modiolus and spiral vessel. Anat Embryol 146:21
Jahnke V (1979) Pränatale Ursachen kindlicher Innenohrschwerhörigkeit. Laryngol Rhinol Otol 58:811–816
Jahnke V, Maas B, Mödder G (1979) Hypakusis bei erworbener Hypothyreose. HNO 27:1–6
Jakobi H, Kuhl KD, Haberland EJ (1979) Verbesserung der Innenohrfunktion nach ATP-Infusion bei Tieren. HNO-Praxis 4:182–187
Jakobi H, Spinar H, Stawinski St, Kleszcz A (1975) Erste Beobachtungen bei kombinierter ATP-Sauerstoff-Überdruckbehandlung von Hörstürzen. Laryngol Rhinol Otol 54:891–895
Jankowski W, Birecki W, Ziemski Z (1971) Einige lokal angewandte Pharmaka und biochemische Störungen des Stoffwechsels der Corti-Zellen. Wiss Z Univ Halle 20:191–198
Jarvis JF (1966) A case of bilateral permanent deafness following acetylsalicylate acid. J Laryngol Otol 80:318–320
Jatho K, Hellmann H (1972) Zur Frage des Lärm- und Klangtraumas des Orchestermusikers. HNO 20:21–29
Jenkins HA, Pollak AM, Fisch U (1981) Polyarteritis nodosa as a cause of sudden deafness. A human temporal bone study. Am J Otolaryngol 2
Jensen JH, Bentzen O, Groes P (1982) Hearing loss in children with abnormal corneal thickness. Audiology 21:177–183
Jensma H (1979) Acute labyrinth-window rupture. Clin Otolaryngol 4:474
Jerger J (1960) Békésy-audiometry in analysis of auditory disorders. J Speech Res 3:275–287
Jerger J (1973) Modern Development in Audiology. 2. Aufl. Academic Press, New York
Jerger J (1973) Audiological findings in aging. Adv Otorhinolaryngol 20:115–124
Jerger J, Alford B, Coats AM, French B (1966) Effects of very low frequency tones on auditory thresholds. J Speech Hear Res 9:150–160
Jerger S, Jerger J (1983) Evaluation of diagnostic audiometric tests. Audiology 22:144–161
Jin KH, Handa T, Ishihara T, Yoshii F (1979) Cockayne syndrome: Report of two siblings and review of the literature in Japan. Brain Develop 1:305–312
Joachims HZ, Eliachar J (1982) Cochlear hearing loss following rubella in an adult. Scand Audiol 11:89–90
Joachims Z, Babisch W, Ising H, Günther T, Handrock M (1983) Dependence of noise-induced hearing loss upon perilymph magnesium concentration. J Acoust Soc Am 74:104–108
Johanson A, Blizzard R (1971) A syndrome of congenital aplasia of the alae nasi, deafness, hypothyreoidism, dwarfism, absent permanent teeth, and malabsorption. J Pediatr 79:982–987
Johnson KR (1970) Audiological manifestations in juvenile-onset diabetes. Thesis for PH D, Michigan State University USA. Zit. n. Strauß (1982)
Johnson RL, Spoendlin HH (1966) Structural evidence of secretion in the stria vascularis. Ann Otol Rhinol Laryngol 75:127–138
Johnsson LG, Hawkins JE Jr (1976) Degeneration patterns in human ears exposed to noise. Ann Otol Rhinol Laryngol 85:725–739

Johnsson LG, Arenberg IK (1981) Cochlear abnormalities in Alport's syndrome. Arch Otolaryngol 107:304–349
Jokinen K (1979) Presbyacusis. III. Perstimulatory threshold adaptation. Acta Otolaryngol (Stockh) 69:324
Jokinen K (1980) Presbyacusis. VI. Masking of speech. Acta Otolaryngol 76:426–430
Juhn SK (1977) Experimental alterations of physiological state of inner ear fluids. Ann Otol Rhinol Laryngol 86:689–697
Juhn SK, Prado S, Rybak L (1979) Effect of urae on osmolality of perilymph. Arch Otolaryngol 105:538–541
Jung WK, Schön FJ (1983) Methoden und Ergebnisse zur Kontrolle der Diuretikawirkung am Innenohr. Arch Otorhinolaryngol. Suppl 1983/II:176–180
Kaaijk CHJ (1977) Longitudinal study of hearing loss in childhood. Relationship between hearing impairment, poor learning and family background. Audiology 16:132–145
Kacker SK, Bajaj JS (1973) Audiometric profile in an Indian family with Alport's syndrome. Audiology 12:28–33
Kaiser-Kupfer MI, Mittal KK, Del Valle LA, Haynes BF (1978) The HLA antigens in Cogan's syndrome. Am J Ophthalmol 86:314–316
Kamei T et al. (1980) Unilateral congenital anomalies of the inner ear. Otolaryngol (Tokyo) 53:7–13; ref Zentralbl Hals-Nas-Ohrenheilk 125 (1981) Nr 1901
Kaneko Y, Nakagawa T, Tanaka K (1970) Reissner's membranes after kanamycin administration. Arch Otolaryngol 92:457–462
Kankkunen A (1982) Pre-school children with impaired hearing in Göteborg 1964–1980. Acta Otolaryngol [Suppl] (Stockh) 391
Kantor TG (1981) Corticosteroids in Cogan's syndrome. Arthrit Rheumat 24:1588
Kanzaki J, O-Uchi T (1981) Bilateral progressive sensorineural hearing loss of unknown etiology. ORL 43:195–203
Kanzaki J, O-Uchi T (1981) Steroid-responsive bilateral sensorineural hearing loss and immune complexes. Arch Otorhinolaryngol 230:5–9
Kanzaki J, O-Uchi T (1983) The progression of hearing loss in the early stages of sudden deafness. Arch Otolaryngol 238:149–156
Kapur YP (1965) Ototoxicity of acetylsalicylic acid. Arch Otolaryngol 81:134–138
Kapur YP, Patt AJ (1967) Hearing in Todas of South India. Arch Otolaryngol 85:400
Kaupp H, Giebel W (1980) Distribution of marked perilymph to the subarachnoidal space. Arch Otorhinolaryngol 229:245–253
Kecht B (1974) Toxoplasmose und Hörstörungen. Laryngol Rhinol Otol (Stuttg) 53:415–421
Kelemen G (1956) Erythroblastosis fetalis: Pathologic report on the hearing organ of newborn infant. Arch Otolaryngol 63:392–398
Kelemen G (1966) Hurler's syndrome and the hearing organ. J Laryngol Otol 80:791–803
Kellerhals B (1972) Acoustic trauma and cochlear microcirculation. Adv ORL 18:91–168
Kellerhals B (1977) Die Behandlung der akuten Innenohrschwerhörigkeit (Hörsturz und akustisches Trauma). Laryngol Rhinol Otol (Stuttg) 56:357–363
Kemp DT (1978) Stimulated acoustic emission from within the human auditory system. J Acoust Soc Am 64:1386–1391
Kemp DT (1979) Evidence of mechanical nonlinearity and frequency selective wave amplication in the cochlea. Arch Otorhinolaryngol 224:37–45
Kemp DT (1982) Cochlear echoes: Implications for noise-induced hearing loss. In: Hamernik RP, Henderson D, Salvi R (eds) New perspectives on noise-induced hearing loss. Raven Press, New York, pp 189–207
Kemper J (1977) Der Hörsturz bei gesundem und vorgeschädigtem Ohr der Gegenseite. Inauguraldissertation Münster; zit n Feldmann 1981
Kerr AG (1980) The effects of blast on the ear. J Laryngol Otol 94:107–110
Kerr AG, Adams DA (1983) Congenital syphilitic deafness – a long term follow up. Adv ORL 31:247–252
Kerr A, Schuknecht HF (1968) The spiral ganglion in profound deafness. Acta Otolaryngol (Stockh) 65:586–598
Kessler L (1968) Akuter Hörsturz im Kindesalter. HNO 16:148–149

Kessler L, Rolfs B, Kessler M, Juntke Ch (1969) Hör- und Sprachstörungen nach Neugeborenen-Bilirubinämie. Laryngol Rhinol Otol (Stuttg) 48:581–590
Kessler L, Tymnik G, Braun HSt (1977) Hereditäre Hörstörungen. JA Barth, Leipzig
Kessler L, Tymnik G, Haferland Chr (1981) Aktuelle Ergebnisse bei der Untersuchung genetisch determinierter Hörstörungen. HNO-Praxis 6:260–264
Khanna SM, Leonard DGB (1982) Basilar membrane tuning in the cat cochlea. Science 215:305–306
Khasanov SA (1982) Hearing function in children with diabetes mellitus. Z Usn Nos Gorlov Bolezn Nr 5, 34–37; ref Zentralbl Hals-Nas-Ohrenheilk 129 (1983) Nr 978
Khasanov SA, Popov IA (1982) Glycogen contents in the organ of Corti in experimental diabetes mellitus. Z Usn Nos Gorlov Bolezn Nr 4, 40–43; ref Zentralbl Hals-Nas-Ohrenheilk 129 (1983) Nr 943
Khasanov SA, Tikhonova IA, Konstantinova NP (1982) Carbohydrate and lipid metabolism in patients with acute neurosensory amblycusis. Vestn ORL (Mosk) Nr 4, 27–29; ref Zentralbl Hals-Nas-Ohrenheilk 129 (1983) Nr 941
Kiang NY-S, Moxon EC, Levine RA (1970) Auditory-nerve findings in cats with normal and abnormal cochleas. In: Wolstenholme O, Knight NJ (eds) Sensorineural hearing loss. Churchill, London, pp 241–273
Kile JE, Wurzbach WF (1980) Temporary threshold shifts induced by vibratory stimulation. Sound Vibr 14:26–29
Kilian PL, Schacht J (1977) Phospholipid labling in the noctuid moth ear: a model for biochemical studies of transduction. Les Colleques de l'Institut National de la Santé et de la Recherche Medicale. In: Portmann M, Aran JM (eds) InSERM 5–7 Sept 1977, 68:167
Kimura RS (1967) Experimental production of endolymphatic hydrops. Internat Sympos Menière's Disease, Mayo Clin Rochester, Minn
Kimura RS, Ota CY, Schuknecht HF, Takahashi T (1976) Electron microscopic cochlear observation in bilateral Menière's disease. Ann Otol Rhinol Laryngol 85:791–801
Kimura RS, Perlman HB (1958) Arterial obstruction of the labyrinth. Part I: Cochlear changes. Ann Otol Rhinol Laryngol 67:5–24
Kimura RS, Schuknecht HF (1965) Membranous hydrops in the inner ear of the guinea pig after obliteration of the endolymphatic sac. Pract Otorhinolaryngol 27:343–354
Kimura RS, Schuknecht HF, Ota CY, Jones DD (1980) Obliteration of the ductus reuniens. Acta otolaryngol (Stochk) 89:295–309
King PF (1976) Otic barotrauma. Audiology 15:279–286
Kirikae J, Nomura Y, Shitara T, Kobayashi T (1962) Sudden deafness due to Buerger's disease. Arch Otolaryngol 75:502–505
Kirikae I, Sato T, Shitara T (1964) A study of hearing in advanced age. Laryngoscope 74:205–220
Kitsera AE, Lyubinets YV (1982) Acoustic vestibular olfactory and gustatory analysers in patient with lung tuberculosis during streptomycin and kanamycin treatment. Z Usn Nos Gorlov Bolezn Nr 5:37–40; ref Zbl Hals-Nas-Ohrenheilk 129 (1983) Nr 979
Kittel G (1963) Pfaundler-Hurlersche Krankheit oder Gargoylismus unter HNO-ärztlicher Sicht. Laryngol Rhinol Otol 42:206–217
Kleinfeldt D (1968) Der doppelseitige Hörverlust unklarer Genese. HNO 16:78–81
Kleinfeldt D, Dahl D (1979) Zur Druckbelastung der runden Fenstermembran im Tierversuch. HNO-Praxis 4:193–195
Klemm E, Altmann E (1983) Die Streptokinase-Behandlung des Hörsturzes. HNO-Praxis 8:209–211
Klemm E, Altmann E, Lange O (1983) Rheologische Probleme der Mikrozirkulation und Konsequenzen medikamentöser Hörsturztherapie. Laryngol Rhinol Otol 62:62–64
Kley E (1951) Zur Herkunft der Perilymphe. Laryngol Rhinol Otol (Stuttg) 30:486–502
Kley HA (1978) Auswirkungen von steroidaler Kontrazeption auf Organe im HNO-Bereich. Arch Otorhinolaryngol 219:474
Kley HA, Werner D (1980) Akute beiderseitige Ertaubung als Folge einer Basilaristhrombose. Arch Otorhinolaryngol 227:376–378
Kligerman AB, Solangi KB, Ventry IM et al. (1981) Hearing impairment associated with chronic renale failure. Laryngoscope 91:583–592
Klinke R, Galley N (1974) Efferent innervation of vestibular and auditory receptors. Physiol Rev 54:316–374
Klinke R, Göttl KH, Roesch A (1981) Testing strategy for ototoxic side effects. Scand Audiol [Suppl] 14:95–101

Klockhoff I, Lindblom U (1966) Endolymphatic hydrops revealed by glycerol test. Preliminary report. Acta Otolaryngol (Stockh) 61:459–462
Klockhoff I, Lyttkens L (1982) Hearing defects of noise trauma type with lack of noise exposure. Scand Audiol 11:257–260
Knight NJ (1977) Severe sensorineural deafness in children due to perforation of the round window membrane. Lancet II:1003–1005
Knight NJ, Phillips MJ (1980) Round window membrane rupture and acquired sensorineural hearing loss in children. Clin Otolaryngol 5:117–128
Knothe J, Flach M, Seidel P (1968) Die Wirkung von Kokain und Tetracain auf die elektrische Aktivität der Meerschweinchencochlea. Laryngol Rhinol Otol (Stuttg) 47:434–341
Knothe J, Flach M, Seidel P (1971) Zur Problematik der Cochlearisschädigung durch lokale Anästhetikumapplikation. Wiss Z Univ Halle 20:199–202
Koburg E, Maass B (1979) Durchblutung des Innenohres. In: Berendes, Link, Zöllner (Hrsg) Hals-Nasen-Ohrenheilkunde in Praxis und Klinik, 2. Aufl, Bd 5, Kap 5. Thieme, Stuttgart
Koehn W, Nickol HJ (1983) Zum Hörsturz von über 60 Jahre alten Patienten. Vortrag Vereinig Westdeutsche HNO-Ärzte Recklinghausen
Koehn W, Nickol HJ (1985) Hörsturz – zur Altersabhängigkeit der Therapieergebnisse unter Berücksichtigung von Naftidrofuryl (Dusodril®). HNO 33:36–39
König E (1957) Pitch discrimination and age. Acta Otolaryngol (Stockh) 48:475
Kohonen A, Jauhiainen T, Liewendahl K, Tarkkanen J, Kaimio M (1971) Deafness in experimental hypo- and hyperthyreoidism. Laryngoscope 81:947–956
Kohonen A, Jauhiainen T, Tarkkanen J (1970) Experimental deafness caused by etacrynic acid. Acta Otolaryngol (Stuttg) 70:187–189
Koide Y, Hata A, Hando R (1966) Vulnerability of the organ of Corti in poisoning. Acta Otolaryngol (Stockh) 61:332–344
Koitchev K, Guilhaume A, Cazals Y, Aran JM (1982) Spiral ganglion changes after massive aminoglycoside treatment in the guinea pig. Acta Otolaryngol (Stockh) 94:431–438
Koizumi S et al. (1980) High frequency sensorineural hearing impairment among senior high-school students. Otolaryngol (Tokyo) 53:27–32; ref Zentralbl Hals-Nas-Ohrenheilk 125 (1981) Nr 1917
Komune S, Snow JB (1981) Ototoxicity of kanamycin sulfate and the barriers in the inner ear. Otolaryngol Head Neck Surg 89:1013
Konigsmark BW (1966) Unpublished data: zit n Konigsmark und Gorlin 1976, S 292
Konigsmark BW, Gorlin RJ (1976) Genetic and metabolic deafness. Saunders, Philadelphia
Konigsmark BW, Mengel MC, Berlin CI (1971) Familial low frequency hearing loss. Laryngoscope 81:759–771
Konishi T (1979) Effects of local application of ototoxic antibiotics on cochlear potentials in guinea pigs. Acta Otolaryngol (Stockh) 88:41–46
Kothe B, Oeken FW (1983) Hörschäden durch Rauchen? HNO-Praxis 8:189–192
Kovar M (1973) The inner ear in diabetes mellitus. ORL 35:42–51
Kozlov MY, Onegova RF, Petrov VS, Sokoloverova M (1976) Diabetes mellitus and hearing impairment. Vestn ORL (Mosk) Nr 5, 21–25; ref Zentralbl Hals-Nas-Ohrenheilk 118 (1979) Nr 3417
Kramer MB, Wood D (1982) Noise-induced hearing loss in rural schoolchildren. Scand Audiol 11:279–280
Kramp B, Dahl D (1978) Das Verhalten der Mikrofonpotentiale bei experimentell lebergeschädigten Meerschweinchen. Arch Otorhinolaryngol 22:153
Kramp B, Schwager A (1978) Zum Einfluß chronischer Lebererkrankungen auf das Innenohr. Dtsch Z Verdau Stoffwechselkr 38:161
Krauer, Pfaltz (1981) Zur Pathogenese des rezidivierenden Hörsturzes. HNO 29:38 (Tagungsbericht)
Krmpotić-Nemanić J (1971) A new concept of the pathogenesis of presbyacusis. Arch Otolaryngol 93:161
Krönig B, Zschiedrich H (1979) Variabilität des Bludrucks: Bedeutung für Diagnostik und Therapie Hochdruckkranker. Nieren-Hochdruckkrankh 4:131
Krüger B (1980) Das Sprachgehör im Alter. Z Gerontol 13:120–148
Krüger B, Bumm P, Lang E (1981) Sprachaudiometrie im Alter. Versuch einer Trennung von primärer und sekundärer Presbyakusis. Laryngol Rhinol Otol (Stuttg) 60:130–134
Kryter KD (1970) The effects of noise on man. Academic Press, New York London

Kubo M, Shida S (1973) Effects if some antibiotics on the acoustic susceptibility of peripheral auditory organ. Internat Congr on Noise as a Public Health Problem Zagreb/Jugoslawien
Kuhl KD, Lotz P, Haberland EJ (1979) Kritische Betrachtungen zur Innenohrtherapie nach tierexperimenteller Überprüfung. HNO-Praxis 4:187–192
Kumagami H, Miyazaki M (1983) Chronological changes of electrocochleogram in experimental endolymphatic hydrops. Special reference with AP outout potential and hair cell cilia. ORL 45:143–153
Kumpf W (1970) Aspekte der Altersschwerhörigkeit. Z Allgemeinmed/Landarzt 16:821
Kumpf W, Wandhöfer A (1972) Zum Hörsturz bei vorgeschädigtem Innenohr der Gegenseite. Laryngol Rhinol Otol (Stuttg) 51:838, 841
Kundell SP, Ochs HD (1980) Cogan syndrome in childhood. J Pediatr 97:96–98
Kusakari J, Kambayashi J, Ise I, Kawamoto K (1978) Reduction of the endocochlear potential by the new "loop" diuretic, Bumetanide. Acta Otolaryngol (Stockh) 86:336–341
Lamm H (1980) Die Wirkung von hyperbarem Sauerstoff auf das Innenohr. Experimentelle Untersuchungen am Meerschweinchen und deren klinische Aspekte. In: Gerstenbrand, Lorenzoni, Seemann (Hrsg) Tauchmedizin. Schlütersche Verlagsanstalt, Hannover
Lamm H, Klimpel L (1971) Hyperbare Sauerstofftherapie bei Innenohr- und Vestibularisstörungen, HNO 19:263
Lamm H, Lehnhardt E, Alm W (1978) Die Wirkung von hyperbarem Sauerstoff (OHP) auf die normale Innenohrfunktion des Meerschweinchens. Simultane Ableitungen von Mikrofonpotentialen und Nervenaktionspotentialen. Arch Otorhinolaryngol 219:397
Lamm H, Lehnhardt E, Lamm K (1984) Instrumental perforation of the round window. Animal experiments using cochleography and ERA. Acta Otolaryngol (Stockh) 98:454–461
Lamore PJJ, Rodenburg N (1980) Significance of the SISI test and its relation to recruitment. Audiology 19:75–85
Lang HP (1970) Das Verhalten der chronischen Lärmschwerhörigkeit nach beendeter Lärmexposition. Inaugural-Dissertation Frankfurt/Main
Larsen HC, Angelborg C, Hultcrantz E (1981) Effect of ethanol and cochlear blood flow. Arch Otorhinolaryngol 233:19–23
Larsen HC, Angelborg C, Hultcrantz E (1982) The effect of uraea and mannitol on cochlear blood flow. Acta Otolaryngol (Stockh) 94:249–252
Lawrence M (1966) Effects of interference with terminal blood supply on organ of Corti. Laryngoscope 76:1318–1337
Lawrence M (1970) Circulation of the capillaries of the basilar membrane. Laryngoscope 80:1364–1375
Lawrence M (1974) Direct visualization of living organg of Corti and studies of its extracellular fluids. Laryngoscope 84:1767
Lawrence M (1980) The flow of endolymph – An unified concept. Otolaryngol Clin North Am 13:577–583
Lawrence M, Nuttall AL, Clapper MP (1974) Electrical potentials and fluid boundaries within the organ of Corti. J Acoust Soc Am 55:122–138
Lawrence W Jr, Kuehn P, Masle ET (1961) An abdominal tourniquet for regional chemotherapy. J Surg Res 1:142–151
Lehnhardt E (1958) Plötzliche Hörstörungen, auf beiden Seiten gleichzeitig oder nacheinander aufgetreten. Laryngol Rhinol Otol (Stuttg) 37:1
Lehnhardt E (1962) Zur einseitigen Taubheit im Kindesalter. Arch Ohr-Nas-Kehlk-Heilk 180:230
Lehnhardt E (1965) Berufsschäden des Ohres. Arch Ohr-Nas-Kehlk-Heilk 185:11, 465
Lehnhardt E (1966) Die c^5-Senke; ihre Deutung auf Grund allgemeingültiger physiologischer Vorstellungen. HNO 14:45
Lehnhardt E (1967) Familiär-progrediente Schwerhörigkeit und subklinische Jodstoffwechselstörung. Laryngol Rhinol Otol 46:260
Lehnhardt E (1970) Zur Ototoxizität der Antibiotika. HNO 18:97–101
Lehnhardt E (1973) Das audiologische Bild der psychogenen Schwerhörigkeit. Arch Klin Exp Ohr-Nas-Kehlk-Heilk 205:226
Lehnhardt E (1974) Zur Abgrenzung der psychogenen Hörstörung von der aggravierten Schwerhörigkeit. HNO 22:134–138
Lehnhardt E (1975) Hörstörungen bei Multipler Sklerose. HNO 23:101–108
Lehnhardt E (1976) Das untere Dynamikplateau der Stapediusreflexschwelle; ein Beitrag zur Duplizitätstheorie der Haarzellen. Arch Klin Exp Ohr-Nas-Kehlk-Heilk 213:471–473

Lehnhardt E (1976) Menière-Krankheit und Hörsturz. Arch Ohr-Nas-Kehlk-Heilk 212:51–362
Lehnhardt E (1977) Granuloma gangraenescens und Wegenersche Granulomatose. In: Berendes, Link, Zöllner (Hrsg) Hals-Nasen-Ohrenheilkunde in Praxis und Klinik, 2. Aufl, Bd 1, Kap 18. Thieme, Stuttgart
Lehnhardt E (1977) Audiometrische Abgrenzung der Altersschwerhörigkeit von der Lärmschädigung des Gehörs. Forschungsbericht Süddeutsche Eisen- und Stahl-Berufsgenossenschaft Mainz
Lehnhardt E (1978) Zur Fragwürdigkeit des Begriffs „Altersschwerhörigkeit". HNO 26:406–413
Lehnhardt E (1978) Praktische Audiometrie. Lehrbuch und synaptischer Atlas, 5. Aufl. Thieme, Stuttgart
Lehnhardt E (1979) Pathophysiologie der Schalleitung einschließlich Ohrtrompete. In: Berendes, Link, Zöllner (Hrsg) HNO-Heilkunde in Praxis und Klinik, 2. Aufl, Bd 6, Kap 1. Thieme, Stuttgart
Lehnhardt E (1981) The sound-intensity related behaviour of the brain stem response P_6 in different forms of hearing disorders. Arch Otorhinolaryngol 232:203–213
Lehnhardt, E, Battmer RD, Becker D (1977) Zum diagnostischen Wert der ipsilateral ausgelösten Impedanzänderung des Trommelfells. Laryngol Rhinol Otol (Stuttg) 56:683–693
Lehnhardt E, Hesch RD (1980) Über verschiedene Typen der Innenohrschwerhörigkeit. Kritisches zur Therapie. HNO 28:73–79
Lehnhardt E, Schmidt W, Franke KD (1982) Aspekts in diagnostics of central neural hearing disorders. Arch Otorhinolaryngol 234:73–95
Leiber B, Olbrich G (1966) Die klinischen Syndrome, 4. Aufl. Urban & Schwarzenberg, München Berlin Wien
Lemieux G, Neemeh JA (1967) Charcot-Marie-Tooth disease and nephritis. Can Med Assoc J 97:1193–1198
Lenarz Th, Gülzow J (1983) Akustisches Innenohrtrauma bei Impedanzmessung. Akutes Schalltrauma? Laryngol Rhinol Otol (Stuttg) 62:58–61
Lenz H, Sluga E, Bernheimner H et al. (1979) Refsum-Krankheit und ihr Verlauf bei diätetischer Behandlung durch 2,5 Jahre. Klinik, biochemische und neuropathologische Daten. Nervenarzt 50:52–60
Leon P, Bonilla JA, Sanchez JR et al (1981) Low frequency hereditary deafness in man with childhood onset. Am J Hum Genet 33:209–214
Lerner SA, Matz GJ (1979) Suggestions for monitoring during treatment with aminoglykoside antibiotics. Otolaryngol Head Neck Surg 87:222–228
Levine MA, Downs RW, Moses AM et al. (1983) Resistance to multiple hormones in patients with pseudohypoparathyroidism. Association with deficient activity of guanine nucleotide regulatory protein. Am J Med 74:545–556
Liberfarb RM, Hirose T, Holmes LB (1981) The Wagner-Stickler syndrome: a study of 22 families. J Petiatr 99:394–399
Likourinas M, Dacou-Voutetakis C, Morfis G et al. (1980) Complexe syndrome in a young girl: Wolfram's syndrome? Eur Urol 6:124–125
Lindquist NG (1973) Accumulation of drugs on melanin. Acta Radiol [Suppl] (Stockh) 321
Lindsay JR (1968) Histopathology of Menière's disease as observed by light microscopy. Otolaryngol Clin North Am 1:319–329
Lindsay J (1973) Histopathology of deafness due to postnatal virus disease. Arch Otolaryngol 98:258–264
Lindsay JR (1973) Profound childhood deafness. Inner ear pathology. Ann Otol Rhinol Laryngol [Suppl] 82:5–121
Livan M (1961) Contributo alla conoscenza delle sordità erediarie. Arch Ital Otol 72:331–339
Lloyd-Mosty RH, Lord IJ (1971) Ototoxicity of intravenous furosemid. Lancet II:1156
Loeb H, Tondeur M, Toppet M, Cremer N (1969) Clinical, biochemical, and ultrastructural studies of an untypical form of mucopolysaccharidosis. Acta paediatr Scand 58:220–228
Löhle E (1980) The influence of a chronic vitamin A deficiency on the acoustic sensory cells and the ganglion spirale cochleae of the rat. An electron microscopic study. Arch Otorhinolaryngol 229:45–53
Löhle E, Schölmerich J, Vuilleumier JP, Köttgen E (1982) Vitamin A-Konzentration im Plasma und das Hörvermögen bei Patienten mit chronischer alkoholischer Leberschädigung. HNO 30:375–380
Logan ThB, Prazma J, Thomas WG, Fischer ND (1974) Tobramycin-ototoxicity. Arch Otolaryngol 99:190–193

Longuebray A, Legros M, Bonnenfant JC (1982) Surdités infantiles post-rubéolique. J Fr Otorhinolaryngol 31:115–120
Lowell SH, Paparella MM (1977) Presbycusis: What is it? Laryngoscope 87:1710–1717
Lucente FE (1971) Aspirin and the otolaryngologist. Arch Otolarnygol 94:443–446
Luetje CM (1979) The CT scan: Pitfalls and posterior fossa cisternography. Otolaryngol Head Neck Surg 87:266–267
Lyons GD, Dodson ML, Casey DA, Melancon BB (1978) Round window rupture secondary to acoustic trauma. South Med J 71:1–73
Lyttkens L, Larsson B, Göller H, Englesson S, Stahle J (1979) Melanin capacity to accumulate drugs in the internal ear. A study on lidocaine, bupivacaine and chlorpromazine. Acta Otolaryngol (Stockh) 88:61–73
Maass B (1982) Innenohrdurchblutung. Anatomisch-funktionelle Betrachtungen. HNO 30:355–364
Maass B, Baumgärtl H, Lübbers DW (1977) Wirkung einer oberen zervikalen Sympathektomie auf den cochleären Sauerstoffpartialdruck (pO_2) unter den Bedingungen einer hämorrhagischen Hypotension. Arch Otorhinolaryngol 216:519–520
Maass B, Baumgärtl H, Lübbers DW (1979) Wirkung einer Sympathektomie auf den Sauerstoffpartialdruck (pO_2) in der Cochlea unter hämorrhagischer Hypotension. Laryngol Rhinol Otol (Stuttg) 58:665–670
Maass B, Ludwig D (1983) Wasserstoff-Clearance-Messungen an der Cochlea-Basis unter akuter Schallbelastung. Arch Otorhinolaryngol Suppl II/1983:163–166
Märtensson B (1960) Dominant hereditary nerve deafness. Acta Otolaryngol (Stockh) 52:270
Mahajan SL, Ikeda Y, Myers TJ, Baldini G (1981) Acute acoustic nerve palsy associated with vincristine therapy. Cancer 47:2404–2406
Maher JF, Schreiner GE (1965) Studies on ethacrynic acid in patients with refractory edema. Ann Intern Med 62:15
Makishima K (1978) Arteriolar sclerosis as a cause of presbycusis. Arch Otolaryngol 98:322–326
Makishima K, Tanaka K (1971) Pathological changes of the inner ear and central auditory pathway in diabetics. Ann Otol Rhinol Laryngol 80:218, 228
Mangabeira-Albernaz PL, Fukuda Y, Chammas F (1981) The Mondini dysplasia. A clinical study. ORL 43:131–152
Mangabeira-Albernaz PL, Fukuda A, Malaasi-Gananca M (1980) Menières disease. ORL 42:91–100
Marangoni F, Barbara M, Fabiani M, Filippo R (1983) Valutazione della funzione uditiva dell'ipotireodismo congenito. Vortrag 2. Intern Symp Audiological Medicine 10.–13. April 1983
Marco J, Lasala FE (1964) Toxicos laberinticos mucopolisacaridos cocleovestibulares. Acta Oto-Rino-Laring Ibero-Amer 15:240–248
Marcus RE, Small H, Emnuel P (1963) Ototoxic medication in premature children. Arch Otolaryngol 77:198–204
Marget W (1977) Infektionskrankheiten. In: Wiskott, Betke, Künzer (eds) Lehrbuch der Kinderheilkunde. G. Thieme, Stuttgart, pp 17.–17.106
Margolis RH, Goldberg SM (1980) Auditory frequency selectivity in normal and presbyacusis subjects. J Speech Hear Res 23:603–613
Marks SC, Schacht J (1981) Effect of ototoxic diuretics on cochlear Na^+/Ka^+ATPase and adenylate cyclase. Scand Audiol [Suppl] 14:131–138
Marshak G (1972) The inner ear in experimental diabetes mellitus. Acta Otolaryngol [Suppl] (Stockh) 300:7–17
Marshak G, Anderson CV (1968) Békésy audiometry with juvenile onset diabetics. J Audit Res 8:323–330
Marshall L (1980) Auditory processing in aging listeners. J Speech Hear Disord 46:226–240
Martin FN, Brunette GW (1980) Loudness and the acoustic reflex. Ear Hear 1:106–108
Martin H, Martin C (1980) Ototoxicité des gouttes auriculaires. J Fr Otorhinolaryngol 29:19–32, 35–37
Martin H, Martin C (1982) Presbyacousie et presbyacousie acélerée. Bull Audiophonol (Besancon) 15:247–253
Maserit A, Severis S, Nes M de (1978) "Variant" angina: one aspect of a continous spectrum of vasospastic myocardial ischemia: pathogenic mechanism estimated incidence and clinics and coronary arteriographic findings in 138 patients. Am J Cardiol 42:1019
Matsumoto I, Morizono T, Paparella MM (1980) Hearing loss following potassium cromate: Two case reports. Otolaryngol Head Neck Surg 88:625–629

Matthias R (1983) Mikrozirkulationsmodulatoren in der Cochlea des Meerschweinchens. Arch Otorhinolaryngol Suppl II/1983:361–362
Matthias R, Handrock M (1980) Zu Wirkung ototoxischer Substanzen bei intratympanaler Applikation. Arch Otorhinolaryngol 227:417–420
Mattox DE (1980) Medical management of sudden hearing loss. Otolaryngol Head Neck Surg 88:111–113
Mattox DE, Simmons SB (1977) Natural history of sudden sensorineural hearing loss. Ann Otol Rhinol Laryngol 86:463–480
Matz GJ (1976) The ototoxic effects of ethacrynic acid in man and animals. Laryngoscope 86:1065–1086
Matz GJ, Beal DD, Krames L (1969) Ototoxicity of ethacrynic acid. Arch Otolaryngol 90:60
Matz GJ, Naunton RF (1968) Ototoxicity of chloroquine. Arch Otolaryngol 88:370–378
Matzker J (1957) Beruht die Altersschwerhörigkeit auf peripheren oder zentralen Veränderungen? Arch Ohr-Nas-Kehlk-Heilk 171:371–373
Matzker J (1958) Ein binauraler Hörsynthesetest zum Nachweis zerebraler Hörstörungen. Thieme, Stuttgart
Matzker J (1959) Two new methods for the assessment of central auditory functions in cases of brain diseases. Ann Otol Rhinol Laryngol 68:1185
Matzker J, Ruckes J (1957) Die Diagnostik morphologisch nachweisbarer Hirnstammerkrankungen durch einen neuartigen Test. Dtsch Med Wochenschr 82:2187
Maxwell ON (1963) Hearing loss in uveitis. Arch Otorhinolaryngol 78:138–142
McCabe BF (1979) Autoimmune sensorineural hearing loss. Ann Otol Rhinol Laryngol 88:585–589
McClure JA, Lycett P (1980) Effect of round window removal on auditory thresholds in cats. J Otolaryngol 9:215–221
McGill TJ (1978) Infection of the temporal bone. Arch Otolaryngol 104:140–144
McKusik VA (1978) Mendelian Inheritance in Man, 5. Aufl. John Hopkins Univ Press, Baltimore
Mees K (1983) Ultrastructural localization of K^+-dependent Ouabain-sensitive NPPase (Na-K-ATPase) in the guinea pig inner ear. Acta Otolaryngol (Stockh) 95:277–289
Mees K (1983) Ultrastrukturelle Lokalisation der Adenylzyklase in der lateralen Schneckenwand. Arch Otorhinolaryngol Suppl II/1983:167–168
Megighian D (1982) Flucturant hearing loss: Pathogenic and clinical considerations. Arch Otorhinolaryngol 236:81–86
Meinecke P (1982) Das Waardenburg-Syndrom Typ I. Autosomal dominant erbliche Kombination multipler fazialer Anomalien mit Innenohrschwerhörigkeit. Klin Paediatr 194:112–116
Mendelsohn M, Katzenberg J (1972) The effect of kanamycin on the cation content of the endolymph. Laryngoscope 82:397–403
Ménégaux A, Pailler JP (1981) Estimation des troubles de l'audition dans la sénescence. Bull Audiophonol (Besancon) 13:29–36
Mengel MC, Konigsmark BW, Berlin CI, McKusik VA (1967) Recessive early onset neural deafness. Acta Otolaryngol (Stockh) 64:313
Menser MA, Forrest JM (1974) Rubella – high incidence of defects in children considered normal at birth. Med J Aust 1:123–126
Mercke U, Nordenfeldt E, Sjöholm A (1980) Die Rolle einer Virusinfektion beim Hörsturz. HNO 28:125–127
Meriwether WD, Mangi RJ, Serpick AA (1971) Deafness following standard intravenous dose of ethacrynic acid. JAMA 216:795
Meurman OH (1953) Studies on the difference limen of intensity and frequence in presbyacusis. Proc 1st Internat Congr Audiol Leiden, pp 59–63
Meyer C, Biedermann M (1980) Immediate alterations in the impulse noise exposed organ of Corti of the guinea pig. Acta Otolaryngol (Stockh) 90:250–256
Meyer zum Gottesberge A (1948) Zur Physiologie der Haarzellen. Arch Ohr-Nas-Kehlk-Heilk 155:308
Meyer zum Gottesberge A (1960) Die Pathologie der C^5-Senke. Acta Otolaryngol (Stockh) 51:250
Meyer zum Gottesberge A, Stupp HF (1969) Streptomycinspiegel in der Perilymphe des Menschen. Acta Otolaryngol (Stockh) 67:171–176
Meyer zum Gottesberge A, Stupp HF (1972) Akute beiderseitige Ertaubung bei Insuffizienz der A. basilaris. Arch Klin Exp Ohr-Nas-Kehlk-Heilk 202:578–581

Meyerhoff WL (1979) "How I do it." Otology and neurology: A specific issue and its solution. The management of sudden deafness. Laryngoscope 89:1867–1868
Meyerhoff WL, Paparella MM, Gudbrandsson FK (1981) Clinical evaluation of Menière's disease. Laryngoscope 91:1663–1668
Meyerhoff WL, Paparella MM, Oda M, Shea D (1979) Myotic infections of the inner ear. Laryngoscope 89:1725–1734
Miayamoto T (1931) Experimentelle Untersuchungen über die Schädigung des Gehörorgans durch Gifteinwirkung. Arb Med Univ Okayama 2:3
Miller GW, Joseph DJ, Cozad RL, McCabe BF (1970) Alport's syndrome. Arch Otolaryngol 92:418–432
Miller MH, Doyle TJ, Geier SR (1981) Acoustic neuroma in a population of noise exposed workers. Laryngoscope 91:363–371
Milne JS (1977) A longitudinal study of hearing loss in older people. Brit J Audiol 11:7–14
Milne JS, Lauder IJ (1975) Pure tone audiometry in older people. Brit J Audiol 9:50–58
Milutinovic PS, Stanbury JB, Wicken JV, Jones EW (1969) Thyroid function in a family with the Pendred syndrome. J Clin Endocrinol Metab 29:962–969
Miriszlai E (1981) Experimental round window membrane ruptures. Acta Paediatr Acad Sci Hung 22:77–81
Misawa T (1981) Two cases of sudden deafness in diabetics. Otorhinolaryngol (Tokyo) 24, Nr. 5; ref Zentralbl Ohr-Nas-Kehlk-Heilk 28 Nr. 2680
Mitschke H (1978) Der Hörsturz, eine mögliche zentrale Manifestation der Zytomegalievirus-Infektion Erwachsener. Laryngol Rhinol Otol (Stuttg) 57:876–881
Mitschke H (1978) Oto-rhino-laryngologische Aspekte der fortgeschrittenen Niereninsuffizienz. Wien Klin Wochenschr 90 [Suppl] 8:1–14
Mitschke H, Schmidt P, Zazgornik J, Kopsa H, Pils P (1977) Effect of renal transplantation on uremic deafness: a long-term study. Audiology 16:530–534
Miyamoto H, Morgenstern C (1979) Potassium level in endolymphatic sac of guinea pigs in vivo. Arch Otorhinolaryngol 222:77–78
Miyamoto H, Morgenstern C (1980) Role of electrolytes in different parts of the endolymphatic sac. Intern Menière-Symposium 12.–14. 5. Düsseldorf
Miyamoto RT, House WF, Brackmann DE (1980) Neurootolotic manifestations of the osteopetroses. Arch Otolaryngol 106:210–214
Møller MB (1981) Hearing in 70 and 75 year old people: Results from a cross sectional and longitudinal population study. Am J Audiol 2:22–29
Mörl Ch, Martusch M, Mörl H (1971) Die Therapie des akuten Hörsturzes mit intraarteriellen Dauerinfusionen. Vorläufige Mitteilung. Laryngol Rhinol Otol (Stuttg) 50:723–729
Moffat DA (1979) Transtympanic electrocochleography in Menière's disease: Variation in the amplitude of the summating potential related to clinical status. Brit J Audiol 13:149–152
Moffat DA, Gibson WPR, Ramsden RT, Morrison AW, Booth JB (1978) Transtympanic electrocochleography during glycerol dehydration. Acta Otolaryngol (Stockh) 85:158–166
Mohr J, Mageroy K (1962) Sex-linked deafness of a possibly new type. Acta Genet (Basel) 10:54–62
Molinari G (1978) Effetto dei gangliosidi di corteccia cerebrale sull'attività elettrica della coclea di cavia trattata con ouabaina. Nuovo Arch Ital Otol 6:293–298
Molvaer OI, Natrud E, Eidsvik S (1978) Diving injuries to the inner ear. Arch Otolaryngol 221:285–288
Moore DC, Best GF (1980) A sensorineural component in chronic otitis media. Laryngoscope 90:1360–1366
Moreira-Filho CA, Neustein I (1979) A presumptive new variant of Norrie's disease. J Med Genet 16:125–128
Moretti A, Arcari G, Pegrassi L (1979) Übersicht über pharmakologische Studien mit Nicerogolin. Arzneim Forsch 29:1223–1227
Moretto G (1958) Ricerche sperimentali sulla possibilità di prevenire l'effetto tossico dell'andride. Minerva Otorinolaring 8:190
Morgans ME, Trotter WR (1958) Association of congenital deafness with goitre; the nature of thyreoid defect. Lancet I:607–609
Morgenstein KM, Manance ED (1969) Temporal bone histopathology in sickle cells disease. Laryngoscope 79:2172–2180
Morgenstern C (1980) Oxygen supply of the middle ear mucosa under normal conditions and after Eustachian tube occlusion. Ann Otol Rhinol Laryngol [Suppl] 89:68–76

Morgenstern C, Amano H, Orsulakova A (1982) Ion transport in the endolymphatic space. Am J Otolaryngol 13:323–327
Morgenstern C, Arnold W (1981) Fluktuierendes Gehör – Eine Analyse wechselnder Schallempfindungsschwerhörigkeiten. Laryngol Rhinol Otol (Stuttg) 60:592–596
Morgenstern C, Kessler M (1978) Oxygen consumption and oxygen distribution in the inner ear. Arch Otorhinolaryngol 220:159–162
Morgenstern C, Lamprecht C, Otterbach J (1983) Das Frequenz-Unterscheidungsvermögen des menschlichen Ohres bei akuten Änderungen des Endolymphraumes. Arch Otorhinolaryngol Suppl II/1983:227–228
Morgenstern C, Laskawi R, Juhn SK (1982) Die Wirkung einer alpha-adrenergen Rezeptorblockade auf die Funktionen des Innenohres. Arch Otorhinolaryngol 234:313–320
Morgenstern C, Lemp C, Lamprecht J (1984) Die Bedeutung des Glyceroltests für die Diagnose unklarer Schallempfindungsstörungen. Tagungsbericht Vereinigung Westdeutscher HNO-Ärzte 1983. HNO 32:439–440
Morgenstern C, Lessmann FJ, Amano H, Orsulakova A, Juhn SK (1981) Inner ear effects of a new loop diuretic (Ozolinon). Scand Audiol Suppl 14:111–118
Morgenstern C, Miyamoto H (1979) DC potential and K^+ activity in experimental endolymphatic hydrops. Arch Otorhinolaryngol 222:273–274
Morgenstern C, Seetz J, Jesdinsky J, Vosteen K-H (1983) Zur Therapie des akuten Hörverlustes. HNO 31:128–131
Mori N, Matsunaga T, Asai H (1980) Clinical application of non invasive electrocochleography. Auris Nasus Larynx 7:111–123
Morimitsu T, Hirashima N, Yasuda K (1975) Amidotrizoate therapy for sudden deafness. J Oto-Rhino-Laryngol Soc Jap 78:591
Morizono T, Paparella M (1978) Hypercholesterolemia and auditory dysfunction. Ann Otol 87:804
Morris TMO (1969) Deafness following acute carbon monoxide poisoning. J Laryngol Otol 83:1219–1225
Morrissey-Walsh E, Barry RGG (1980) Familial diabetes mellitus and optic atrophy. I Med J 73:211–212
Morrison A, Moffat DA, O'Connor AF (1980) Clinical usefulness of electrocochleography in Menière's disease: An analysis of dehydrating agents. Otolaryngol Clin North Am 13:703–721
Morse MJ, Lirenman DS, Johnson HW et al. (1981) The association of renal pelviocaliceal dysmorphism and sensorineural deafness: A new syndrome. J Urol 125:625–627
Moser F, Winkler U (1971) Unterbindung der A. carotis externa bei akutem Hörsturz. Wiss Z Univ Halle 20:38–41
Moser HW, Braine H, Pyeritz RE et al. (1980) Therapeutic trial of plasmaphereses in Refsum disease and in fabry disease. Birth Defects 16:491–497
Mozzo W, Santoni P, Calvelli C (1978) La nefrosi cronica come causa di perditá auditiva neurosensorale. Studio clinico sperimentale. Nuovo Arch Ital Otol 6:307–335
Muckle TJ, Wells M (1962) Urticaria, deafness, and amyloidosis: A new heredo-familial syndrome. Q J Med 31:235–248
Müller O (1937) Die feinsten Blutgefäße des Menschen. Enke, Stuttgart
Münker G (1977) Knochenleitungsveränderungen beim Sero-Mukotympanon. Laryngol Rhinol Otol (Stuttg) 56:591–594
Mulch G, Handrock M (1979) „Hörsturz beidseits" nach akuter Heroinintoxikation. Laryngol Rhinol Otol (Stuttg) 58:435–437
Murakami Y (1979) Routes of viral infection into the inner ear. ORL Tokyo 22 Nr 6, Abst 2–3; ref Zentralbl Hals-Nas-Ohrenheilk 124 (980/81) Nr 5451
Myers EN, Stool S (1968) Cytomegalic inclusion disease of the inner ear. Laryngoscope 78;1904–1915
Myers RM, Bernstein JM (1965) Salicylate ototoxicity. A clinical and experimental study. Arch Otolaryngol 82:483–493
Nadol JB (1978) Hearing loss as a sequela of meningitis. Laryngoscope 88:739–755
Nadol JB, Burgess B (1982) Cochleosaccular degeneration of the inner ear and progressive cataracts inherited as an autosomal dominant trait. Laryngoscope 92:1028–1037
Nagahara K, Fisch U, Yagi N (1983) Perilymph oxygenation in sudden and progressive hearing loss. Acta Otolaryngol (Stockh) 96:57–68

Nagi NA (1979) Diabetes insipidus, diabetes mellitus, optic atrophy and deafness. A clinical and genetic study. Postgrad Med J 55:377–380
Nakai Y (1971) Electronmicroscopic study of the inner ear after ethacrynic acid intoxication. Pract Oto-Rhino-Laryngolog (Basel) 33:366–376
Nakai Y (1977) Combined effect of 3′4′dideoxykanamycin B and potent diuretics on cochlea. (A scanning and transmission electron microscopic evaluation.) Laryngoscope 87:1548
Nakai Y, Chang KC, Onashi K, Marisako N (1983) Ototoxic effect of an aminoglycoside drug on an immature ear. Acta Otolaryngol [Suppl] (Stockh) 393:1–5
Nakai Y, Konishi K, Chang KC et al. (1982) Ototoxicity of the anticancer drug cisplatin. An experimental study. Acta Otolaryngol (Stockh) 93:227–232
Nakai Y, Morimoto A, Chang KC et al. (1980) Inner ear damage induced by bacterial endotoxin. Arch Otorhinolaryngol 229:209–220
Nakai Y, Yamane H, Minowa K et al. (1982) Application of loop diuretics for treatment of sensorineural hearing impairment. Acta Otolaryngol (Stockh) 94:37–43
Nakai Y, Zushi K, Chang KC et al. (1981) An experimental study on the progressiveness of cochlear damage by aminoglykoside drug. Acta Otorhinolaryngol (Stockh) 91:199–206
Nance WE (1971) Genetic counseling for the hearing impaired. Audiology 10:222–233
Nance WE (1980) The genetic analysis of profound prelingual deafness. Birth Defects 16:263–269
Nance WE, Setleff R, McLeod A et al. (1971) X-linked mixed deafness with congenital fixation of the stapedial footplate and perilymph gusher. Birth Defects 7:64–69
Nance WE, Sweeney A (1971) Evidence for autosomal recessive inheritance of the syndrome of renal tubular acidosis and deafness. Birth Defects 7:(4) 70–72
Nassuphis P (1951) Die Wirkung des Atoxyls auf das Innenohr. Arch Ohr-Nas-Kehlk-Heilk 157:594
Natali R, Puyat PM, Rachinel J et al. (1980) Rupture de la fenêtre ronde d'origine traumatique au decours d'une plongée en apnee. Ann Oto-Laryngol (Paris) 97:883–887
National Center for Vital Health Statistics 1967, 1968; zit n Konigsmark u Gorlin (1976)
Nedzelski JM, Barber HO (1976) Round window fistula. J Otolaryngol 5:379–385
Neveling R (1967) Die akute Ertaubung. Kölner Universitäts-Verlag
Niemeyer W (1971) Relations between the discomfort level and the reflex threshold of the middle ear muscles. Audiology 10:172–176
Niemeyer W, Sesterhenn G (1974) Calculating the hearing threshold from the stapedius reflex threshold for different sound stimuli. Audiology 13:421
Nilsson LR, Borgfors N, Gamstorp J, Holst H, Lidén G (1964) Nonendemic goitre and deafness. Acta Paediatr Scand 53:117–131
Nishida HJ (1977) Electrocochleographic study of sudden deafness. Otolaryngol (Tokyo) 49:93–104
Nomoto M, Tsukamoto K, Nagamatsu K (1981) Case of Cogans's syndrome. Clin Neurol 21: 574–580
Nomura Y (1982) A study of the round window. Univ of Tokyo Press
Nomura Y, Kitamura K (1979) Abrupt (sharp cut) type sensorineural hearing loss. A human temporal bone study. Auris Nasus Larynx 6:13–21
Nomura Y, Okuno T, Kawataba I (1983) The round window membrane. Adv Oto-Rhino-Laryngol 31:50–58
Nomura Y, Tsuchida M, Mori S, Sakurai T (1982) Deafness in cryoglobulinemia. Ann Otol Rhinol Laryngol 91:250–255
Norre ME, Jessurun EL (1980) Glycerol test and fluctuating sensorineural hearing loss. Acta otorhinolaryngol Belg 34:262–269
Novotny GM (1980) "Cochlear bends". J Laryngol Rhinol Otol 9:395–398
Novotny O (1975) Altersfaktor bei Gehörmüdigkeit bei professioneller Schwerhörigkeit durch Lärm. Cesk Otolaryngol 24:5
Nowinski GJ (1977) Presbyacusis among the population of the Tenere desert. Centr Afr Med 23:124–126
Nutall L, Lawrence M (1979) Intracellular potential changes of Corti's organ with anoxia. Arch Otolaryngol 105:574–578
Oda M, Preciado MC, Quick CA et al. (1974) Labyrinthine pathology of chronic renal failure patients treated with hemodialysis and kidney transplantation. Laryngoscope 84:1489–1506
Öckermann PA (1967) A generalized storage disorder resembling Hurler's syndrome. Lancet II:239–241

Ödkvist LM, Bergholtz LM, Ählfeldct H, Andersson B, Edling CH, Strand E (1982) Otoneurological and audiological findings in workers exposed to industrial solvents. Acta Otolaryngol [Suppl] (Stockh) 386:249–251

Ohlsson L (1963) Congenital renal disease, deafness and myopia in one family. Acta Med Scand 174:77

Ohtani I, Ohtsuki K, Aikawa T, Omata T, O-Uchi J, Saito T (1982a) Individual variation and mechanism of kanamycin ototoxicity in rabbits. Acta Otolaryngol (Stockh) 94:413–419

Ohtani I, Ohtsuki K, Aikawa T, Sato Y, O-Uchi J, Saito T (1982b) Evalution of ototoxicity of aminoglycoside antibiotics in rabbits. Auris Nasus Larynx 9:67–74

Oosterveld WJ (1981) Ziekte van Ménière: een oderzoek bij 457 patienten. Ned Tijdschr Geneeskd 125:582–585

Opitz H, Schmidt F (1967) Handbuch der Kinderheilkunde, Bd VI, S 309 ff. Springer, Berlin Heidelberg New York

Orchik DJ, Dunn JS (1977) Sickle cell anemia and sudden deafness. Arch Otolaryngol 103:369–370

Orsulakova A, Schacht J (1982) A biochemical mechanism of the ototoxic interaction between neomycin and ethacryn acid. Acta Otolaryngol 93:43–48

Osterhammel D (1979) High-frequency audiometry and noise-induced hearing loss. Scand Audiol 8:85–90

Osterhammel D (1980) High frequency audiometry. Clinical aspects. Scand Audiol 9:249–256

Osterhammel D, Christau B (1982) High frequency audiometry and stapedius muscle reflex thresholds in juvenile diabetics. Scand Audiol 9:13–18

Osterhammel D, Osterhammel P (1979) High frequency audiometry. Age and sex variations. Scand Audiol 8:73–81

Ott, Felten v (1981) Therapieresultate der Oxycarboninhalation beim Knalltrauma. HNO 29:39–39 (Tagungsbericht)

Oudot J, Martin H (1979) Approches d' une étude plus aprofondie de la micro-angiopathie. J Franc ORL 28:303–306

Oudot J, Martin H (1980) Róle des plaquettes dans la pathologie de l'audition. J Fr Otorhinolaryngol 29:315–320

Qudot J, Pignat JC, Martin H (1979) Intoxication aigue à l'aspirine et surdité. A propos de 1 cas. J Fr Otorhinolaryngol 28:687–693

Pagani JJ, Thomson JW, Hanafee WN (1980) Pitfalls in the radiographic diagnosis of the internal auditory canal. Laryngoscope 90:322–325

Paloheimo S, Thalmann R (1977) Influence of „loop" diuretics upon Na^+K^+-ATPase and adenylate cyclase of the stria vascularis. Arch Otorhinolaryngol (NY) 217:347–359

Palva T, Dammert K (1969) Human cochlear aquaeduct. Acta Otolaryngol [Suppl] (Stockh) 246:1–58

Palva T, Raunio P, Karma P, Ylikoski J (1979) Fluid pathways in temporal bones. Acta Otolaryngol (Stockh) 87:210–316

Pang LQ (1974) Sudden sensorineural loss following diving and treatment by recompression: Report of two cases. Trans Am Acad Ophthalmol Otolaryngol 436–443. Zit. n. Novotny (1980)

Panning B, Mehler D, Lehnhardt E (1983) Transient low-frequency hypoacousia after spinal anaesthesia. Lancet I:582

Paparella MM (1978) Differential diagnosis of hearing loss. Laryngoscope 88:1710–1717

Paparella MM (1980) Mondini's deafness. A review of histopathology. Ann Otol Rhinol Laryngol [Suppl] 67, Nr 2, Part 3, 1–10

Paparella MM, Goycoolea MV, Meyerhoff WL, Shea D (1979) Endolymphatic hydrops and otitis media. Laryngoscope 89:43–58

Pappas DG, Mundy MR (1982) Sensorineural hearing loss: infectious agents. Laryngoscope 92:752–754

Parker FI, James GWL (1978) The effect of various topical antibiotic and antibacterial agents on the middle and inner ear of guinea pigs. J Pharmacol 30:236

Parker A, Elberling C, Warburg M (1978) Electrophysiological study of Norrie's disease. An X-linked recessive trait with hearing loss. Audiology 17:293–298

Parving A, Johnsen NJ, Holm-Jensen S (1978) Dominantly inherited low-frequency hearing loss. Audiology 17:165–172

Parving A, Parving HH, Lyngsøe J (1983) Hearing sensitivity in patients with myxoedema before and after treatment with L-thyroxine. Acta Otolaryngol (Stockh) 95:315–321

Parving A, Warburg M (1977) Audiological findings in Norrie's disease. Audiology 16:124–131

Passwell JH, David R, Boichis H, Herzfeld S (1981) Hereditary nephritis with associated defects in proximal renal tubular function. J Pediatr 98:85–87
Patterson JH, Burdick CK, Mozo BT, Camp RT Jr (1977) Temporary threshold shift in man resulting from four-hour exposure to octave bands of noise centered at 63 and 1,000 Hz. J Acoust Soc Am 62:595(A)
Paulsen K, Hundhausen Th (1971) Hörschäden durch Boxen. Laryngol Rhinol Otol (Stuttg) 50:297–324
Paulson OB, Strandgaard S (1978) Physiologie und Pathophysiologie der Hirndurchblutung. Pharmakotherapie 1:121–128
Pausch J, Jäckle B, Schmidt D, Mann W (1982) Systemerkrankung mit enger Beziehung zum Cogan-I-Syndrom. Dtsch Med Wochenschr 107:1143–1147
Pearlman RC (1982) Presbycusis: The need for a clinical definition. Am J Otol 3:183–186
Pearson JCG (1977) Prediction of presbyacusis. J Soc Occup Med 27:125–133
Peckham CS (1972) Clinical and laboratory study of children exposed in utero to maternal rubella. Arch Dis Childh 47:571–577
Peckham CS, Martin JAM, Marshall WS, Dudgeon JA (1979) Congenital rubella deafness: a preventable disease. Lancet I/8110:258–261
Pedersen CB (1974) Brief-tone audiometry in persons treated with salicylate. Audiology 13:311–319
Pedersen U, Elbrond O (1979) Surgical findings and results of stapedectomy in patients with osteogenesis imperfecta. J Laryngol Otol 93:1229–1233
Pellegrini A (1966) Aetiology of deafness in children. Proc 8. Internat Congr Tokyo, pp 410–411
Pendred V (1896) Deafmutism and goitre. Lancet II:532
Pérez-Garrigues H, Garcia-Ibanez JL, Fernández-Moscoso A (1982) Malfomaciones de oido interno tipo Mondini. A propósito de un caso. Acta ORL esp 33:315–321; ref Zentralbl Hals-Nas-Ohrenheilk 129 (1983) Nr 1549
Perin D, Jungers P, Grunfeld JP (1980) Perimacular changes in Alport's syndrome. Clin Nephrol 13:163–167
Petmezakis J, Anagnostakis D, Georgopoulos G, Matsaniotis N (1980) Lärmschädigungsaspekte bei Frühgeborenen. Arch Otorhinolaryngol 223:477
Peytral C, Henin JM, Vacher SA et al. (1981) Ototoxicité du cisplatinum. Ann Oto-Laryngol (Paris) 98:85–88
Pfalz R (1983) Efferentes, auditorisches System: Evidenz für seine Mitwirkung bei Adaptation, Habituation, Ermüdung? Vortrag Arbeitstagung 1983 der Arbeitsgemeinschaft Deutscher Audiologen und Neurootologen, 17.–19. 3. 1983 in Münster
Pfander F (1975) Das Knalltrauma. Analyse, Vorbeugung, Diagnose, Behandlung, Prognose und Begutachtung. Springer, Berlin Heidelberg New York
Pfander F (1978) Wird die lärmbedingte Hörgefährdung bei gleichzeitiger Vibration im Infraschallgebiet verstärkt? Arch Otorhinolaryngol 219:411–412
Pfeiffer RA, Jünemann G, Polster J, Bauer H (1973) Epiphysal dysplasia of the femoral head, severe myopia, and perceptive hearing loss in three brothers. Clin Genet 4:141–144
Pietersen E, Carlsen BH (1966) Hearing impairment as the initial sign of polyarteritis nodosa. Acta Otolaryngol (Stockh) 61:189–195
Pillsbury HC (1981) Metabolic causes of hearing loss and vertigo. Otolaryngol Clin North Am 14:347–354
Pillsbury HC, Shea JJ (1979) Luetic hydrops: Diagnosis and therapy. Laryngoscope 89:1135–1144
Pirsig W, Rollin H (1969) Akute Ertaubung nach Gentamycinbehandlung bei Anurie. HNO 17:274–278
Plasse HM, Spencer FC, Mittleman M et al. (1980) Unilateral sudden loss of hearing. An unusual complication of cardiac operation. J Thorac Cardiovasc Surg 79:822–826
Plath P (1974) Differentialdiagnose zur Abgrenzung der Lärmschwerhörigkeit von anderen Hörfunktionsstörungen. Arbeitsmed Tgg über die berufliche Lärmschwerhörigkeit Bad Reichenhall 30./31. 5.; Schriftenreihe des Hauptverbandes der gewerblichen Berufsgenossenschaften eV
Plath P (1975) Hörschäden als Symptom von Funktionsstörungen des Kreislaufs. Therapiewoche, pp 4748–4753
Plath P (1980) Passagere Taubheit bei Enzephalomyelitis disseminata. HNO 27:348–350
Plath P (1982) Beziehungen zwischen Gehör und Sprachverständnis im Alter. Audiophonol (Besançon) 15:261–265

Plath P (1983) Sensorineurale Schwerhörigkeit bei Funktionsstörungen des Mittelohres. Arch Otorhinolaryngol Suppl II/1984:222–224
Plester D (1962) Audiometrische Untersuchungen bei einem Naturvolk. Arch Ohr-Nas-Kehlk-Heilk 180:765–771
Plester D (1978) Die einseitige Hörstörung. Arch Otorhinolaryngol (NY) 219:451–464
Plochl E, Tasser C (1980) Untersuchungen an 104 Kindern eines Institutes für Hörbehinderte. Pädiatr Padol 15:375–384
Podvinec S, Stefanovic P (1966) Surdité par la streptomycine et prédisposition familiale. J Fr Otorhinolaryngol 15:61–67
Pollard TJ, Smith CA, Brummett R (1981) The effects of low dose ethacrynic acid on the guinea pig with special reference to normal variations in the stria vascularis. Acta Otolaryngol (Stockh) 92:249–258
Praml GJ, Sonnabend E (1980) Lärmschwerhörigkeit durch Dentalturbinen. Dtsch Zahnärztl Z 35:400–406
Pratt H, Sohmer H, Barazani N (1978) Surface-recorded cochlear microphonic potentials during temporary threshold shifts in man. Audiology 17:204–212
Prazić M, Salaj H (1975) Ototoxicity in children caused by streptomycin. Audiology 14:173–176
Prazić M, Salaj B, Subotić R (1964) Familial sensitivity to streptomycin. J Laryngol Otol 78:1037–1043
Prazma J (1981) Effect of glycerol on cochlea microcirculation. Acta Otolaryngol (Stockh) 92:459–461
Prazma J, Thomas WG, Fischer ND, Preslar MJ (1972) Ototoxicity of ethacrynic acid. Arch Otolaryngol 16:448
Precerutti G (1968) Considerazioni di genetica su alcune di ipoacusia ereditaria semplice. Minerva Otorinolaringol (Torino) 18:176
Probst R (1983) Otoneurologische Befunde bei Wernicke-Korsakoff-Syndrom. HNO 31:123–127
Pruszewicz A, Kruk-Zagajewska A, Szyfter W, Smolińska K (1983) Lipid levels in patients with sudden deafness of unknown aetiology. Audiology 22:63–72
Pruszewicz A, Obrebowski A, Swindziński P et al. (1980) Cochleare Gehörbeschädigungen bei Kindern mit serologischer Unverträglichkeit. Folia Phoniatr (Basel) 32:274–284
Pullen FW (1972) Round window membrane rupture: A cause of sudden deafness. Trans Am Acad Ophthalmol Otolaryngol 76:1444
Pullen FW, Rosenberg GJ, Cazeba CH (1979) Sudden hearing loss in divers and fliers. Laryngoscope 89:1373–1377
Purriel B, Drets M, Pascale E et al. (1973) Familial hereditary nephropathy (Alport's syndrome). Ann J Med Assoc 49:1469–1482
Pyykkö J, Stark J (1982) Vibration syndrome in the etiology of occupational hearing loss. Acta Otolaryngol [Suppl] (Stockh) 386:296–300
Quante M (1973) Die Wirkung von Lärm und ototoxischen Substanzen auf vorgeschädigte Ohren. Arch Klin Exp Ohr-Nas-Kehlk-Heilk 205:266–269
Quaranta A, Amoroso C, Violante F (1980) Studio eziopatogenetico delle sorditá improvvise idiopatiche. Minerva Otorinolaringol 39:157–160
Quick CA, Duvall AJ (1970) Early changes in the cochlear duct from ethacrynic acid: An electronmicroscopic evaluation. Laryngoscope 80:954
Quick CA, Fish A, Brown C (1973) The relationship between cochlea and kidney. Laryngoscope 83:1469–1482
Radecke H (1984) Klinische und biochemische Befunde beim Pseudohypoparathyreoidismus. Dissertation Hannover (in Vorbereitung)
Radü HJ (1980) Hörsturz bei Kindern. Arch Otorhinolaryngol 227:373–376
Rahm WE, Strother WF, Crump JF, Parker DeE (1962) The effects of anaesthetics upon the ear. IV. Lidocain hydrochloride. Ann Otol Rhinol Laryngol 71:116–123
Rake M, Saunders M (1966) Refsum's disease. A disorder of lipid metabolism. J Neurol Neurosurg Psychiatr 29:417–422
Ramsden RT, Wilson P, Gibson WPR (1980) Immediate effects of intravenous tobramycin and gentamycin on human cochlear function. J Laryng Otol 94:521–531
Ranke OF (1953) Das Wesen des Rekruitment. Vortrag. 1. Deutscher Audiologenkursus, Freiburg 5.–9. 10., p 37
Ransome J, Ballantyne JC, Shaldon S, Bosher SK, Hallpike CS (1966) Perceptive deafness in subjects with renale failure treated with haemodialysis and polybrene. J Laryng Otol 80:651–677

Rauch S (1964) Biochemie des Hörorgans. Thieme, Stuttgart, pp 224–226, 278–386
Redell RC, Lebo CP (1972) Ototraumatic effects of hard rock music. Calif Med 116:1–4
Refetoff A, DeWind LT, DeGroot LJ (1967) Familial syndrome combining deaf-mutism, stippled epiphyses, goyter and abnormally high PBI: Possible target organ refractoriness to thyroid hormone. J Clin Endocrinol 27:279–294
Refsum S (1945) Heredoataxia hemerologia polyneuriformis – et tidligere ikke beskrevet familiaert syndrom? Nord Med 28:2682–2685
Refsum S (1946) Heredopathia atactica polyneuritiformis: A familial syndrome not hitherto described. A contribution to the clinical study of the hereditary disease of the nervous system. Acta Psychiatr Scand [Suppl] 38
Refsum S (1977) Heredopathia atactica polyneuritiformis phytanic acid storage disease (Refsum's disease) with particular reference to ophthalmological disturbances. Metab Ophthalmol 22:73–79
Reiter D, Konkle DF, Myers AR et al. (1980) Middle ear immittance in rheumatoid arthritis. Arch Otolaryngol 106:114–177
Rejtö K, Pálfalvi L, Komora V (1982) Pure-tone and speech intelligibility disturbances in patients with ototoxic disorders. Audiology 2:159–176
Rempt E (1970) Gehörschäden bei Kanamycinlangzeittherapie. Laryngol Rhinol Otol (Stuttg) 49:504–509
Renou G, Sénéchal G, Sterks JM (1978) Surdité bilatérale due à la Framycétine utilisée par voie locale. Ann Otolaryngol (Paris) 95:691–694
Reynier JP de (1964) Les surdités brusques chez l'enfant. Pract Oto-Rhino-Laryngol 26:63–70
Reynier JP de (1979) La surdité de l'enfant. Cah ORL Chir Cervico-Fac 14:25–37
Riedner ED, Leven LS, Holliday MJ (1980) Hearing patterns in dominant osteogenesis imperfecta. Arch Otolaryngol 106:737–740
Rietema SJ (1979) The clinical significance of electrocochleography. Thesis, Leiden 1979. Zit n. Hoke u. Lütkenhöner (1981)
Ristow W (1968) Zur Behandlung der Meniére-Krankheit mittels temporärer Labyrinthanästhesie. Laryngol Rhinol Otol (Stuttg) 47:441–447
Ristow W (1980) Innenohr-Funktionsstörungen durch Tauchen. Arch Otorhinolaryngol 223:258
Ristow W, Röser D, Juraske P (1978) Zur Behandlung und Prognose der akuten Innenohrstörungen. Arch Otorhinolaryngol 219:336–367
Ritter K (1975) Angioarchitektur der Gefäßstrombahn der Cochlea. Arch Otorhinolaryngol 210:266
Ritter K (1978) Die Gefäße des Innenohres. Arch Otorhinolaryngol 219:155–177; 309–310
Rizvi SS, Gibbin KP (1979) Effect of transverse temporal bone fracture on the fluid compartment of the inner ear. Ann Otol Laryngol 88:741–748
Rizvi SS, Holmes RA (1980) Hearing loss from hemodialysis. Arch Otolaryngol 106:751–756
Roach RE (1973) Response of the diabetic to Békésy audiometry. Arch Otolaryngol 98:349–353
Robertson D (1974) Cochlear neurons frequency selectivity altered by perilymph removal. Science 186:153–155
Robin PE (1981) Deafness and diabetes. Clin Otolaryngol 6:309
Robinson DW (ed) (1971) Occupational Hearing Loss. Academic Press, London New York
Robinson DW, Sutton GJ (1979) Age effect in hearing – a comparative analysis of published threshold data. Audiology 18:320–334
Rösler G, Anderson H (1978) Maximum steepness of slopes in hearing threshold courves. Audiology 17:299–316
Ronis ML, Roser CL, Ronis BJ (1966) Otologic manifestations of Waldenström's macroglobulinemia. Laryngoscope 76:513–523
Rosen S, Bergmann M, Plester D, El-Mofty A, Satti MH (1962) Presbycusis study of a relatively noise-free population in the Sudan. Ann Otol Laryngol 71:727–743
Rosen S, Olin P (1965) Hearing loss and coronary heart disease. Arch Otolaryngol 82:236–243
Rosen S, Olin P, Rosen H (1970) Dietary prevention in hearing loss. Acta Otolaryngol (Stockh) 70:242
Rosenhall U, Kankkunen A (1981) Hearing alterations following meningitis. 2. Variable hearing. Ear Hear 2:170–176
Rossi M, Ferlito A, Polidoro F (1980) Maternal rubella and hearing impairment in children: Considerations in 66 cases. J Laryng Otol 94: 281–289
Rowson KHK, Hinchcliffe R, Gable DR (1975) A virological and epidemiological study of patient with acute hearing loss. Lancet 471–473

Rubinstein M, Muchnik C, Hildesheimer M, Shartov W (1977) In: Inner Ear Biology. INSERM, Bordeaux
Rüedi L (1954) Actions of vitamin A on the human and animal ear. Acta Otolaryngol (Stockh) 44:502
Rüedi L, Furrer W (1946) Das akustische Trauma. Pract Oto-Rhinol-Laryngol (Basel) 8:177
Rumpelt HJ, Langer KH, Schärer K, Straub E, Thoenes W (1974) Split et extremely thin glomerular basement membranes in hereditary nephropathy (Alport's syndrome). Virchows Arch path Anat 364:225
Russell NJ, Fox KE, Brummett RE (1979) Ototoxic effects of the interaction between kanamycin and ethacrine acid. Cochlear ultrastructure correlated with cochlear potentials and kanamycin levels. Acta Otolaryngol (Stockh) 88:369–381
Russell IJ, Sellick PM (1978) Intracellular studies of hair cells in the mammalian cochlea. J Physiol 284:261–290
Russolo M, Poli P (1980) Acute idiopathic auditory failure: Prognosis. A review of 65 cases. Audiology 19:422–433
Ryan A, Dallos P (1975) Effect of absence of cochlear outer hair cells on behavorial auditory threshold. Nature 253:44–45
Ryan AF, Wicham MG, Bone RC (1979) Element content of intracochlear fluids, outer hair cells, and stria vascularis as determined by energydispersive roentgen ray analysis. Otolaryngol Head Neck Surg 87:659–665
Rybak LP (1981) Cis-platinum associated hearing loss. J Laryngol Otol 95:745–747
Rybak LP (1982) Pathophysiology of furosemide ototoxicity. J Otolaryngol 11:127–133
Rybak LP, Green TP, Juhn SK, Morizono T, Mirkin BL (1979) Elimination kinetics of furosemide in perilymph and serum of chinchilla. Acta Otolaryngol (Stockh) 88:382–387
Saigal S, Lunyk O, Larke RPB, Chernesky MA (1982) The outcome in children with congenital cytomegalovirus infection. Am J Dis Child 135:896–901
Saito HR, Daly JF (1971) Quantitative analysis of acid mucopolysaccharides in the normal and kanamycin intoxicated cochlea. Acta Otolaryngol (Stockh) 71:22–26
Salami A, Mora E, Brera S, Stura M (1983) Influenza delle turbe del metabolismo tireoideo sulla via acustica. Vortrag 2. Internat. Sympos on Audiological Medicine, Sirmione 10–13 April
Salt AN, Stopp PE (1979) The effect of cerebrospinal fluid pressure on perilymphatic flow in the opened cochlea. Acta Otolaryngol (Stockh) 88:198–202
Sanders JW, Bess FH (1981) Special auditory testing: Review and update. Am J Otol 3:172–176
Sando I, Egami T (1977) Inner ear hemorrhage and endolymphatic hydrops in a leukemic patient with sudden hearing loss. Ann Otol Rhinol Laryngol 86:518–524
Sando I, Harada T, Loehr A, Sobel JH (1977) Sudden deafness: Histopathological correlation in temporal bone. Ann Otol Rhinol Laryngol 86:269–279
Sato K (1983) Ototoxicity of aminoglycoside antibiotics in animal study. Adv Otorhinolaryngol 29:145–150
Sauer RC, Kammerle A (1981) Reporting results in Menière's disease. The prospective of the clinical audiologist. Am J Otol 2:211–215
Savastano M, Molinari G, Aporti F et al. (1982) ERA in congenital and alloxan induced diabetic mice. Effect of gangliosides treatment. Riv Ital ORL Audiol Foniat 2:115–121; ref Zentralbl Hals-Nas-Ohrenheilk 129 (198) No 408
Saxén A (1952) Inner ear in presbyacusis. Acta Otolaryngol (Stockh) 41:213–227
Schachern PA, Paparella MM, Goycoolea M, Goldenberg B, Schlievert P (1981) The round window membrane following application of staphylococcal exotoxin: An electron microscopic study. Laryngoscope 91:2007–2017
Schacht J (1979) Isolation of an aminoglycoside receptor from guinea pig inner ear tissues and kidney: Arch Otorhinolaryngol 224:129–134
Schätzle W (1971) Histochemie des Innenohres. Urban & Schwarzenberg, München Berlin Wien
Schätzle W, Haubrich J (1967) Histochemische Veränderungen der Meerschweinchencochlea bei experimenteller Hypothyreose. Arch Klin Exp Ohr-Nas-Kehlk-Heilk 188:224–231
Schätzle B, Schnieder EA (1979) Stoffwechsel der Kochlea. In: Berendes, Link, Zöllner (Hrsg) Hals-Nasen-Ohrenheilkunde in Praxis und Klinik, 2. Aufl Bd 5, Kap 6. Thieme, Stuttgart
Schätzle W, Westernhagen B v (1970) Experimentelle Untersuchungen zum Einfluß des Endotoxinschocks auf das Innenohr. Arch klin-exp Ohr-Nas-Kehlk-Heilk 196:172–177

Scheie HG, Hambrick GW Jr, Barness LA (1962) A newly recognized forme fruste of Hurler's disease (Gargoylism). Am J Ophthalmol 53:753–769
Schindler O (1962) L'addattamento uditivo nell'età senile. Minerva Otorinolaringol (Torino) 12:532
Schmidt CL, Stange G (1976) Die Aktivität motorischer Einheiten des M. splenicus capitis bei peripheren vestibulären Läsionen. Arch Otorhinolaryngol 214:175–180
Schmidt CL, Stange G (1977) Akuter Hörsturz nach Dialyse. Arch Otorhinolaryngol 216:645–646
Schmidt PH (1967) Presbyacusis. Audiology [Suppl] 1
Schmidt PH (1976) Electrocochleographic diagnosis. Arch Otorhinolaryngol 212:315–320
Schmidt PH (1981) Low-tone perceptive hearing loss. Acta Otolaryngol (Stockh) 91:463–468
Schneider WJ, Becker EL (1966) Acute transient hearing loss after ethacrynic acid therapy. Arch Intern Med 117:715–717
Schnieder EA (1973) Innenohr- und Hirndurchblutung. Über die Wirkung gefäßerweiternder Mittel auf die Hirndurchblutung. Laryngol Rhinol Otol (Stuttg) 52:186–195
Schönenberger U, Streit CH, Hoigne R (1981) Nephro- und Ototoxizität von Aminoglykosid-Antibiotika unter besonderer Berücksichtigung von Gentamycin. Schweiz Rundsch Med (Praxis) 70:169
Scholtz H, Barolin GS (1981) Abnormales Zellbild bei normaler Zellzahl im Liquor cerebrospinalis. Wien Klin Wochenschr 93:398–400
Schorn K (1981) Difference limen for intensity in patients with sudden deafness and other inner ear disorders. Adv Otorhinolaryngol 27:100–109
Schreiber K (1979) Renale tubuläre Azidose. In: Schreiber K (Hrsg) Die angeborenen Stoffwechselanomalien, 2. Aufl, S 271 ff. Thieme, Stuttgart
Schüssler U, Handrock M, Matthias R (1982) Die Ruptur der runden Fenstermembran – eine Ursache des akuten Hörsturzes. Laryngol Rhinol Otol (Stuttg) 61:207–210
Schuknecht HF (1964) The pathology of several disorders of the inner ear which cause vertigo. Sth med J 57:1161–1167
Schuknecht HF (1968) Pathology of Menière's disease. Otolaryngol Clin North Am 1:331–337
Schuknecht HF (1974) Pathology of the ear. Harvard Univ Press, Cambridge
Schuknecht HF (1979) Cochlear otosclerosis. A continuing fantasy. Arch Otorhinolaryngol 222:79–84
Schuknecht HF (1982) Cochleosacculotomy for Menière's disease: Theory, technique and results. Laryngoscope 92:854–858
Schuknecht HF, Benitez JT, Beekhuis J (1962) Further observations on the pathology of Menière's disease. Ann Otol Rhinol Laryngol 71:1039
Schuknecht HF, Churchill JA, Doran R (1959) The localization of acetylcholine in the cochlea. Arch Otolaryngol 69:549–559
Schuknecht HF, Igarashi M, Chasin WD (1965) Inner ear hemorrhage in leukemia. A case report. Laryngoscope 75:662–668
Schuknecht HF, Kimura RS, Naufal PM (1973) The pathology of sudden deafness. Acta Otolaryngol (Stockh) 76:75–97
Schuknecht HF, Northrop C, Igarashi M (1968) Cochlear pathology after destruction of the endolymphatic sac in the cat. Acta Otorhinolaryngol (Stockh) 65:479–487
Schuknecht HF, Richter E (1980) Apical lesions of the cochlea in idiopathic hydrops and other disorders: pathophysiological implications. ORL (Basel) 42:46–76
Schuknecht HF, Woellner RC (1955) Experimental and clinical study of deafness from lesions of cochlear nerve. J Laryngol Otol 69:75–97
Schultz-Coulon HJ (1973) Über die Bedeutung des Umweltgeräusches für den Hochtonschwerhörigen. HNO 21:26–32
Schultz-Coulon HJ (1983) Das Hören in fortgeschrittenem Alter. Vortrag Jahrestagung 1983 der Vereinigung Westdtsch HNO-Ärzte Recklinghausen
Schwandt P (1980) Hyperlipoproteinämien, Diät und Medikamente. In: Schwandt P (Hrsg) Fettstoffwechselstörungen. MMW Medizin Verlag München, S 7 ff
Schwetz F, Doppler U, Schewczik R, Welleschick B (1980) The critical intensity for occupational noise. Acta Otolaryngol (Stockh) 89:358–361
Seinsch W, Matthias R, Handrock M (1982) Haben Hyper- oder Hypovitaminosen (A und D) einen Einfluß auf die Funktion des Innenohres? Arch Otorhinolaryngol 235:590–592
Sekula J, Wlodyka J (1979) Perilymphatic fistulas. J Otolaryngol 33:469–474; ref Zentralbl Hals-Nas-Ohrenheilk 124 (1980) Nr 4620
Sekula J, Wlodyka J (1982) The round window in acute hearing loss. Audiology 21:55–60

Sellick PM, Johnstone BM (1975) Production and role of inner ear fluid. Neurobiol 5:337–362
Sellick PM, Russell IJ (1980) The response of inner hair cells to basilar membrane velocity during low frequency auditory stimulation in the guinea pig cochlea. Hearing Res 2:439–445
Serjeant GR, Norman W, Todd GB (1975) The internal auditory canal and sensorineural hearing loss in homozygous sickle cell disease. J Laryngol Otol 89:453–455
Shaia FT, Sheehy JL (1976) Sudden sensori-neural hearing impairment: a report of 1.220 cases. Laryngoscope 86:389–397
Shapiro MJ, Purn JM, Rakin C (1981) A study of the effects of cardiopulmonary bypass surgery on auditory function. Laryngoscope 91:2046–2052
Sharp M, Orchik DJ (1978) Auditory function in sickle cell anemia. Arch Otolaryngol 104:322–324
Shea J (1979) Eversion of the lining of the vestibule. Laryngoscope 84:1122–1134
Shea JJ, Kitabchi AE (1973) Management of fluctuant hearing loss. Arch Otolaryngol 97:118–124
Sheehy JL (1976) Treatable sensori-neural hearing impairment. J Otolaryngol Soc Aust 4:3–7
Sheehy JL, Robinson JV, Bush JE (1980) Intravenous histamine in otologic practice. Side effects in 2,347 administrations. Arch Otolaryngol 106:159–160
Shneerson JM, Chattopadhyay B, Murphy MFG, Fawcett IM (1980) Permanent perceptive deafness due to streptococcus suis type II infection. J Laryngol Otol 94:425–427
Sieger A, White NH, Skinner MW, Spector GJ (1983) Auditory function in children with diabetes mellitus. Ann Otol Rhinol Laryngol 92:237–241
Silman F, Gelfand SA (1979) Prediction of hearing levels from acoustic reflex thresholds in persons with high-frequency hearing losses. J Speech Hear Res 22:697–707
Silverstein H, Bernstein JM, Davies D (1967) Salicylate ototoxicity; a biochemical and electrophysiological study. Ann Otol Rhinol Laryngol 76:118–128
Silverstein H, Yules RB (1971) The effect of diuretics on cochlear potentials and inner ear fluids. Laryngoscope 83:873
Simmons FB (1968) Theory of membrane breaks in sudden hearing loss. Arch Otolaryngol 88:541–548
Simmons FB (1980) Patterns of deafness in newborn. Laryngoscope 90:448–453
Simmons FB, Burton RD, Beatty D (1962) Round window injury: auditory behavioural and electrophysiological consequences in the cat. Trans Am Acad Ophthalmol Otolaryngol 66:715–722
Simon H, Orive B, Zamora I, Medizabal S (1979) The acidification defect in the syndrome of renal tubular acidoses with nerve deafness. Acta Pädiatr Scand 68:291–295
Singer SJ (1974) The molecular organization of membranes. Annu Rev Biochem 43:805–833
Sittoni V, Bonanni C, Crosara C, Colletti V, Maschio G, Lupo A (1983) Audiometric evaluation in patients with severe renal disease before and after haemodialysis. Vortrag 2. Internat Sympos on Audiological Medicine, Sirmione 10–14 April
Skinner BA, Greist MC, Norins AL (1981) The keratitis, ichthyosis, and deafness (KID) syndrome. Arch Dermatol 117:285–289
Smith BM, Myers MG (1979) The penetration of gentamicin and neomycin into perilymph across the round window membrane. Otolaryngol Head Neck Surg 87:888–891
Smith CA (1957) Capillary areas of the membranous labyrinth. Ann Otol Rhinol Laryngol 66:521
Smith FR, Goodman DS (1971) The effects of diseases of the liver, thyroid, and kidneys on the transport of vitamin A in human plasma. J Clin Invest 50:2426–2436
Smith FR, Goodman SD, Zaklama MS, Gabr MK, El Magaghy S, Patwardhan VN (1973) Serum vitamin A, retinol-binding protein, and prealbumin concentrations in protein-calorie malnutrition. I. A functional defect in hepatic retinol release. Am J Clin Nutr 26:973–981
Smith KE, Spaulding JS (1972) Ototoxic reaction to propylthiouracil. Arch Otolaryngol 96:369–370
Smyth GDL, Hassard TH (1976) Eighteen years of experiences in stapedectomy. Ann Otol Rhinol Laryngol 49 [Suppl] 1–36
Snow JB, Komune S (1981) Ototoxicity of kanamycin sulfate and the barriers in the inner ear. Otolaryngol Head Neck Surg 89:1013–1018
Snow JB Jr, Suga F (1973) Labyrinthine vasodilatators. Arch Otolaryngol 97:365–370
Sohar E (1956) Renal disease, inner ear deafness, and ocular changes; new heredofamilial syndrome. Arch Int Med 97:627–630
Soldatov JB, Khrappo NS (1979) Fluctuating hypoacusis. Z usn os vorlev boezn Nr 2, 1–6; ref Zentralbl Hals-Nas-Ohrenheilk 122 (1980) Nr 1290
Speaks CH, Nelson D, Ward WD (1970) Hearing loss in rock-and-roll musicians. J Occup Med 12:216–219

Spears GS, Whitworth JM, Konigsmark BW (1970) Hereditary nephritis with nerve deafness. Am J Med 49:52–63
Spiter B, Ventry JM (1980) Central auditory dysfunction among alcoholics. Arch Otolaryngol 106:224
Spoendlin H (1975) Neuroanatomical basis of cochlear coding mechanisms. Audiology 14:383–407
Spoendlin H (1979) Anatomisch-pathologische Aspekte der Elektrostimulation des ertaubten Innenohres. Arch Otorhinolaryngol 223:1–75
Spoendlin H (1980) Akustisches Trauma. In: Berendes, Link, Zöllner (Hrsg) HNO-Heilkunde in Praxis und Klinik, 2. Aufl, Bd 6, Kap 42. Thieme, Stuttgart
Spoor A (1967) Presbycusis values in relation to noise induced hearing loss. Audiology 6:48–57
Spranger J, Gehler J, Cantz M (1976) The radiographic features of mannosidosis. Radiology 119:401–407
Spreng M (1982) Auswirkungen des Lärms auf das Hören. Audiolog Akustik 21:66–75, 94–113
Stagno S, Reynolds DW, Amos CS, Dahle AJ, McCollister FP, Mohindra I, Ermicilla R, Alford CA (1977) Auditory and visual defects resulting from symptomatic and subclinical congenital cytomegalovirus and toxoplasma infections. Pediatrics 59:669–678
Stahle J, Wilbrand HF (1983) The temporal bone in patients with Menière's disease. Acta Otolaryngol 95:81–94
Stange F, Neveling R (1980) Hörsturz. In: Berendes, Link, Zöllner (Hrsg) Hals-Nasen-Ohren-Heilkunde in Praxis und Klinik, 2. Aufl, Bd 6, Kap 45. Thieme, Stuttgart
Stebbins WC, Hawkins JE, Johnsson LG, Moody DB (1979) Hearing thresholds with outer and inner hair cell loss. Am J Otolaryngol 1, Fall 1, 15–27
Steele MW (1981) Genetics of congenital deafness. Pediatr Clin North Am 28:973–980
Stehr K, Epp C, Spiess H (1975) Erste Ergebnisse mit einer kombinierten Lebendimpfung gegen Masern, Mumps und Röteln. Monatschr Kinderheilk 123:410–412
Steinert R, Mester W (1982) Welchen Einfluß hat die Unterbindung der großen Halsschlagader auf die Kochleapotentiale? Laryngol Rhinol Otol 61:477–480
Steinert R, Spath JA Jr. (1984) Kochleapotentiale und Mangeldurchblutung. HNO 32:160–164
Stephens SDG (1970) Temporary threshold shift in myxoedema. J Laryngol Otol 84:317
Stephens SDG, Luxon L, Hinchcliffe R (1982) Immunological disorders and auditory lesions. Audiology 21:128–148
Sterkers JM, Renou CG (1979) Neurotonie et troubles otologiques. Ann Otolaryngol (Paris) 96:281–290
Sterkes JM, Vignaud J, Ponsot G et al. (1980) Syndrome de Mondini. Mèningites récidivantes. Cure chirurgicale. Ann Otolaryngol (Paris) 97:559–568
Stevenson PW (1975) Responses to speech audiometry and phonemic discrimination patterns in the elderly. Audiology 14:185–231
Strauss M, Davis GL (1973) Viral disease of the labyrinth. Ann Otol Rhinol Laryngol 82:577–594
Strauss M, Towfighi J, Lord S, Lipton A, Harvey HA, Brown B (1983) Cis-platinum ototoxicity: clinical experience and temporal bone histopathology. Laryngoscope 93:1554–1559
Strauß P, Chüden H (1974) Ist das Gehör Jugendlicher durch Diskolärm gefährdet? Klinikarzt 3:77–82
Strauß P, Herrig M, Rick W, Faßbender-Balg S (1982) Der Einfluß des Diabetes mellitus auf das Hörorgan. A. Experimenteller Streptozotocin-Diabetes bei der Ratte. Laryngol Rhinol Otol (Stuttg) 61:319–324
Strauß P, Kunkel A (1977) Grenzstrang- und Infusionsbehandlung beim Hörsturz. Laryngol Rhinol Otol (Stuttg) 56:366–371
Strauß P, Schmittner S (1982) Innenohr und Diabetes mellitus vom Erwachsenentyp. Vergleich eines Tiermodells mit klinischen Beobachtungen. HNO 30:116 (Tagungsbericht)
Strauß P, Schmittner S, Rick W, Faßbender-Balg S (1982) Der Einfluß des Diabetes mellitus auf das Hörorgan. B. Spontaner Diabetes bei der Maus. Laryngol Rhinol Otol (Stuttg) 61:325–330
Strauß P, Schneider K, Terriulo V, Sachsse B (1982) Der Einfluß des Diabetes mellitus auf das Hörorgan. C. Juveniler Diabetes und Diabetes mellitus vom Erwachsenentyp beim Menschen. Laryngol Rhinol Otol (Stuttg) 61:331–338
Strauß P, Strahl M (1976) Spätergebnisse nach über 15 Jahren Stapedektomie. Laryngol Rhinol Otol (Stuttg) 55:761–764
Strohm M (1980) Erfahrungen mit der Gabe von Urografin bei Innenohrschwerhörigkeit. Laryngol Rhinol Otol (Stuttg) 59:159–162
Strohm M (1982) Verletzungen der Membran des runden Fensters. Laryngol Rhinol Otol (Stuttg) 61:297–301

Strother WS, Parker DE, Rahm W, Crump JF (1964) The effect of anaesthetics upon the ear. V. Cochlear potentials and behaviour thresholds. Ann Otol Rhinol Laryngol 73:141–152
Stroud MH, Calcaterra TC (1970) Spontaneous perilymph fistulas. Laryngoscope 80:479–487
Strubinski A, Malicka K (1966) Localization of changes in the organ of hearing in diabetics. Otolaryngol Pol 20:443–448; ref Zentralbl Hals-Nas-Ohrenheilk 93:374 (1967)
Stupp HF (1970) Untersuchung der Antibiotikaspiegel in den Innenohrflüssigkeiten und ihre Bedeutung für die spezifische Ototoxizität der Aminoglykosidantibiotika. Acta Otolaryngol [Suppl] (Stockh) 262:5–78
Stupp H, Küpper K, Lagler F, Sous H, Quante M (1973) Inner ear concentrations and ototoxicity of different antibiotics in local and systemic application. Audiology 12:350–363
Subotić R (1976) Histopathological findings in the inner ear caused by measles. J Laryngol Otol 90:174–181
Suga F, Lindsay JR (1976) Histopathological observations of presbycusis. Ann Otol Rhinol Laryngol 85:169–184
Sulkowsky WJ (1980) Industrial Noise Pollution and Hearing Impairment. Problems of Prevention, Diagnosis, and Certification Criteria. Available from the U.S. Department of Commerce, National Technical Information Service, Springfield, Virginia 22161; Copyrigth 1980 by WJ Sulkowski
Sutherland HC, Gasaway DC (1978) Current hearing treshold levels for noise-exposed US Air Force personnel: one year's reportings. SAM-Tr 78–39, Dec 1978; zit n Chung et al. 1983
Suzuki M (1982) The effect of artery ligation and asphyxia on auditory evoked brain stem response. Auris Nasus Larynx (Tokyo) 9:119–131
Svatkoc LG, Kovgalyuk (1979) Audiometric studies in widened frequency range in patients with tuberculosis treated with antibiotics of the aminoglycoside group. Vestn ORL (Mosk) Nr. 5, 29–31; ref Zentralbl Hals-Nas-Ohrenheilk 123: (1980) Nr 2941
Sweeney PJ, Douglas JF, McCavert M (1979) Muckle-Wells syndrome – first Irish case. J Ir Coll Physicians Surg 9:68
Sykora GF, Kaufman B, Katz RL (1980) Congenital defects of the inner ear in association with meningitis. Radiology 135:379–382
Tanaka K et al. (1983) A case of the traumatic inner ear damage. Otolaryngol (Tokyo) 55:121–125; ref Zentralbl Hals-Nas-Ohrenheilk 129:Nr 3221
Tanaka K, Motomura S (1981) Permeability of the labyrinthine windows in guinea pigs. Arch Otorhinolaryngol 233:67–75
Tato JM, Rainville MJ (1976) Utilisation du réflexe stapédien pour l'adaptation des prothèses auditives. Audiology 15:428–432
Taylor IG (1980) The prevention of sensori-neural deafness. J Laryngol Otol 94:1327–1343
Taylor IG, Irwin J (1978) Some audiological aspects of diabetes mellitus. J Laryngol Otol 92:99–113
Terkildsen K, Osterhammel P, Bretlau B (1973) Acoustic middle ear muscle reflexes in patients with otosclerosis. Arch Otolaryngol 98:152
Terrahe K (1979) Schwindel und Gleichgewichtsstörungen beim oberen Zervikalsyndrom. Therapiewoche 1392
Thalmann I, Kobayashi T, Thalmann R (1982) Arguments against a mediating role of the adenylate cyclase: Cyclic AMP system in the ototoxic action of loop diuretics. Laryngoscope 92:589–593
Thalmann R (1981) Effects of loop diuretics, mercurials, and other diuretic substances upon the physiological chemistry of the cochlea. Scand Audiol [Suppl] 14:119–129
Thalmann R, Ise I, Bohne BA, Thalmann I (1977) Action of "loop" diuretics and mercurials upon the cochlea. Acta Otolaryngol (Stockh) 83:221–232
Thalmann R, Miyoshi T, Kusukari J, Thalmann I (1973) Quantitative approaches to the ototoxicity problem. Audiology 12:364–382
Theisen JM, Mann W, Ino T et al. (1980) Anmerkung zur Infusiontherapie beim akuten Hörsturz. Arch Otorhinolaryngol 223:241–243
Thomas JE, Cody DTR (1981) Neurologic perspectives of otosclerosis. Mayo Clin Proc 56:17–21
Thompson P, Wood RP, Bergstrom L (1980) Erythromycin ototoxicity. J Otolaryngol 9:60–62
Thomsen J, Vesterhauge S (1979) A critical evaluation of the glycerol test in Menière's disease. Adv Otorhinolaryngol 25:49–53
Thomson AJ, Searles M, Russell G (1977) Quality of survival after severe birth asphyxia. Arch Dis Child 52:620–626
Thould AK, Scowen EF (1964) The syndrome of congenital deafness and simple goiter. J Endocrinol 30:69–77

Thuemler R, Atzpodien W, Kremer GJ, Haferkamp G (1977) Refsum-Syndrom (Heredopathia atactica polyneuritisformis). Klinik, Diagnostik und diätetische Behandlung. Dtsch Med Wochenschr 102:1454–1457
Tiedemann R (1978) Totaler beidseitiger Innenohrverschluß nach Gentamycin. Arch Otorhinolaryngol 219:434–435
Tjernström Ö, Denneberg T, Harris S, Nordström L, Toremalm NG (1982) Ototoxicity of Netilmycin. Acta Otolaryngol (Stockh) 94:421–429
Todd GB, Serjeant GR, Larson MR (1973) Sensori-neural hearing loss in Jamaicans with SS disease. Acta Otolaryngol (Stockh) 76:268–272
Tonkin JP, Fagan P (1975) Rupture of the round window membrane. J Laryngol Otol 89:733–756
Tonndorf J (1968) Pathophysiology of hearing loss in Menière's disease. Otolaryngol Clin North Am 1:375–388
Tonndorf J (1976) Endolymphatic hydrops: Mechanical causes of hearing loss. Arch Otorhinolaryngol 212:293–299
Tonndorf J (1979) A rational approach to the traveling wave phenomen. Am J Otolaryngol 1:83–93
Tonndorf J (1981) Stereociliary dysfunction, a cause of sensory hearing loss, recruitment, poor speech discrimination and tinnitus. Acta Otolaryngol (Stockh) 91:469–479
Townsend TH, Bes FH (1980) Effects of age and sensorineural hearing loss on word recognition. Scand Audiol 9:245–248
Tran Ba Huy P, Manuel C, Meulemans A (1979) Pharmacokinetics of gentamicin in perilymph and endolymph studied in the rat by radioimmunassay. Arch Otorhinolaryngol (NY) 224:135–136
Tran Ba Huy P, Meulemans A, Manuel Ch et al. (1981) Critical appraisal of the experimental studies on the ototoxic interaction between ethacrynic acid and aminoglycoside antibiotics. A pharmacokinetical study. Scand Audiol [Suppl] 14:225–232
Tsuiki T, Murai S (1971) Familian incidence of streptomycin hearing loss and hereditary weakness of the cochlea. Audiology 10:315–322
Tumarkin A (1957) On Menière's syndrome. Proc Roy Soc Med 54:907
Turner G (1970) A second family with renal, vaginal, and middle ear anormalities. J Pediatr 76:641
Turner JS Jr (1970) Hereditary hearing loss with nephropathy (Alport's syndrome). Acta Otolaryngol 271:7–33
Uddman R, Ninoyu O, Sundler F (1982) Adrenergic and peptidergic innervation of cochlear blood vessels. Arch Otorhinolaryngol 236:7–14
Ulehlová L (1982) Stria vascularis in acoustic trauma. Arch Otorhinolaryngol 237:133–138
Ulrich K (1926) Verletzungen des Gehörorgans bei Schädelbasisfrakturen. Acta Otolaryngol [Suppl] (Stockh) 6:1–50
Upfold LJ (1970) Deafness following rubella in pregnancy. Med J Aust 1:420–424
Urban GE (1973) Reversible sensori-neural hearing loss associated with sickle cell crises. Laryngoscope 83:633–638
Vanderbilt University Hereditary Deafness Study Group (1968) Dominantly inherited low-frequency hearing loss. Arch Otolaryngol 88:242–250
Veltri RW, Wilson WR, Sprinkle PM et al. (1981) The implication of viruses in idiopathic sudden hearing loss: primary infection of reactivation of latent viruses? Otolaryngol 89:137–141
Venkateswaren PS (1971) Transient deafness from high doses of furosemid. Brit Med J 4:113
Ventura FP (1978) Counselling the hearing-impaired geriatric patient. Patient Couns Health Educ 1:22–25
Vertes D, Axelsson A, Miller J, Lidén G (1979) Some vascular effects of noise exposure in the chinchilla cochlea. Acta Otolaryngol (Stockh) 88:47–55
Vick HP (1981) Beitrag zur Koinzidenz von pathologischen Augenhintergrundspigmentierungen und Taubheit. HNO-Praxis 6:282–288
Vick HP, Eichler J, Vick U (1979) Beitrag zu Befunden und Ätiologie der Makuladystrophie bei hochgradig hörgeschädigten Kindern (Syndrom nach Diallinas-Amalric). Folia Ophthalmol (Jena) 4:105–108
Villar J, Garza C, Bosch J (1981) Resultados en el tratamiento de la sordera brusca. Acta ORL Esp 32:329–331
Virgiliis S de, Argiolu F, Sanna G et al. (1979) Auditory involvement in thalassemia major. Acta Haematol 61:209–215
Virolainen E, Puhakka H, Rahko T (1980) The cochlear component in operated otosclerosis after a mean period of 16 years. A follow-up study. Audiology 19:101–104

Visencio LH, Gerber SE (1979) Effect of hemodialysis on pure-tone thresholds and blood chemistry. J Speech Res 22:756–764
Vogt K, Bödefeld R (1982) Untersuchungen zur Druckfestigkeit der Innenohrfenster. HNO-Praxis (Leipzig) 7:187–190
Vos JA de (1963) Deafness in hypothyreoidism. J Laryngol Otol 77:390–414
Vosteen KH (1976) Die Produktion von Endo- und Perilymphe und die Durchlässigkeit der Innenohrmembranen. Arch Otorhinolaryngol 212:219
Walter B, Blegvad B (1981) Identification of wave I by means of atraumatic ear canal electrode. Scand Audiol [Suppl] 13:63–64
Waltzman SB, Cooper JS (1981) Nature and incidence of misonidazoleproduced ototoxicity. Arch Otolaryngol 107:52–54
Wandhöfer A (1971) Der einseitige akute Hörverlust im Vergleich mit dem konsekutiven Hörverlust des zweiten Ohres. Inauguraldiss. Münster 1971; zit n Feldmann 1981
Wandhöfer A (1979) Der Hörsturz. Akt Neurol 6:13–26
Ward PH, Honrubia V (1969) The effects of local anesthetics on the cochlea of the guinea pig. Laryngoscope 79:1605–1617
Watanabe Y (1963) Influence of diamox upon inner ear and histochemical study of carbonic anhydrase. J Oto-Rhino-Laryngol Soc Japan 66:657–670
Watanuki K, Kashiwazaki H, Kawamoto K, Katagiti S (1968) The effects of kanamycin intoxication on the RNA metabolism in the cells of Reissners membrane. Arch Ohr-Nas-Kehlk-Heilk 192:369–375
Weber I (1960) Ein Beitrag zu den kryptogenen Hörstörungen des Innenohres. Laryngol Rhinol Otol (Stuttg) 39:589–595
Wedel H v (1979) Untersuchungen zum zeitlichen Auflösungsvermögen beim dichotischen Hören. Arch Otorhinolaryngol 222:133–144
Wedel H v, Opitz HJ (1980) The time resolution of changes in short duration signal changes – psychoacoustical and electrophysiological studies. Hear Res 2:387–395
Wedel H v, Tegtmeier W (1980) Der Einfluß der Presbyakusis auf das soziale Hörvermögen. Arch Otorhinolaryngol 223:399–402
Wegener F (1967) Die pneumogene allgemeine Granulomatose – sog. Wegenersche Granulomatose. In: Staemmler, Kaufmann (Hrsg) Lehrbuch der speziellen pathologischen Anatomie. de Gryuter, Berlin, Ergänzungsband I/1, S 225–299
Weidauer H (1971) Fermenthistochemische Untersuchungen am Innenohr des Meerschweinchens nach Applikation von Aminobenzol. Arch Klin Exp Ohr-Nas-Kehlk-Heilk 199:590–595
Weidauer H (1972) Fermenthistochemische Veränderungen am Innenohr des Meerschweinchens nach Nitrobenzol. Arch Klin Exp Ohr-Nas-Kehlk-Heilk 202:681–686
Weidauer H (1974) Histochemische Veränderungen am Innenohr des Meerschweinchens nach Schwefelkohlenstoffexposition. Arch Klin Exp Ohr-Nas-Kehlk-Heilk 207:462
Weidauer H (1975) Hör- und Gleichgewichtsstörungen durch gewerbliche Intoxikationen. Dtsch Ärztebl 72:747–749
Weidauer H, Arnold W (1976) Strukturelle Veränderungen am Hörorgan beim Alport-Syndrom. Laryngol Rhinol Otol (Stuttg) 55:6–16
Weidauer H, Arnold W, Seelig HP (1977) Nachweis von Basalmembran-Antikörpern im Innenohr bei experimenteller Masugi-Nephritis. Laryng Rhinol Otol (Stuttg) 56:500–507
Weidauer H, Bröker HJ, Grusendorf M et al. (1981) Ein unbekanntes hereditäres Syndrom: Innenohrschwerhörigkeit, Hypokalzämie, Vitiligo. Arch Otorhinolaryngol 231:677–679
Weidauer H, Lenarz Th (1982) Verhalten des Stapediusreflexes bei akustischer Langzeitstimulation. Laryngol Rhinol Otol (Stuttg) 61:674–677
Weidauer H, Lenarz Th (1984) Das Kearns-Sayre-Syndrom aus hals-nasen-ohrenärztlicher Sicht. Laryngol Rhinol Otol (Stuttg) 62:141–146
Weidauer H, Tenner A (1973) Hörsturz beiderseits in Verbindung mit doppelseitigem transitorischen Astarterienverschluß des Auges. Laryngol Rhinol Otol (Stuttg) 52:121–128
Weinaug P (1982) Untersuchungen zur Spontanremission beim akuten Hörsturz. HNO-Praxis (Leipzig) 7:86–93
Weinaug P (1984) Die Spontanremission beim Hörsturz. HNO 32:346–351
Welleschik B, Körpert K (1980) Ist das Lärmschwerhörigkeitsrisiko für Männer größer als für Frauen? Laryngol Rhinol Otol (Stuttg) 59:681–689

Westernhagen B v (1968) Histochemische Untersuchungen zur Wirkung der Salicylsäure auf das Innenohr. Arch klin-exp Ohr-, Nas-, Kehlk-Heilk 190:86
Westmore GA, Everdsen ID (1981) Noise-induced hearing loss and orchestral musicians. Arch Otolaryngol 107:761–764
Wetmore SJ, Abramson M (1979) Bullous myringitis with sensorineural hearing loss. Otolaryngol Head Neck Surg 87:66–70
Wigand ME, Heidland A (1970) Akute, reversible Hörverluste durch rasche, hochdosierte Furosemid-infusionen bei terminaler Niereninsuffizienz. Arch Otorhinolaryngol 196:314–319
Wigand ME, Meents O, Hennemann H, Heidland A (1982) Kochleo-vestibuläre Störungen bei Urämie in Beziehung zum Elektrolytstoffwechsel und Glomeruluminfiltrat. Schweiz Med Wochenschr 102:477–482
Wilke H, Großgerge H, Haubold E et al. (1977) Häufigkeit und Verteilung von Risikofaktoren beim Hörsturz. Fortschr Med 95:1757–1764
Willemse C (1952) Protection contre la surdité professionelle – Role de la vitamine A. Acta Med Belg 6:319
Wilmes E, Deinhardt F (1983) Virale Krankheiten im HNO-Bereich. Arch Otorhinolaryngol [Suppl] 1:1–112
Wilmes EH, Roggendorf M (1979) Zur Virusätiologie des Hörsturzes. (Serologische Untersuchungen.) Laryngol Rhinol Otol (Stuttg) 58:817–821
Wilson KS, Juhn SK (1970) The effect of ethacrynic acid on perilymph Na^+ and K^+ (preliminary report). Pract Oto-Rhino-Laryng (Basel) 32:279–287
Wilson WR, Byl FM, Laird N et al. (1980) The efficacy of steroids in the treatment of idiopathic sudden hearing loss. A double-blind clinical study. Arch Otolaryngol 106:772–776
Wilson WR, Laird N, Moo-Young G et al. (1982) The relationship of idiopathic sudden hearing loss to diabetes mellitus. Laryngoscope 92:155–160
Windle-Taylor PC, Emery PJ, Phelps PD (1981) Ear deformities associated with the Klippel-Feil syndrome. Ann Otol Rhinol Laryngol 90:210–216
Witter HL, Deka RC, Lipscomb DM et al. (1980) Effects of prestimulatory carbogen inhalation on noise-induced temporary threshold shift in humans and chinchilla. Am J Otol 1:227–232
Wittmaack K (1936) Betrachtungen über die Erkrankungen des Innenohres auf der Grundlage der Tonuslehre. Arch Ohr-Nas-Kehlk-Heilk 141:25
Wittmaack K (1903) Der Angriffspunkt des Chinins im Nervensystem des Gehörorganes. Arch Ges Physiol 95:234
Wittmaack K (1956) Die Ortho- und Pathobiologie des Labyrinths. Thieme, Stuttgart
Wlodyka J (1978) Studies on cochlear aquaeduct patency. Ann Otol Rhinol Laryngol 87:22–28
Wolff D, Bernhard WG, Tsutsumi S, Ross IS, Nussbaum HE (1965) The pathology of Cogan's syndrome causing profound deafness. Ann Otol Rhinol Laryngol 74:507–520
Wolfowitz B (1979) Spontaneous CSF otorrhea simulating serous otitis. Arch Otolaryngol 105:496–499
Wolfram DJ, Wagene HP (1938) Diabetes mellitus and simple optic atrophy among siblings: Report of four cases. Proc Mayo Clin 13:715–718
Wright ChG, Schaefer StD (1982) Inner ear histopathology in patients treated with cis-platinum. Laryngoscope 92:1408–1413
Wurtle P (1981) Traumatic rupture of the eardrum with round window fistula. J Otolaryng 10:309–312
Yamada O, Kodra K, Yagi T (1979) Cochlear processes affecting wave V latency of the auditory evoked brain stem response. A study of patients with sensory hearing loss. Scand Audiol 8:67–70
Yamakawa K (1929) Die Wirkung der arsenigen Säure auf das Ohr. Arch Klin Exp Ohr-Nas-Kehlk-Heilk 123:238–296
Yassin A, Badry A, Fatt-Hi A (1970) The relationship between electrolyte balance and cochlear balances in cases of renal failure. J Laryngol Otol 84:429–436
Yoo TJ, Stuart J, Kang AH, Cremer M, Townes A (1982) Collagen-induced autoimmune sensorineural hearing loss, vestibular dysfunction and otosclerosis in rodents. In: Abstracts of the fifth midwinter research meeting, January 18–21. St. Petersburg Beach, Florida
Yoshie N (1968) Auditory nerve action potential responses to clicks in man. Laryngoscope 78:198–215
Young NJA, Hitchings RA, Sehmi K, Bird AC (1979) Stickler's syndrome and neovascular glaucoma. Br J Ophthalmol 63:826–831
Young WG Jr, Lesage AM, Dillon ME, Lee JM, Collaway HA Jr, Reeves JW (1961) Chemotherapy of intrathoracic neoplasms employing different pelvic perfusion hypothermia. Ann Surg 154:372–381

Zadory K, Palfalvi L, Bacsa L et al. (1982) Computer evaluation of acute hearing impairment. Fül-Orr-Gége-Gyóyászat 28:92–97; ref Zentralbl Hals-Nas-Ohrenheilk 129 (1983) Nr 399
Zajtchuk JT, Falor WH, Rhodes MF (1979) Hypercoagulability as a cause of sudden neurosensory hearing loss. Otolaryngol Head Neck Surg 87:268–273
Zangemeister HE (1953) In: Kietz H, Zangemeister HE (Hrsg) Einführung in die Audiometrie. Verlag angewandte Wissenschaften, Wiesbaden
Zechner G (1973) Zur Pathohistologie des Ductus und Saccus endolymphaticus. Acta Otolaryngol (Stockh) 75:232–238
Zechner G (1974) Die Innenohrflüssigkeiten und ihre Bedeutung für die Funktion der Sinnesorgane. Arch Otorhinolaryngol 207:539–542
Zechner G (1976) Pathohistologie des Ductus und Saccus endolymphaticus beim Innenohrhydrops. Arch Otorhinolaryngol 212:277–286
Zechner G (1977) Kapselotosklerose und Innenohrstrukturen (Morphologische Befunde). Laryngol Rhinol Otol (Stuttg) 56:57–63
Zechner G (1980) Zum Cogan-Syndrom. Acta Otolaryngol (Stockh) 89:310–316
Zechner G (1980) Innenohrhydrops als Folge gestörter Endolymphzirkulation. Laryngol Rhinol Otol (Stuttg) 59:829–833
Zechner G (1980) Pathohistology by endolymphatic hydrops in man: Morphological details on disturbed longitudinal endolymph circulation. In: Menière's disease. Pathogenesis, diagnosis, and treatment. Internat. Sympos. Düsseldorf Mai 1980, Thieme, Stuttgart
Zechner G, Altmann (1968) The temporal bone in Hunter's syndrome (gargoylism) Arch Klin Exp Ohr-Nas-Kehlk-Heilk 192:137–144
Zenner HP, Zenner B (1979) Vasopressin and isoproterenol activate adenylate cyclase in the guinea pig inner ear. Arch Otorhinolaryngol 222:275–283
Ziemski Z, Jankowski V (1972) Ototoxicity of sodium salicylate. Otolaryngol Pol 26:391–392; ref. Zentralbl Hals-Nas-Ohrenheilk 107 (1973) Nr 1886
Zwicker E, Schorn K (1978) Psychoacoustical tuning curves in audiology. Audiology 127:120–140
Zwislocki JJ (1975) Phase opposition between inner and outer hair cells and auditory sound analysis. Audiology 14:443–455

Subject Index

MIX
Papier aus verantwortungsvollen Quellen
Paper from responsible sources
FSC® C105338

If you have any concerns about our products,
you can contact us on
ProductSafety@springernature.com

In case Publisher is established outside the EU,
the EU authorized representative is:
Springer Nature Customer Service Center GmbH
Europaplatz 3, 69115 Heidelberg, Germany

Printed by Libri Plureos GmbH
in Hamburg, Germany